GW00691885

BASIC CLINICAL RADIOBIOLOGY
for Radiation Oncologists

Edited by

G. Gordon Steel

Edward Arnold
A member of the Hodder Headline Group
LONDON   BOSTON   MELBOURNE   AUCKLAND

© 1993 Edward Arnold Publishers

First published in Great Britain 1993

Distributed in the Americas by Little, Brown and Company
34 Beacon Street, Boston, MA 02108

British Library Cataloguing in Publication Data

Steel, G. G.
  Basic Clinical Radiobiology
  I. Title
  616.9940642

  ISBN 0–340–60144–2

Whilst the advice and information in this book is believed to be
true and accurate at the date of going to press, neither the author
nor the publisher can accept any legal responsibility or liability
for any errors or omissions that may be made. In particular
(but without limiting the generality of the preceding disclaimer)
every effort has been made to check drug dosages; however,
it is still possible that errors have been missed. Furthermore,
dosage schedules are constantly being revised and new side
effects recognised. For these reasons the reader is strongly
urged to consult the drug companies' printed instructions before
administering any of the drugs recommended in this book.

Typeset in 10/11 pt Times by Anneset, Weston-super-Mare, Avon.
Printed and bound in Great Britain for Edward Arnold, a division
of Hodder Headline PLC, Mill Road, Dunton Green, Sevenoaks,
Kent TN13 2YA by Butler & Tanner Limited, Frome and London.

Preface

Developments in cancer therapy are increasingly arising out of studies in basic science and it is best for their implemetation to be in the hands of clinicians who are familiar with the relevant scientific areas. This book deals with the biological aspects of radiotherapy. It seeks to present in a concise and interesting way the main ideas and significant scientific developments that underlie current attempts to improve the radiotherapeutic management of cancer.

The book is directed at an international audience. It has arisen out of teaching courses organised by the European Society for Therapeutic Radiation Oncology (ESTRO) and the material will also be of use to readers in North America and the rest of the world.

For the benefit of readers who have a visual memory, and particularly for those whose first language is not English, we have chosen to use a high ratio of charts to text. We have also added a substantial glossary of scientific terms. At the end of each chapter is a list of prominent published material, mainly books and reviews, that are recommended for further reading. Citations in the text sometimes refer to these works.

The early chapters deal with growth and cell proliferation in tumours and normal tissues. The concept of cell survival is fundamental to this field and it leads on to the discussion of models of cell killing, isoeffect relationships, and developments in fractionation. Later chapters deal with biologically based developments in other areas of radiotherapy. Discussion of molecular aspects of radiation biology is left to the final chapter, in order not to frighten new-comers to the field: clinical radiobiology does not yet *require* a knowledge of molecular biology but work in this area helps to throw light on basic aspects of the subject and may well be the shape of things to come.

G. Gordon Steel
1993

List of contents

List of authors

Dr. A.C. BEGG,
Dr. F.A. STEWART and
Dr. N. van ZANDWIJK

Netherlands Cancer Institute
Antoni van Leeuwenhoek Huis
Plesmanlaan 121
1066 CX Amsterdam
The Netherlands

Dr. M.C. JOINER

CRC Gray Laboratory
PO Box 100
Mount Vernon Hospital
Northwood
Middlesex HA6 2JR
United Kingdom

Prof. A. van der KOGEL and
Dr. A.C.C. RUIFROK

St Radboud University Hospital
Institute for Radiotherapy
Geert Grooteplein Zuid 32
6525 GA Nijmegen
The Netherlands

Prof. J. OVERGAARD,
Dr. S. BENTZEN and
Dr.M.R. HORSMAN

Aarhus Kommunehospital
Radiumstationen
Cancer Research Institute
8000 Aarhus
Denmark

Prof. G.G. STEEL and
Dr. T.J. McMILLAN

Radiotherapy Research Unit
Institute of Cancer Research
Sutton
Surrey SM2 5NG
United Kingdom

Dr. T.E. WHELDON

Department of Radiation Oncology
University of Glasgow
CRC Beatson Laboratories
Garscube Estate
Glasgow G61 1BD
United Kingdom

1

Introduction: The significance of radiobiology for radiotherapy

G. Gordon Steel

1.1 The role of radiotherapy in the management of cancer

Radiotherapy is one of the two most effective treatments for cancer. Surgery, which of course has the longer history, is in the majority of cases the primary form of treatment and it leads to good therapeutic results in a range of early non-metastatic tumours. Radiotherapy has replaced surgery for the long-term control of many tumours of the head and neck, cervix, bladder, prostate and skin, in which it often achieves a reasonable probability of tumour control with good cosmetic result. Wide-field irradiation is also successful in Hodgkin's disease and other lymphomas. In addition to these examples of the curative role of radiation therapy, a large proportion of patients with a wide variety of types of malignant disease receive valuable palliation by this approach.

Chemotherapy is the third most important treatment modality at the present time. Following the early use of nitrogen mustard during the 1920s it has emerged to the point where upwards of 30 drugs are available for the management of cancer, although no more than 10 – 15 are in common use. A large proportion of patients receive chemotherapy at some point in their management and useful symptom relief and disease arrest are often obtained.

Reliable information about the relative roles of surgery, radiotherapy and chemotherapy is difficult to obtain, but is necessary whenever priorities for research funding in this area are under review. Often-quoted is the analysis by DeVita et al (1979) of the probable outcome of treatment of the 700,000 newly-diagnosed cases in the USA in 1977. DeVita estimated that local treatment, which includes surgery and/or

radiotherapy, could be expected to be successful in approximately 280,000 ($\approx$40%) of these cases. In perhaps 15% of the total, radiotherapy would be the principal form of treatment. In contrast, of the cases where chemotherapy was the main-line treatment, DeVita estimated that only around 2% (of the total 700,000 cases) were likely to achieve long-term survival. Similar figures from a review by Souhami and Tobias (1986) are shown in Figure 1.1. They estimated that apart from skin cancers and *in situ* cervical carcinomas probably 30% of cancers are cured by surgery, radiotherapy, or both. Many patients (perhaps 40%) do receive chemotherapy but their contribution to the overall cure rate may be only around 2%, with some prolongation of life in perhaps another 10%.

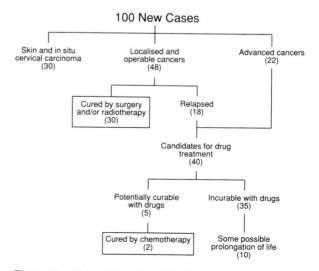

Figure 1.1 The relative roles of local and systemic treatment in the management of cancer. From Souhami and Tobias (1986), with permission.

If these figures are correct, it may be that around 7 times as many patients currently are cured by radiotherapy as by chemotherapy. This is not to undervalue the important benefits of chemotherapy in a number of chemosensitive diseases, but to stress the greater role of radiotherapy as a curative agent (Tubiana, 1992).

Considerable efforts are being devoted at the present time to the improvement of radiotherapy and chemotherapy. Wide publicity is given to the newer areas of drug development such as lymphokines, growth factors, anti-oncogenes, etc. But if we were to imagine aiming to increase the results shown in Figure 1.1 to the point where, say, 2% more patients are cured, it would seem on a realistic estimation that this would more likely be achieved by increasing the results of radiotherapy from 15% to 17% than by *doubling* the results achieved by chemotherapy.

There are three main ways in which such an improvement in radiotherapy might be obtained:

(i)   by raising the standards of radiation dose delivery to those currently in use in the best radiotherapy centres;
(ii) by improving radiation dose distributions, either using techniques of conformal radiotherapy with photons, or ultimately by the use of proton beams;
(iii) by exploiting radiobiological initiatives.

It is the last of these approaches that is the subject of this book.

1.2 The role of radiation biology

Experimental and theoretical studies in radiation biology contribute to the development of radiotherapy at three different levels:

Ideas – providing a conceptual basis for radiotherapy, identifying mechanisms and processes that underlie the response of tumours and normal tissues to irradiation and which help to explain observed phenomena. Examples are knowledge about hypoxia, reoxygenation, tumour cell repopulation, mechanisms of repair of DNA damage.

Treatment Strategy - development of specific new approaches in radiotherapy. Examples are hypoxic cell sensitizers, high-LET radiotherapy, accelerated radiotherapy, hyperfractionation.

Protocols – advice on the choice of schedules for clinical radiotherapy. For instance, conversion formulae for changes in fractionation or dose rate, or advice on whether to use a chemical radiosensitizer at the start or at the end of a course of radiotherapy. We may also include under this heading methods for predicting the best treatment for the individual patient (*individualized radiotherapy*).

There is no doubt that radiobiology has been very fruitful in the generation of new ideas and in the identification of potentially exploitable mechanisms. A variety of new treatment strategies have been produced, but unfortunately few of these have so far led to demonstrable clinical gains. In regard to the third of the levels listed above, the newer conversion formulae based on the linear-quadratic equation seem to be successful and there are encouraging signs that some approaches to the individualization of radiotherapy may be working. But beyond this, the ability of laboratory science to guide the radiotherapist in the choice of specific protocols is limited by the inadequacy of the theoretical and experimental models: it will always be necessary to rely on clinical trials for the final choice of a protocol.

1.3 The time-scale of effects in radiation biology

Irradiation of any biological system generates a succession of processes that differ enormously in time-scale. This is illustrated in Figure 1.2 where these processes are divided into three phases (Boag, 1975):

The Physical Phase consists of the interactions between charged particles and the atoms of which the tissue is composed. A high-speed electron takes about 10^{-18} seconds to traverse the DNA molecule and about 10^{-14} seconds to pass across a mammalian cell. As it does so it interacts mainly with orbital electrons, ejecting some of them from atoms (*ionization*) and raising others to higher energy levels within an atom or molecule (*excitation*). If sufficiently energetic, these secondary electrons may excite or ionise other atoms near which they pass, giving rise to a cascade of ionisation events. For 1 gray of absorbed radiation dose, there are in excess of

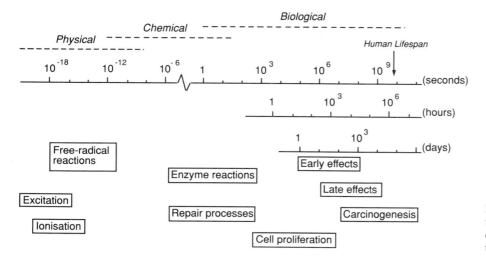

Figure 1.2 Time-scale of the effects of radiation exposure on biological systems.

10^5 ionizations within the volume of every cell of diameter 10 microns.

The Chemical Phase describes the period in which these damaged atoms and molecules react with other cellular components in rapid chemical reactions. Ionization and excitation lead to the breakage of chemical bonds and the formation of broken molecules (*free radicals*). These are highly reactive and they engage in a succession of reactions that lead eventually to the restoration of electronic charge equilibrium. Free-radical reactions are complete within approximately 1 millisecond of radiation exposure. An important characteristic of the Chemical Phase is the competition between *scavenging* reactions, for instance with sulphydryl compounds that inactivate the free radicals, and *fixation* reactions that lead to stable chemical changes in biologically-important molecules.

The Biological Phase includes all subsequent processes. These begin with enzymatic reactions that act on the residual chemical damage. The vast majority of lesions, for instance in DNA, are successfully repaired. Some rare lesions fail to repair and it is these that lead to eventual cell death. Cells take time to die; indeed after small doses of irradiation they may undergo a number of mitotic divisions before dying. It is the killing of stem cells and the subsequent loss of the

cells that they would have given rise to that causes the early manifestations of normal-tissue damage during the first weeks and months after radiation exposure. Examples are breakdown of the skin or mucosa, denudation of the intestine and haemopoietic damage (Section 13.2). A secondary effect of cell killing is compensatory cell proliferation, which occurs both in normal tissues and in tumours. At later times after the irradiation of normal tissues the so-called *late reactions* appear. These include fibrosis and telangiectasia of the skin, spinal cord damage and blood-vessel damage (Section 13.2). An even later manifestation of radiation damage is the appearance of second tumours (*radiation carcinogenesis*), thus illustrating the fact that the time-scale of the observable effects of ionizing radiation may extend up to many years after exposure.

1.4 Response of normal and malignant tissues to radiation exposure

Much of the text of this book will focus on effects of radiation exposure that become apparent to the clinician or the patient during the weeks, months and years after radiotherapy. These effects are seen both in tumour tissues and in the normal tissues that surround a tumour and which are unavoidably exposed to radiation. The primary tasks of radiation biology as applied to radiotherapy are to *explain* observed phenomena, and to suggest improvements to existing therapies (as set out in Section 1.2).

The response of a tumour is seen by *regression*, often followed by *regrowth* (or *recurrence*), but perhaps with failure to regrow during the normal lifespan of the patient (which we term *cure* or *local control*). These italicized terms describe the tumour responses that we seek to understand. The relationship between regression and regrowth are illustrated graphically in Figure 2.8. The cellular basis of tumour response, including tumour control, is dealt with in Section 5.6.

The responses of normal tissues to therapeutic radiation exposure range from those that cause mild discomfort to others that are life-threatening. The speed at which the response develops varies widely from one tissue to another and depends on the dose of radiation which the tissue receives. Generally speaking, the haemopoietic and epithelial tissues manifest radiation damage within weeks of radiation exposure, while damage to connective tissues becomes important at later times. A major development in the radiobiology of normal tissues during the 1980s was the realization that *early* and *late* normal-tissue responses are differently modified by a change in dose fractionation and this has given rise to the current interest in hyperfractionation (Section 9.2).

The first task of a radiobiologist is to *measure* a tissue response accurately and reliably. The term *assay* is used to describe such a system of measurement. Assays for tumour response are described in Section 14.3. For normal tissues, the following three general types of assay are available:

Scoring of gross tissue effects. It is possible to grade the severity of damage to a tissue using an arbitrary scale as is done in Figures 4.4 and 12.3. In superficial tissues this approach has been remarkably successful in allowing isoeffect relationships to be determined.

Assays of tissue function. For certain tissues, functional assays are available that allow radiation effects to be documented. Examples are the use of breathing rate as a measure of lung function in mice (Figures 13.4, 13.8), EDTA clearance as a measure of kidney damage (Figure 8.3), or blood counts as an indicator of bone marrow function.

Clonogenic assays. In some tumours and some normal tissues it has been possible to develop methods by which the colony of cells that derive from a single irradiated cell can be observed. In tumours this is particularly important because of the belief that regrowth of a tumour after sub-curative treatment is caused by the proliferation of a small number of tumour cells that retain colony-forming ability. This important area of radiation biology is introduced in Chapter 5.

1.5 Response curves, dose-response curves and isoeffect relationships

The response that is measured in an irradiated tissue increases over a certain time period and it may subsequently decline (Figure 1.3A). How should we quantify the level of response produced by a given dose of radiation? We could use the measured response at some chosen time after irradiation, such as the time of maximum response, but the timing of the peak may change with radiation dose and this would lead to some uncertainty in the interpretation of the results. A common device is to calculate the *cumulative* response (Figure 1.3B). Some normal-tissue responses give a cumulative curve that rises to a plateau, and the height of the plateau is quite a good measure of the total effect of that dose of radiation on the tissue. Other normal-tissue responses, in particular the late responses seen in connective and nervous tissues, are progressive and the cumulative response curve will continue to rise (Figure 13.3). In such cases there is no satisfactory alternative to choosing a fixed time at which to evaluate a response.

The next stage in a study of the radiation response of a tissue will be to vary the radiation dose and thus investigate a *dose-response relationship* (Figure 1.3C). Many examples of such curves are given in this book (for instance, Figures 12.1, 13.7, 14.1); cell survival curves (Section 5.3) are further examples of dose-response curves that are widely used in radiobiology. The position of the curve on the dose scale indicates the sensitivity of the tissue to radiation; its *steepness* also gives a direct indication of the change in response that will accompany an increase or decrease in radiation dose (Section 14.1).

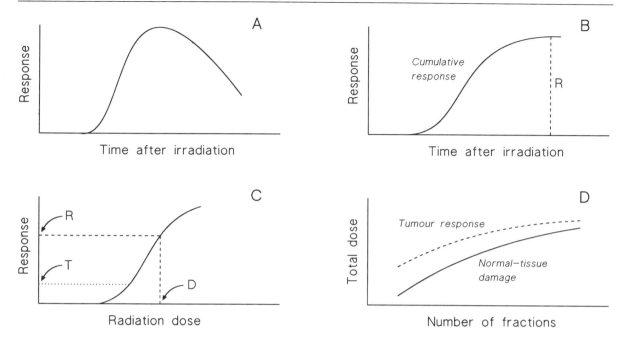

Figure 1.3 Four types of chart leading to the construction of an isoeffect plot. A: Time-course of development of radiation damage in a normal tissue. B: The cumulative response. C: A dose-response relationship, constructed by measuring the response (R) for various radiation doses (D). D: Isoeffect plot for a fixed level of normal-tissue damage (also a similar plot for tumour response).

The foregoing paragraphs have for simplicity referred to 'dose' as though we are concerned only with single radiation exposures. It is a well-established fact that multiple radiation doses given over a period of a few weeks generally give a better curative response than can be achieved with a single dose (Chapter 7). Diagrams similar to Figures 1.3A, B, and C can also be constructed for fractionated radiation treatment, although the results are easiest to interpret when the fractions are given over a time that is short compared with the time-scale of development of the response. If we change the schedule of dose fractionation, for instance by giving a different number of fractions, changing the fraction size or radiation dose rate, we can then investigate the therapeutic effect in terms of an *isoeffect plot* (Figure 1.3D). Experimentally this is done by performing multiple-dose studies for each chosen schedule and calculating a dose-response curve. We then select some particular level of effect (T in Figure 1.3C) and read off the total radiation dose that gives this effect. For effects on normal tissues the isoeffect will

often be some upper limit of *tolerance* of the tissue, perhaps expressed as a probability of tissue failure (Sections 12.2, 13.4). The isoeffect plot shows how the total radiation dose for the chosen level of effect varies with dose schedule. Examples are Figures 7.1, 7.3, 9.1, 9.4, and recommendations for tolerance calculations are set out in Chapter 10. The dashed line in Figure 1.3D illustrates how therapeutic conclusions may be drawn from isoeffect curves. If the curve for tumour response is flatter than for normal-tissue tolerance, then there is a therapeutic advantage in using large fraction numbers: a tolerance dose given using small fraction numbers will be far short of the tumour-effective dose, whereas for large fraction numbers it may be closer to an effective dose.

1.6 The concept of therapeutic index

Discussion of the possible benefit of a change in treatment strategy must always consider simultaneously the effects on tumour response and on normal-tissue damage. A wide range of factors enter into this assessment. In the clinic, in addition to quantifiable aspects of tumour response and toxicity, there may be a range of poorly-quantifiable factors such as new forms of toxicity or risks to the patient, or practicability and convenience to hospital staff; also cost implications. These must be balanced in the clinical setting. The function of radiation biology is to address the *quantifiable biological aspects* of a change in treatment.

In the laboratory this can be done by considering dose-response curves. As radiation dose is increased, there is always a tendency for tumour response to increase, and the same is true of normal-tissue damage. If, for instance, we measure tumour response by determining the proportion of tumours that are controlled, then we may expect a sigmoid relationship to dose (for fractionated radiation treatment we could consider the total dose or any other measure of treatment intensity). This is illustrated in the upper part of Figure 1.4. If we quantify normal-tissue damage in some way for the same treatment schedule, there will also be a rising curve of toxicity (lower panel). The shape of this curve is unlikely to be the same as that for tumour response and we probably will not wish to determine more than the initial part of this curve (since a high frequency of damage is unacceptable). By analogy with what must be done in the clinic, we can then fix a notional upper limit of *tolerance*. This fixes, for that treatment schedule, the upper limit of radiation dose that can be tolerated, for which the tumour response is indicated by the point labelled **A**.

Consider now the effect of adding to radiation therapy a cytotoxic drug. We expect that this will increase the tumour response for any radiation dose, and this will be seen as a movement to the left of the curve for tumour control (Figure 1.4). There will probably also be an increase in damage to normal tissues which again will consist of a left-ward movement of the toxicity curve. The relative displacement of the curves for the tumour and normal tissues will usually be different. But in this simple case there is a straightforward way of asking whether the combined treatment is better than radiation alone: for the same tolerance level of normal-tissue damage the maximum radiation dose will be lower and the corresponding level of tumour control is indicated by point **B**. If **B** is higher than **A** then the combination is

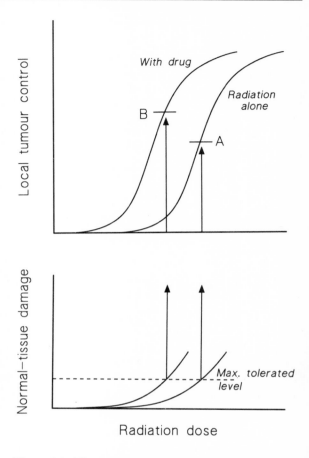

Figure 1.4 The procedure by which an improvement in *therapeutic index* might be identified, as a result of adding chemotherapy to radiotherapy. *See also* Figures 12.3, 18.1.

better than radiation alone. Improvement in therapeutic index has often been achieved in studies on experimental tumours in animals but the confirmation of this in the clinic is unfortunately rare (Section 18.5).

This example indicates the radiobiological concept of *therapeutic index*: it is the tumour response for a fixed level of normal-tissue damage. The concept can in principle be applied to any therapeutic situation or to any appropriate measures of tumour response or toxicity; the application of this in the clinic is not a straightforward matter, as indicated in Section 18.1. Therapeutic index carries the notion of 'cost-benefit' analysis. It is impossible to discuss the potential benefit of a new treatment without reference to its effect on therapeutic index.

Key points

1. Radiotherapy is an important curative and palliative modality in the treatment of cancer. Significant gains are still to be made by the optimization of biological and physical factors.
2. Therapeutic index is 'the name of the game' in curative cancer therapy.
3. The effects of radiation on mammalian tissues should be viewed as a succession of processes extending from microseconds after exposure to months and years thereafter. In choosing one end-point of effect, it is important not to overlook the rest of this whole process.

1.7 The importance of radiation biology for the future development of radiotherapy

Many developments in radiotherapy have resulted from new technologies or have been made empirically by clinicians; there are few examples of developments that have begun in the radiobiological laboratory and been carried through to the point where patient survival has significantly improved. The role of oxygen is one positive example that has led to some benefits with hyperbaric oxygen and chemical radiosensitizers. Current developments in fractionation and predictive testing also show considerable promise.

Compared with chemotherapeutic agents, radiation is now a well understood cytotoxic agent. Its access to tumour cells is just a matter of dosimetry, independent of the transport mechanisms that largely determine the effectiveness of chemical agents. The sequence of processes listed in Section 1.3 above are well described for radiation; some of them are equally relevant to the response of tissues to cytotoxic drug treatment, and thus research into radiation biology has brought benefits to other areas of therapeutic cancer research.

The future is likely to require greater and greater dependence on basic science. The simple empirical things have mostly been fully exploited and increasing knowledge about the cellular and molecular nature of radiation effects will undoubtedly lead to developments for which the radiotherapist will require a grounding in fundamental mechanisms. That is the purpose of this book.

Bibliography

Boag JW (1975). The time scale in radiobiology. 12th Failla memorial lecture. In: *Radiation Research*. (Eds) Nygaard OF, Adler HI and Sinclair WK. Academic Press.

DeVita VT, Goldin A, Oliverio VT *et al* (1979). The drug development and clinical trials programs of the Division of Cancer Treatment, National Cancer Institute. *Cancer Clinical Trials* 2:195-216.

Souhami R and Tobias J (1986). *Cancer and its Management*. Blackwells; Oxford.

Tubiana M (1992). The role of local treatment in the cure of cancer. *Eur J Cancer* 28A:2061-2069.

Further reading

Awwad HK (1990). *Radiation Oncology: Radiobiological and Physiological Perspectives*. Kluwer Academic Publishers; Dordrecht, The Netherlands.

Hall EJ (1988). *Radiobiology for the Radiologist*. JB Lippincott Co.; Philadelphia.

Steel GG, Adams GE and Horwich A (1989). *The Biological Basis of Radiotherapy*, second edition. Elsevier; Amsterdam.

2

The growth rate of tumours

G. Gordon Steel

2.1 Introduction

The speed of development of the disease process in patients with cancer depends to a large extent on the growth rate of primary and metastatic tumours. In patients in whom treatment is unsuccessful the speed of recurrence and the survival of the patient also depend on tumour growth rate. Growth rate is not the *only* determinant of the time-course of cancer: the location and the biochemical properties of the lesions may also play a part.

2.2 Measurement of tumour size

The precision and frequency with which tumour size can accurately be measured varies widely from one anatomical site to another. At the time of surgery a single measurement can often be made. The size of superficial lesions can be measured with engineer's calipers, within the constraints of skin thickness and depth of the lesion. Chest x-rays, CT and NMR scanning, and other imaging techniques also allow repeated measurements of tumours in some sites. The greatest amount of published data on tumour growth has been on primary and metastatic tumours in the lung. However, even in this site where the difference of tissue density between tumour and surrounding tissues is considerable, the size of lesion that can be discriminated is limited. Spratt *et al* (1963) tested the acuity of radiologists by placing plastic balls of different sizes over various parts of the chest of patients before taking x-rays and summarized the results of their studies as follows:

"The radiologists could locate the opacities of lucite balls 10–12 mm in diameter regularly regardless of their location. They could locate the radiopacities of balls 6 mm in diameter only when they were located in intercostal spaces contrasted against aerated lung. They could distinguish the radiopacities of 3 mm diameter balls from normal pulmonary shadows in these same areas of favourable contrast only when they were shown precisely where to look."

Careful studies of the growth and regression of lung metastases were made by Breur (1966) using a series of circles engraved on perspex, increasing in diameter by 0.5 or 1.0 mm. Thomlinson (1982) made very precise measurements of primary breast tumours using calipers. Various formulae have been used to transform linear dimensions into volumes, for instance:

$$V = \pi /6 \times (\text{mean diameter})^3$$

$$V = 0.5 \times \text{length} \times (\text{width})^2 \; [\text{taking } \pi \approx 3]$$

and provided the same formula is used consistently there is probably little to choose between them. For the measurement of tumours in laboratory animals, the calibration curve method (Steel, 1977) has a lot to commend it. Animals are taken with tumours of widely-varying size. The external dimensions of each tumour are measured, after which it is excised and weighed. Tumour weight is then plotted against an external measurement (for instance the product of length and width) and a smooth curve through these data comprises a calibration curve that can be used to interpret any further external measurements on non-excised tumours. This approach does not depend on any assumptions about the geometric form of the tumours, nor about the effect of skin thickness, and the scatter of points around the calibration curve also gives a direct indication of precision.

The size and growth rate of tumours can

be measured indirectly by quantifying tumour products in blood: CEA for choriocarcinomas, immunoglobulins for plasmacytomas, AFP or HCG in testicular tumours (Price *et al*, 1990 a and b).

2.3 Exponential and non-exponential growth

Exponential growth is where tumour volume increases by a constant *fraction* in equal intervals of time. Thus, the time for tumour volume to double (the *volume doubling time*, T_d) is the same for lesions of size 1–2 g or 10–20 g or 100–200 g, etc. The equation of exponential growth is:

$$V = \exp \left(0.693 \times \frac{time}{T_d} \right)$$

where 0.693 is $\log_e 2$. The logarithm of tumour volume increases linearly with time. It is therefore conventional to plot tumour growth curves on a logarithmic scale of volume.

Why is the idea of exponential growth so important? This is, in fact, the *simplest* mode of growth. If cells are allowed to proliferate under constant conditions, with no loss or infertility, their number will increase exponentially. It is *departure* from exponential growth that we have to explain! As indicated in Section 3.2, there are two principal processes that cause tumours to grow with a doubling time that is longer than the cell cycle time: cell loss and decycling (i.e. proliferating cells moving into a non-proliferating state). Non-exponential growth can thus arise by any combination of 3 factors: increasing cell cycle time, decreasing growth fraction, increasing rate of cell loss (Steel, 1977).

The nomogram in Figure 2.1 indicates the relation between tumour volume, cell number and the number of doublings, starting from a single cell. Cells are assumed to have a mass of 10^{-9} g. The nomogram is correct for any mode of growth; exponential is the special case where the doubling time is constant.

Figure 2.2 illustrates an important feature of exponential growth. The same exponential line is drawn on a *linear* scale of volume (above) or on a *logarithmic* scale (below). On the linear scale (which is what a clinical observer will tend to see) there appears to be a long 'silent interval' or latent

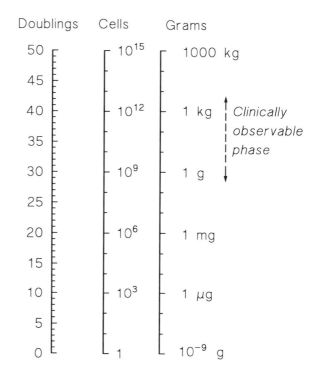

Figure 2.1 The relationship between the weight of a tumour, the number of cells it contains (assuming 10^9 per gram), and the number of doublings from a single cell.

period where no growth is seen. But during this time the tumour is growing regularly and with a constant doubling time. Once the tumour becomes detectable (at a size of perhaps 1 g) its size on a linear scale appears to sweep upwards, steeper and steeper. This is only a subjective and misleading impression, for growth is in fact perfectly regular and exponential.

Exponential growth of tumours in laboratory animals is uncommon. It is more usual to find that the doubling time increases progressively as the tumour gets bigger. This is illustrated in Figure 2.3 which shows a number of well-measured growth curves for tumours in rats and mice. The points are averages for a group of similar tumours. In each case the curves (on the logarithmic scale of volume) bend downwards, showing that the tumours grew progressively more slowly. The volume doubling time can be judged at any point by drawing a tangent to the curve and reading off its doubling time.

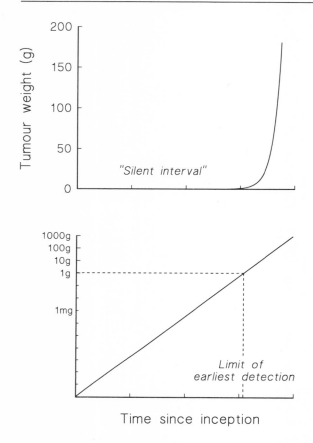

Figure 2.2   An exponential growth curve plotted on a linear scale (above) or on a logarithmic scale (below). The 'clinical' phase of growth is a minor part of the whole 'life history' of the tumour.

Growth curves of the type shown in Figure 2.3 have often been described by the Gompertz equation:

$$V = V_0 \exp[A/B \{1 - \exp(-B.t)\}]$$

Here V_0 is the volume at time zero and A and B are parameters that determine the growth rate. At very early time intervals (*t* small) the equation becomes exponential: $V = V_0 \exp(A.t)$. At long time intervals $\exp(-B.t)$ becomes small compared to 1.0 and the volume tends to a maximum value of $V_0 \exp(A/B)$. It can be seen in Figure 2.3 that the curves for the two rat tumours (fibroadenomas and Walker tumours) tend towards a larger maximum than for the mouse tumours, suggesting that this maximum size bears some relation to the host body weight. The Gompertz equation is not a unique description of such growth curves. For a fuller discussion see Steel (1977).

2.4 The growth rate of human tumours

Some examples of carefully measured human lung tumours are shown in Figure 2.4; the lines are straight or nearly so and these represent good examples of exponential tumour growth. Some human lung tumours show a Gompertzian pattern of growth, and irregular growth (sudden increase or decrease in growth rate) is not uncommon.

Published data on the growth rate of tumours

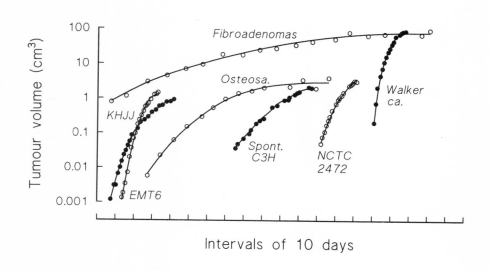

Figure 2.3   Growth curves for tumours in rats and mice. The primary breast fibroadenomas and the Walker tumours were in rats, the others in mice. The fitted curves are Gompertz equations. From Steel (1977), with permission.

Tumour volume (cm³)
10000
1000
100
10
1
0.1
MM
AR
RP
LH
NC
JS
Intervals of 100 days

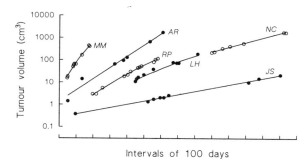

Figure 2.4 Growth curves for primary human lung tumours. Data of Schwartz, redrawn by Steel (1977), with permission.

Number of tumours
40
30
20
10
0
10 20 50 100 200 500 1000
Volume doubling time (days)

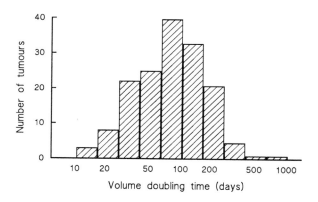

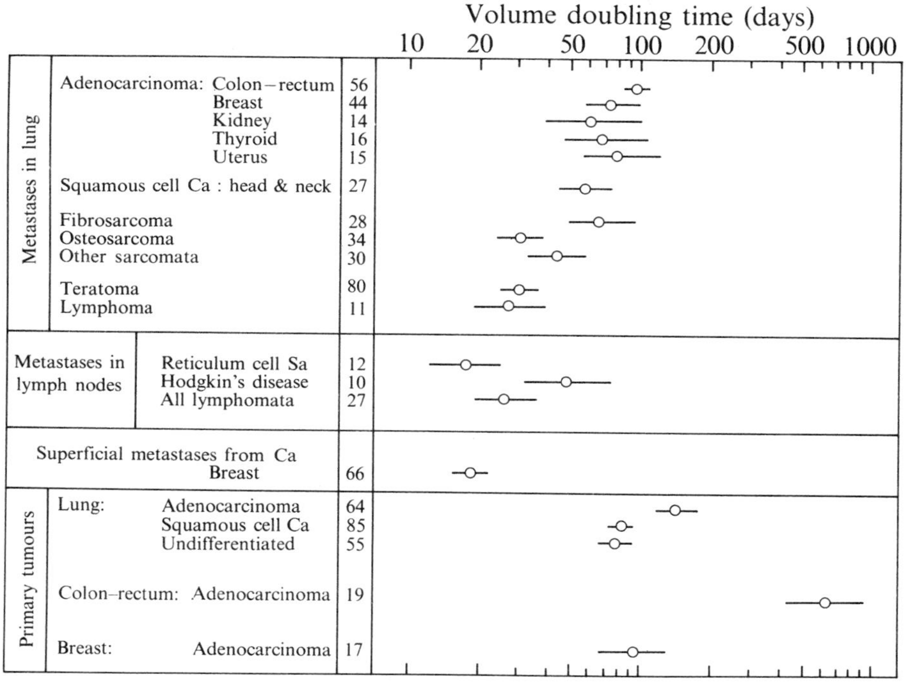

Figure 2.5 The distribution of volume doubling times for 159 lung metastases of adenocarcinoma from various primary sites. From Steel (1977) with permission.

was reviewed by Steel (1977). Within any one tumour type there is a wide range of volume doubling times. For instance, the range of values for lung metastases of adenocarcinoma is shown in Figure 2.5. Some double their volume in a week, some in a year or more, and the median is around 90 days. This median value is typical of other classes of human tumour. Figure 2.6 shows the geometric mean values of doubling time for tumours of various types. Lymphomas, teratomas, and superficial breast metastases grow faster than the average; primary colon tumours grow more slowly.

Volume doubling time (days)
10 20 50 100 200 500 1000
Metastases in lung
Adenocarcinoma: Colon–rectum 56
Breast 44
Kidney 14
Thyroid 16
Uterus 15
Squamous cell Ca : head & neck 27
Fibrosarcoma 28
Osteosarcoma 34
Other sarcomata 30
Teratoma 80
Lymphoma 11
Metastases in lymph nodes
Reticulum cell Sa 12
Hodgkin's disease 10
All lymphomata 27
Superficial metastases from Ca Breast 66
Primary tumours
Lung: Adenocarcinoma 64
Squamous cell Ca 85
Undifferentiated 55
Colon–rectum: Adenocarcinoma 19
Breast: Adenocarcinoma 17

Figure 2.6 A summary of data on the volume doubling times of human tumours. The points show geometric mean values, with standard errors. From Steel (1977) with permision.

2.5 The speed of tumour regression

After treatment, some tumours show a rapid volume response and others respond much more slowly. It is important to distinguish between *speed of shrinkage* and the *probability of local tumour control*, for some rapidly shrinking tumours recur early. Some clinical studies have shown a correlation between shrinkage rate and local control, but this is not the case in all clinical situations. Careful studies by Thomlinson (1982) showed that among primary breast tumours there was a 50-fold range of regression halving times (Figure 2.7). The rapidly shrinking tumours tended to be highly cellular, while those that shrank slowly had a large amount of connective tissue. He also found that in tumours that were treated by radiotherapy as well as by chemotherapy the rate of regression was independent of the treatment: it was characteristic of the biology of the tumour.

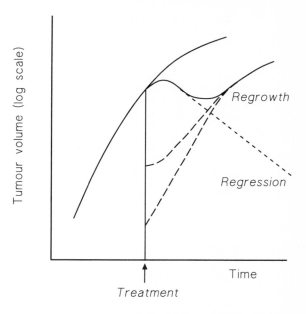

Figure 2.8. The volume response of an uncontrolled tumour is the resultant of two processes: regression and regrowth. Repopulation during the period of regression may take place at a rate that may differ from the growth rate of the untreated tumour.

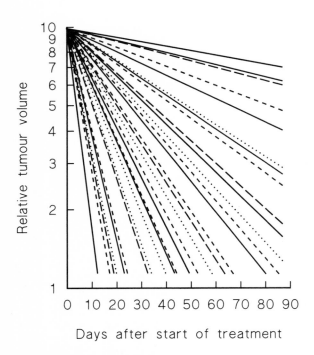

Figure 2.7 The range of regression rates of some of the 78 primary human breast tumours studied by Thomlinson (1982).

The overall volume response of a tumour to treatment is illustrated in Figure 2.8. There are two components of response: regression and regrowth. The nadir (i.e. minimum tumour volume) will depend upon both. For judging the effectiveness of tumour treatment it is therefore wise to choose a measure that reflects the regrowth component rather than the speed of regression. *Partial remission* is an unsatisfactory criterion. *Duration of disease-free interval* is to be preferred. For measurable lesions the preferred parameter is the *tumour growth delay*: this indicates the difference between the times that treated or untreated tumours reach a fixed multiple of the pretreatment tumour size (e.g. twice the size at the start of treatment, *see* Section 14.3).

Key points

1. The accurate measurement of tumour size greatly helps clinical judgement on the rate of progression or response to treatment of tumours.
2. Tumour growth curves should always be plotted on a logarithmic scale in order to compare the data with exponential growth. Think logarithmically!
3. The rate of regression following treatment often varies widely among tumours of the same histopathological type. Slow regression does not necessarily mean little response.
4. The growth rate of tumours can vary widely among tumours of the same type. Volume doubling times in the region of 3 months are common.

Bibliography

Breur K (1966). Growth rate and radiosensitivity of human tumours. *Eur J Cancer* 2:157-171.

Price P, Hogan SJ and Horwich A (1990 a). The growth rate of metastatic non-seminomatous germ cell testicular tumours measured by marker production doubling time. I: Theoretical basis and practical application. *Europ J Cancer* 26:450-453.

Price P, Hogan SJ, Bliss JM and Horwich A (1990 b). The growth rate of metastatic non-seminomatous germ cell testicular tumours measured by marker production doubling time. II: Prognostic significance in patients treated with chemotherapy. *Europ J Cancer* 26:453-456.

Spratt JS, Ter-Pogossian M and Long RTL (1963). The detection and growth of intrathoracic neoplasms. *Archs Surg* 86:283-288.

Thomlinson RH (1982). Measurement and management of carcinoma of the breast. *Clin Radiol* 33:481-493.

Further reading

Steel GG (1977). *The Growth Kinetics of Tumours*. Oxford University Press; Oxford.

3

Cell proliferation in tumours

Adrian C. Begg

3.1 Cell kinetic compartments of a tumour

The neoplastic cells within a tumour can be divided into four compartments based on their kinetic properties (Figure 3.1). The most important compartment is that of actively dividing cells. All cells in this compartment are going through the cell cycle and can be distinguished using cell labelling techniques. All new tumour cells are produced from this compartment which is therefore the major contributor to growth of the tumour volume. This compartment is called the *growth fraction*, and the cells within it are sometimes called 'P' (for proliferating) cells.

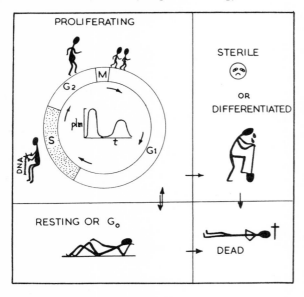

Figure 3.1 The neoplastic component of a tumour comprises four categories of cells: proliferating, resting, differentiated, and dead cells.

In addition to actively dividing cells, there are two other compartments in the majority of tumours which contain non-proliferating cells. These are the resting (or G_0) compartment and the sterile (or differentiated) compartment. The major difference between them is that G_0 cells are capable of re-entering the cell cycle (or P compartment), while sterile or differentiated cells are no longer capable of division. G_0 cells are often called 'Q' (for quiescent) cells. Some G_0 cells may be clonogenic (capable of repopulating a tumour) and are therefore dangerous and need to be killed by the applied therapy. It is often not easy to distinguish G_0 cells from sterile cells based on kinetic techniques, although terminally differentiated cells can sometimes be distinguished morphologically in well differentiated tumours. Differentiated cells are no longer a serious danger to the patient, although if present in large numbers, their bulk can cause problems. The other main contributor to tumour bulk is the *stroma*: normal-tissue cells such as blood cells and fibroblasts that in some cases can exceed the number of neoplastic cells.

Fourthly, there exists in most tumours a compartment consisting of dead and dying cells. This is a characteristic of tumours and is the result of an inadequate blood supply. This compartment contains pyknotic cells and regions of necrosis, sometimes quite large.

The arrows in Figure 3.1 indicate that transfer of cells can take place from one compartment to another. Movement of cells from the Q to the P compartment, which can occur after or during some treatments, is called *recruitment*. Transfer from P to Q must occur, for otherwise the proportion of Q-cells would decline towards zero in a growing tumour due to the multiplication of P cells. Some cells may have an inadequate supply of nutrients such as oxygen and may fail to divide further. Cells can enter the differentiated compartment due to natural differentiation processes. Finally, cells can leave the volume of a primary tumour mass, either as viable cells (this can lead to metastases), or by death followed by the resorption of their constituents. This process is called *cell loss*.

3.2 Factors affecting tumour growth rate

The volume doubling time of a tumour (T_d, Section 2.3) is determined by three main factors: the cell cycle time (T_c), the growth fraction (GF) and the rate of cell loss. Tumours grow faster if: the cycle time is short, the growth fraction is high, and cell loss is low (Table 3.1). The *potential doubling time*, or T_{pot}, is defined as the time within which the cell population of the tumour would double if there were no cell loss (Steel, 1977). It depends on the cell cycle time and the growth fraction.

Table 3.1 Kinetic parameters of a typical human tumour

Cell cycle time ($\approx$ 2 d)	Potential doubling time ($\approx$5d)	Volume doubling time ($\approx$ 70 d)
Growth fraction ($\approx$40%)		
Cell loss ($\approx$90%)		

The potential doubling time can be obtained from a thymidine labelling index (LI) or S-phase fraction by the relation:

$$Potential\ doubling\ time\ (T_{pot}) = \lambda \frac{T_s}{LI} \quad (Eqn\ 3.1)$$

where T_s is the duration of the S-phase and λ is a parameter that corrects for the non-rectangular age distribution of growing cell populations, usually between 0.7 and 1.0. The S-phase duration can be measured by the labelled mitoses technique (Section 3.4). The volume doubling time (T_d) is found using calipers, from radiographs or from CT scans. The rate of cell loss from a tumour can be estimated from the *cell loss factor*:

$$Cell\ loss\ factor = 1 - \frac{T_{pot}}{T_d} \quad (Eqn\ 3.2)$$

(Steel, 1977). This factor is simply the cell loss rate

as a fraction of the cell birth rate. The slow growth of many human tumours is largely the result of a high rate of cell loss. The principal mechanisms of cell loss are necrosis and differentiation: well-differentiated carcinomas (by definition) maintain some features of the hierarchical tissue structure of the tissue of origin (Section 4.1) and cell turnover by this normal pathway probably continues in the malignant state.

Evidence from studies on tumours in mice and rats suggests that the slowing of growth rate as tumours increase in size (Section 2.3) is associated with a progressive increase in the rate of cell loss, a decrease in the growth fraction, and a lengthening of the mean cell cycle duration (Steel, 1977).

3.3 Values of kinetic parameters in human tumours

Studies have been carried out in which ³H-thymidine was given to patients and multiple biopsies taken in order to measure cell cycle parameters. Radioactive thymidine is specifically incorporated into DNA, although some of it is catabolised and lost from the tissue. Many early studies of cell proliferation were based on thymidine labelling of S-phase cells. Cell cycle times for human tumours from these studies ranged from 15 hours to more than 100 hours with an average of $\approx$ 2.3 d (Steel, 1977). These values are similar to cell number doubling times found for human tumour cells grown in culture. As shown in Section 2.4, the *volume* doubling times for human tumours are much longer, ranging from 4 days to over a year, around a median of roughly 3 months. There are large differences between individual tumours, even within a particular histological type. Growth fractions for the relatively few human tumours studied range between 6% and 90%, with most solid tumours having values well below 50%. Cell loss factors are almost always high, usually ranging from 70% to over 90% (Table 3.2). This is apparent from average T_{pot} values of a few days compared with T_d values of a few months: for instance, if T_{pot} = 5 d and T_d = 70d, cell loss factor = 1–(5/70) = 0.93 or 93%.

Table 3.2   Cell loss calculations for human tumours

	Thymidine labelling index (%) *(median and range)*	Volume doubling time (days) *(median and range)*	T_{pot} (days)	Cell loss factor (per cent)
Colorectal carcinoma	15 (10–22)	90 (60–170)	3.1	96
Squamous cell carcinoma of head and neck	6.9 (5–17)	45 (33–150)	6.8	85
Undifferentiated bronchial carcinoma	19 (8–23)	90 (40–160)	2.5	97
Melanoma	3.3	52 (20–150)	14	73
Sarcomas	2.0 (0.3–6)	39 (16–78)	23	40
Lymphomas	3.0 (0.4–13)	22 (15–70)	16	29
Childhood tumours	13 (10–25)	20	3.6	82

From Steel (1977)

3.4 Cell kinetic methods

Percent Labelled Mitoses

With this technique, all phases of the cell cycle can be determined. Cells are pulse labelled with ³H-thymidine (³H-TdR), a radioactively labelled nucleoside that is specifically incorporated into DNA, not RNA. The labelling is done either by injection into an animal or patient (which as a result of the rapid metabolism of thymidine gives almost instantaneous labelling of cells in the S-phase), or for cells in tissue-culture by washing the tracer out after a few minutes. Samples of the cell population are taken at a range of times after labelling. Autoradiographs are then prepared: photographic emulsion is laid over the cells to detect electron emission from the ³H decays and the slides are left in the dark for an appropriate exposure time. Recognizable mitotic figures can then be scored as labelled (black grains over the nucleus) or unlabelled. The ³H-TdR labels only cells which at the time of administration were in the S-phase. This cohort of cells then moves through the cell cycle, reaching mitosis (M) after a period equal to the duration of the G_2-phase (stage b in Figure 3.2). At this time the first labelled mitotic figures will be observed. After a further period of T_s the last few labelled cells will be passing through mitosis and the fraction of labelled mitoses will drop, theoretically to zero (stage e). The result is that the fraction of labelled mitoses when plotted against time shows a series of waves, each separated by one cell cycle time (T_c, Figure 3.2); the width of each wave is the DNA synthesis duration (T_s). The length of G_2 can be obtained from the time between labelling and when labelled mitoses start to appear. The disadvantages of the method for studies on cancer patients are the need to administer radioactivity, the requirement for repeated biopsies, the long exposure times of the autoradiographs and the labour and skill required for the scoring. An alternative more rapid method using a thymidine analogue and flow cytometry is described below.

Continuous Thymidine Labelling

Cells are given a continuous supply of ³H-TdR, either by repeated injection or a continuous infusion in animals, or by a continuous exposure of cells *in vitro*. The fraction of labelled cells rises progressively with time as G_1 cells enter S and become labelled (Figure 3.3A). After a period of (T_c-T_s) all cells in the cell cycle should be labelled. Variation in the durations of cell-cycle phases will tend to smooth out the continuous labelling curve. It has sometimes been thought that the level at which a continuous labelling curve flattens out gives an indication of the growth fraction. However, in any growing cell population whose growth fraction is constant there must be a continual production of Q-cells by *decycling* of P-cells. This will lead to the progressive labelling of some Q-cells during continuous labelling, a process that will be enhanced if Q-cells have a limited lifespan (Steel, 1977). In tumour cell populations it is thus not possible to estimate the growth fraction from a continuous labelling curve. The steepness of such a curve nevertheless

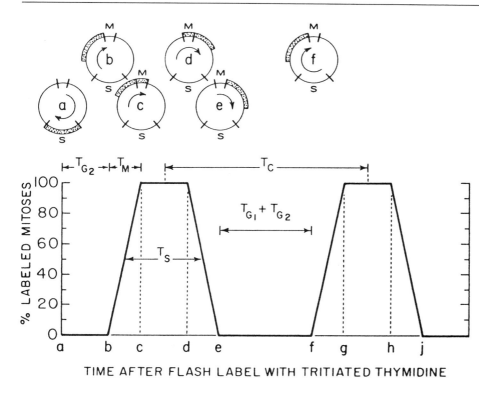

Figure 3.2 Illustrating the movement of cells through the cell cycle in the technique of labelled mitoses. The stippled blocks indicate cells labelled by a brief exposure to ³H-thymidine.

TIME AFTER FLASH LABEL WITH TRITIATED THYMIDINE

provides a way of evaluating the proliferation rate of a cell population.

Double Labelling

This technique can be used to measure the duration of DNA synthesis (T_s) from a single biopsy. Two labelled forms of thymidine are used, one labelled with ³H and the other with ¹⁴C. These can be distinguished in an autoradiograph by the distance of the black grains away from the nucleus: ³H grains lie over the nucleus while longer-range emissions from ¹⁴C lie around as well as over the nucleus. Administration of the two labels is separated by an interval (t) which must be shorter than G_2. Late S-phase cells labelled with the first isotope will enter G_2 and will not therefore be labelled with the second isotope (Figure 3.3B). The fraction of cells with only one label is proportional to the time between labels, while the fraction with the second label (with or without the first) is proportional to the S-phase duration:

$$\frac{\text{cells with }^3\text{H only}}{\text{all cells with }^{14}\text{C}} = \frac{t}{T_s} \quad \text{(Eqn 3.3)}$$

T_s can therefore be calculated from cell counts made on the autoradiograph of a single tissue specimen. This method can also be carried out using two different non-radioactive thymidine analogues instead of ³H-TdR and ¹⁴C-TdR (see below).

The Stathmokinetic Technique

This technique uses compounds which block cells in mitosis, such as colchicine, colcemid, vincristine or vinblastine. Under this block, the fraction of cells in metaphase rises with time (Figure 3.3C). If the dose of the blocking agent is correctly chosen, the rate of increase of the metaphase index gives a measure of the *mitotic rate*, i.e. the rate at which cells are entering mitosis. Satisfactory accumulation only continues for a limited time, after which some arrested cells begin to degenerate. If every mitosis produces 2 daughter cells, the mitotic rate equals the cell birth rate. It is thus possible to calculate the potential doubling time from the relation:

$$T_{pot} = \log_e(2) \ / \ mitotic \ rate \quad \text{(Eqn 3.4)}$$

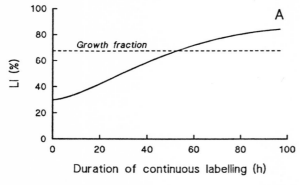

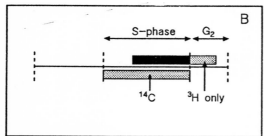

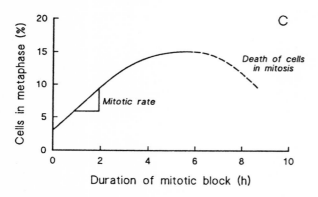

Figure 3.3 Three further cell kinetic techniques. A: continuous thymidine labelling in a tumour cell population; B: the principle of the double-labelling technique; C: the stathmokinetic method.

In addition, the duration of mitosis, T_m, can also in principle be obtained. The advantage of this technique is that no radioactivity or special staining is required.

Thymidine Analogues

Replacement of the methyl group of thymidine (Figure 3.4) with halogen atoms of similar

size such as iodine or bromine creates the analogues iodo- or bromo-deoxyuridine (IUdR, BrUdR). Enzymes responsible for DNA synthesis cannot easily distinguish between thymidine and its analogues and so these are incorporated into DNA via the same pathway as thymidine. Once in the DNA, they can be detected with specific antibodies which recognize the small distortions in the DNA molecule caused by their incorporation. The development of these antibodies has led to their widespread use for cell kinetic studies. The antibodies can in turn be labelled with an enzyme (usually a peroxidase) which allows immunocytochemical staining, or a fluorescent label (usually the green fluorescent molecule FITC) for flow cytometry. In this way, all cells that have incorporated the analogue and were therefore in the S-phase, can be detected by a brown colour on immunoperoxidase-stained sections or green fluorescence for flow cytometry.

Flow Cytometry

For cell kinetic studies using flow cytometry, BrUdR labelled cells are stained with a mouse antibody specific for the DNA-incorporated analogue, followed by an anti-mouse antibody conjugated with FITC (Figure 3.5). Cells are counter-stained for total DNA content using propidium iodide (PI, a red fluorescent stain). In the flow cytometer, the stained cells flow through

5-IODO-2'-DEOXYURIDINE   THYMIDINE

I = 2.15Å CH_3 = 2.00Å

Figure 3.4 The structure of thymidine and its analogue, IUdR. The comparative diameters of the iodine atom and the methyl group are indicated.

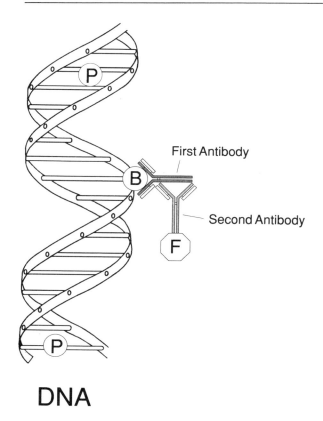

DNA

Figure 3.5 The principle of BrUdR staining of DNA. B = an incoporated BrUdR molecule; P = an intercalated propidium iodide molecule; F = FITC conjugated to the second antibody.

a laser beam which excites the fluorochromes, giving green fluorescent emissions from FITC and red from the PI (Hall, 1988). These colours can be separated using optical filters and their intensities measured for each cell using photomultiplier tubes (Figure 3.6). The data are displayed as two-parameter cytograms, for instance green *versus* red fluorescence intensities. Three subpopulations representing G_1 cells (low green and low red), G_2/M cells (low green and high red) and S-phase cells (high green) can readily be seen. Up to 10,000 cells per second can be analyzed in this way by modern flow cytometers, making this a rapid and quantitative method, without the use of radioactivity.

An example of the flow cytometer output is shown in Figure 3.7. This shows green (IUdR) *versus* red (DNA) fluorescence cytograms for A549 human lung carcinoma cells at different times (1–15 h) after pulse labelling *in vitro* with IUdR. Movement of labelled and unlabelled cells through the cell cycle can be seen from the changing patterns. At time zero, i.e. immediately after pulse labelling, the labelled cells should be distributed equally between the G_1 and G_2 positions. In Figure 3.7, some movement of the cells through the S phase has already occurred by 1 h (top left) as seen by the 'leaning' to the right of the dot pattern. This becomes more pronounced with increasing times. By 6–7 h (middle column), all the unlabelled cells that were in G_1 have moved into the S phase, and all the labelled cells have moved out of S and are now in G_2 or G_1. This gives an almost inverted picture compared with that at 1 h. All phases of the cell cycle can be obtained from these pictures, in a manner similar to the analysis of percent labelled mitoses curves, except that the fraction of labelled cells in mid-S is measured instead of the fraction of labelled cells in mitosis.

Obtaining Kinetic Information from One Sample

The Relative Movement method allows T_s, LI and T_{pot} to be estimated from one tissue sample (Begg *et al*, 1985). This is useful for clinical application where it is often difficult to take more than one biopsy (Waldman *et al*, 1988; Wilson *et al*, 1988). Several hours after i.v. injection of BrUdR or IUdR a tumour biopsy is taken, fixed in ethanol, and subsequently stained and analyzed by flow cytometry. The average position (red fluorescence) of the labelled cells which have not yet divided, relative to the positions of G_1 and G_2, is measured using computer-drawn windows around the appropriate subpopulations (Figure 3.8A). The Relative Movement parameter (RM) is a DNA-content parameter defined to be zero for cells in G_1 and 1.0 for cells in G_2. Since on average the labelled cells immediately after staining will be homogeneously distributed within the S-phase, it is assumed that RM at that time is 0.5. Subsequently, the cells progress towards G_2 and RM increases. The procedure is to measure RM in a sample taken a few hours (t) after labelling, then draw a curve between RM = 0.5 at $t = 0$ and the measured RM at time t. This is extrapolated to the time required for RM to reach 1.0, which gives the estimate of T_s (Figure 3.8B). The relation between

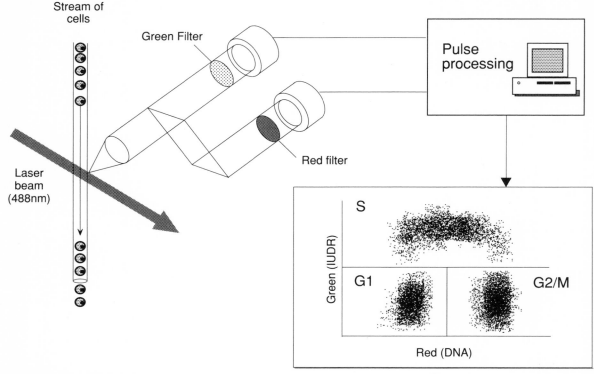

Figure 3.6   The principle of flow cytometry.

RM and time is approximately linear (though theoretically slightly curved). Panel C in Figure 3.8 shows an example of data obtained in this way for cells growing at different rates due to different culture temperatures. It can be concluded that the duration of the S-phase approximately doubled as a result of lowering the temperature.

Human Tumour Kinetics in vivo by Thymidine Analogue Labelling

As described above, some basic kinetic information can be obtained by labelling human tumour biopsy material *in vitro* with ^{3}H-TdR or a thymidine analogue, thus obtaining the labelling index. More information can be obtained by *in vivo* labelling, and this avoids some potential artefacts of the *in vitro* procedure. Human tumours can be labelled by *in vivo* injection of IUdR or BrUdR because these analogues produce little or no toxicity at the low doses required for

pulse-labelling kinetic studies. An example of the flow cytometer outputs following *in vivo* labelling of a human tumour with IUdR and biopsy a few hours later is shown in Figure 3.9. Panel B shows the distribution of DNA content; the peak on the left is a diploid peak that indicates the presence of non-malignant stromal cells. The large peak is due to G_1 cells and the smallest peak to G_2 tumour cells. Panel A shows IUdR uptake plotted vertically, against DNA content. The normal cells are again visible as the left-hand cluster of dots. These are not included in the analysis. Two subpopulations of labelled cells can be seen, as expected, several hours after labelling, one small one at the tumour G_1 position and a larger one covering most of the S-phase. The kinetic parameters labelling index (LI), DNA synthesis time (T_s), and the potential doubling time ($= \lambda \times T_s/LI$) can be obtained from these data. This method is now being used as a predictive test for rapidly and slowly repopulating tumours (Section 23.4).

It is not yet possible to measure T_c from one biopsy, although if the growth fraction were known it could be calculated from T_{pot}. Several antibodies exist that have been reported to be specific for cycling cells (e.g. Ki67, PCNA, anti-DNA polymerase), although these have not yet been validated as reliable growth-fraction markers in human tumours.

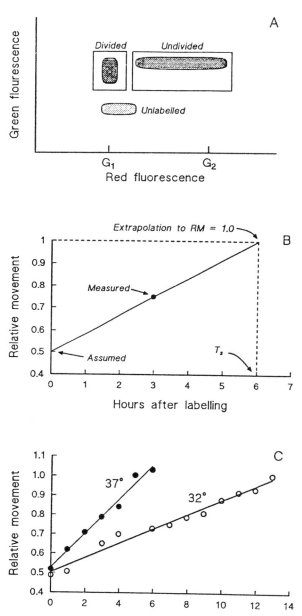

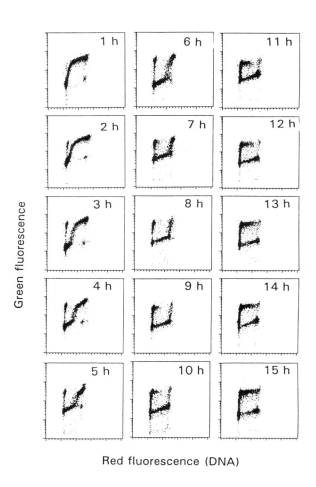

Figure 3.7 Flow cytometer traces from samples taken at hourly intervals from an *in vitro* cell population that was labelled with IUdR at time zero. Green fluorescence (IUdR content) is plotted vertically; red fluorescence (DNA content) horizontally.

Figure 3.8 Principle of the relative movement method. A: the 2-dimensional flow-cytometer display; B: the principle of the method; C: an example of a study on cells at two different temperatures, the difference in slopes indicates different S-phase durations.

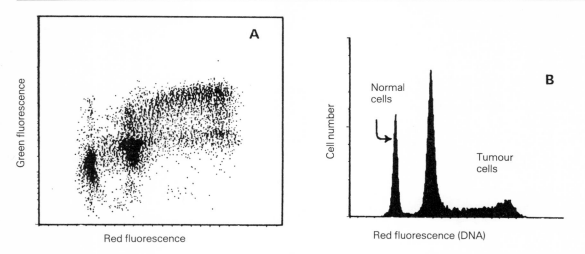

Figure 3.9   Flow cytometry output from a human tumour biopsy a few hours after labelling with IUdR. A: the 2-dimensional display of red-green fluorescence; B: the derived distribution of DNA contents.

Key points

1. Tumour growth rate is determined by the cell cycle time, the growth fraction, and the rate of cell loss. Potential doubling time indicates the cell proliferation rate and is the predicted doubling time of the cell population in the absence of cell loss.
2. Cell cycle times average around two days in human tumours, compared with volume doubling times of over two months. Cell loss is high in many human tumours, particularly in carcinomas.
3. There is a wide variation of kinetic parameters among human tumours, even between those of the same histological type.
4. The movement of cells through the cell cycle can be measured using ^{3}H-thymidine or the thymidine analogues bromo-deoxyuridine or iodo-deoxyuridine. Methods include autoradiography, immunocytochemistry and flow cytometry.
5. Human tumour cell kinetics can be measured by *in vitro* labelling of biopsies or by injecting the patient with low doses of thymidine analogues. Flow cytometric analysis methods allow calculation of the potential doubling time from one biopsy.

Bibliography

Begg AC, McNally NJ, Shrieve DC and Karcher H (1985). A method to measure the duration of DNA synthesis and the potential doubling time from a single sample. *Cytometry* 6:620-626.

Hall EJ (1988). *Radiobiology for the Radiologist.* 3rd Edition. Chapter 11. Lippincott Co.; Philadelphia.

Waldman FM, Dolbeare F and Gray J (1988). Clinical application of the bromodeoxyuridine assay. *Cytometry* 3:65-72.

Wilson GD, McNally NJ, Dische S *et al* (1988). Measurement of cell kinetics in human tumours *in vivo* using bromodeoxyuridine incorporation and flow cytometry. *Br J Cancer* 58:423-431.

Further reading

Steel GG (1977). *The Growth Kinetics of Tumours.* Oxford University Press; Oxford.

Tannock IF and Hill RP (1992). *The Basic Science of Oncology,* 2nd edition chapter 10. McGraw-Hill, New York.

4

Cell proliferation in normal tissues

Albert J. van der Kogel

4.1 Proliferative organization of tissues

Cell proliferation in normal tissues is, in contrast to tumours, highly organized with cell production homeostatically controlled. In adult tissues under non-pathological conditions the production of cells is exactly balanced by the loss of differentiated mature cells; the cell loss factor is thus 1.0. The degree of organization of cells within proliferative and functional compartments has been used to distinguish between two categories of tissues, *hierarchical* and *flexible* (Michalowski, 1981):

Hierarchical (H-type) tissues – tissues with a clearly recognizable separation between the stem-cell compartment, an amplification compartment (usually proliferating rapidly), and a post-mitotic compartment of mature functional cells (Figure 4.1A);

Flexible (F-type) tissues – tissues without a recognizable separation between these compartments,

in which some at least of the functional cells also have the capacity of cell renewal (Figure 4.1B).

H-type tissues are mostly the rapidly renewing cell systems, such as skin, mucosae, intestinal epithelia, and the haemopoietic system. The self-renewing stem cells in these tissues may comprise only a small percentage (less than a few percent) of the total of proliferating cells, while the bulk of the proliferating cells that make up the amplification compartment are involved in production of the cells that are needed for the final maturation into functional cells. The rate of cell production is determined by the life-span of the mature cells, which may vary from a few days (in the case of granulocytes or intestinal villus cells) to more than 100 days (for instance erythrocytes). Schematic examples of tissue organization in epithelial tissues are shown in Figure 4.2: in skin the stem cells are confined to the flat basal layer; in the small intestine they are to be found in roughly the lower half of the crypt.

Tissues that are not clearly identified as having a hierarchical organization are usually classified as flexible (*F-type*). The tissues in this category are all slowly renewing (e.g. liver, kidney, lung and central nervous system); some degree of proliferative hierarchy may exist but not as well defined and recognized as in the rapidly renewing tissues. The next sections deal with the proliferative organization of tissues and its impact on response to radiation.

4.2 Radiation response of hierarchical tissues

The most important mode of cell death following irradiation results from damage to the proliferative process. Irradiation therefore tends not

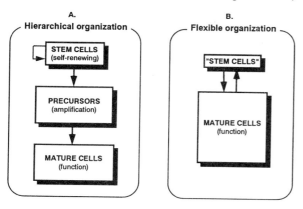

Figure 4.1 Schematic outline of the proliferative organization of **A**: hierarchical and **B**: flexible normal-tissue systems.

Epidermis

Intestinal crypt

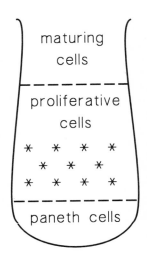

Figure 4.2 Proliferative organization of the skin and the intestinal mucosa. In the basal layer of the skin, about 1 in 10 basal cells are considered to be stem cells (*), the others as transit cells. The proliferative activity is confined to the basal layer. In the crypts of the small intestine the proliferative cells occupy roughly the bottom two-thirds of the crypt, with stem cells near the bottom (*). Most of the proliferative cells are in the amplification zone; they mature near the top of the crypt and then migrate up on to the villus. From Thames and Hendry (1987), with permission.

to damage the mature functional cells in H-type tissues. Lymphocytes are an exception to this. They undergo interphase death after irradiation, the phenomenon known as *apoptosis*. The time between irradiation and tissue response is mostly determined by the life-span of the mature cells

and is generally independent of the radiation dose. This is schematically illustrated in Figure 4.3A, showing the loss of functional cells at the normal rate of attrition and the lack of replacement because of cell death in the precursor and stem-cell pool. After a relatively low dose (D_1) the

A: HIERARCHICAL TISSUE

B: FLEXIBLE TISSUE

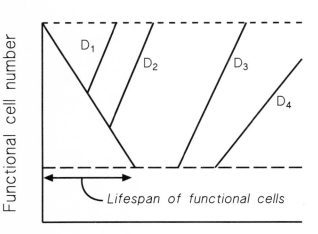

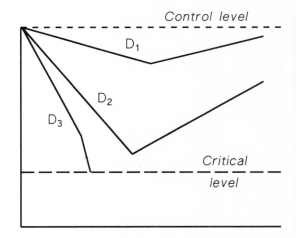

Time after irradiation

Figure 4.3 The distinction between hierarchical (H-type) and flexible (F-type) tissues, as illustrated by the predicted changes in functional cell number after increasing radiation doses (D1 - D4). The 'critical level' is the level below which tissue breakdown will occur. Modified from Michalowski (1981), with permission.

proliferating pool is rapidly restored and replenishment of the functional cells occurs. After a higher dose (D_2) more functional cells are lost and the onset of repopulation takes longer. After both doses the number of mature cells is still sufficient to maintain tissue integrity and no major damage is observed. This is not so after a higher dose (D_3), when the functional cell pool falls to a critical level and the tissue breaks down, followed eventually by recovery. The rate of recovery may become slower when, after an even higher dose (D_4), the rapidly proliferating precursor pool is emptying and first needs to be replenished by the more slowly proliferating stem cells. Also, other factors may start to play a role, such as an impaired blood supply which may slow down tissue recovery or perhaps lead to permanent tissue necrosis.

These principles of the response of H-type tissues are clearly demonstrated in the skin. The loss of the differentiating layers is reflected by the occurrence of various degrees of dry and moist desquamation. An example in the mouse skin is shown in Figure 4.4A. These curves form a mirror-image of the theoretical curves of Figure 4.3A, and the time-course of the reactions can be related to the cycle time of the basal cells (≈ 4.5 days), to the radiation-induced division delay, and to the number of cell layers in the mouse skin ($\approx 3 - 4$). When the cycle time of the proliferating basal cells is reduced to 2 days by plucking of the hair, the skin reactions develop much faster (Figure 4.4B). Note also that recovery, especially after the higher doses, is delayed compared with the unperturbed skin, suggesting a sensitization of the more rapidly dividing basal cells.

Morris and Hopewell (1988) made direct counts of the change in cell density of basal cells forming the proliferative compartment of pig skin. Figure 4.5 shows the effects of different radiation doses in two strains of animal. The results show a pattern similar to Figure 4.3A, but with the difference of a more rapid restoration after the higher dose level. This probably reflects a shortening of the cell cycle in response to a more severe depletion of the basal layer after higher radiation doses, as the tissue attempts to restore the more severe injury more rapidly. It is also of interest that the timing of changes in the basal layer is different for different pig strains, reflecting slight differences in cell kinetics.

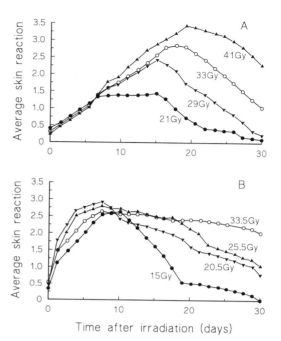

Figure 4.4 The time-course of radiation-induced desquamation in the dorsal skin of the mouse foot. **A**: normal skin; **B**: plucked skin, showing a faster development of reactions due to a shorter cycle time. From Hegazy and Fowler (1973), with permission.

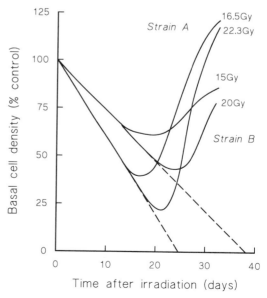

Figure 4.5 Radiation-induced changes in basal cell density in the epidermis of pig skin. Results are shown for two different strains of pig. From Morris and Hopewell (1988), with permission.

4.3   Radiation response of flexible tissues

The strict hierarchy in proliferation and differentiation is mostly observed in rapidly renewing cell systems, in which the timing of the acute radiation response relates directly to the turnover rate of the mature cells. Tissues or organs with a slow rate of renewal are usually not as well characterized, and vascular and parenchymal components may both contribute to the development of organ failure after irradiation. In addition, for several parenchymal cell types the existence of stem cells in the slowly renewing tissues has been demonstrated (e.g. glial progenitors in CNS; satellite cells in muscle; oval cells in the liver). Therefore these *flexible* tissues may at least partly be classified as hierarchical. The model of the radiation response of flexible tissues as proposed by Michalowski (1981) and shown in Figure 4.3B is thus not as generally applicable as the H-type model; it varies from one tissue to another depending on which *target cells* are responsible for a specific radiation effect (Section 13.2). In this model the rate of cell loss increases with radiation dose, as the mature cells are also the proliferating cells that die in mitosis. The model predicts a *dose-dependent* latency to loss of organ function; this has been shown for lung, kidney, and the CNS. However, this could also be predicted by adopting a late *H-type* response in which the variable and long latent times are wholly based on the characteristics of a (small) stem-cell compartment (Tucker and Hendry, 1990). A particular feature of the F-type model is the

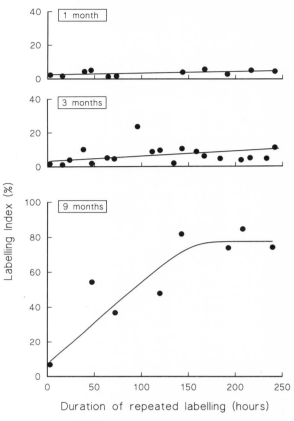

Figure 4.7   Cell proliferation in the epithelium of the mouse bladder at 1, 3 and 9 months after irradiation with 25 Gy electrons. In this slowly renewing tissue the proliferation rate only increases significantly between 3 and 9 months after irradiation, coinciding with the histological appearance of hyperplasia and the occurrence of functional deficit. From Stewart (1986), with permission.

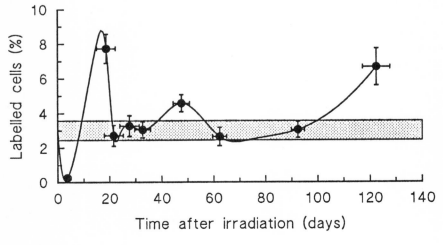

Figure 4.6   Kinetics of glial-cell proliferation in the cervical spinal cord after a single dose of 20 Gy. In spite of the late radiation response (5 - 6 months) of this tissue, an early wave of proliferation is observed. From Hornsey *et al* (1981), with permission.

prediction of an *avalanche* of cell loss when a critical number of functional cells is depleted. The idea is that homeostatic mechanisms might increase the proliferation rate of irradiated cells and therefore lead to enhancement of mitotic cell death. However, this aspect of the F-type model has not yet clearly been demonstrated in any tissue.

Changes in cell proliferation after irradiation of late-responding tissues are illustrated here for two tissues, spinal cord and the bladder. In the rat spinal cord two waves of proliferation have been noted (Hornsey *et al*, 1981): an early wave after about 20 days and a much later wave after more than 100 days (Figure 4.6). The early wave may be related to an initial response of glial stem cells (Section 13.2), while the late wave occurs at a time preceding the occurrence of necrosis. A similar late increase in proliferation at more than 6 months after irradiation is noted in the mouse bladder (Figure 4.7), and is thought to reflect the beginning of epithelial denudation. This epithelial response in the bladder is not related to the development of late fibrosis, as early chemical stimulation of proliferation does not precipitate fibrosis in the irradiated bladder. Thus, proliferative responses do occur in slowly renewing tissues, but are usually not as clearly related to the occurrence of functional injury as is the case in acutely responding tissues.

Key points

1. The time of appearance and dose-dependence of radiation damage in a normal tissue depends upon its proliferative organisation.
2. Rapid renewal systems are organized in a hierarchical way (H-type), with 3 compartments: stem cells, a proliferating amplification compartment, and mature functional cells.
   H-type tissues are characterized by:
   A) *Time-to-response* is *dose-independent* and related to the life-span of the functional cells.
   B) *Rate of recovery* is *dose-dependent* and related to the number of surviving stem cells.
3. Slowly renewing cell systems have been termed *flexible* (F-type) because they have a less recognizable separation of proliferative compartments, and the functional cells maintain the capacity of proliferation. However, some so-called late-responding tissues may be more hierarchical than has previously been thought.

Bibliography

Hegazy MAH and Fowler JF (1973). Cell population kinetics and desquamation skin reactions in plucked and unplucked mouse skin. II. Irradiated skin. *Cell Tissue Kinet* 6:587-602.

Hornsey S, Myers R, Coultas PG *et al* (1981). Turnover of proliferative cells in the spinal cord after x-irradiation and its relation to time-dependent repair of radiation damage. *Br J Radiol* 54:1081-1085.

Michalowski A (1981). Effects of radiation on normal tissues: hypothetical mechanisms and limitations of *in situ* assays of clonogenicity. *Rad Environm Biophys* 19:157-172.

Morris GM and Hopewell JW (1988). Changes in the cell kinetics of pig epidermis after single doses of X-rays. *Br J Radiol* 61:205-211.

Stewart FA (1986). Mechanisms of bladder damage and repair after treatment with radiation and cytostatic drugs. *Br J Cancer* 53 (Suppl VII): 280-291.

Thames HD and Hendry JH (1987). *Fractionation in Radiotherapy*. Taylor & Francis; London.

Tucker SL and Hendry JH (1990). Predicted dose-latency relationships for early- and late-responding hierarchical tissues. *Int J Radiat Biol* 57:163-184.

Further reading

Appleton DR, Sunter JP and Watson AJ (1980). *Cell Proliferation in the Gastrointestinal Tract*. Pitman Medical, Tunbridge Wells.

Potten CS (Ed) (1983). *Stem Cells, their Identification and Characterisation*. Churchill Livingstone, Edinburgh.

Potten CS and Hendry JH (Eds) (1983). *Cytotoxic Insult to Tissue*. Churchill Livingstone, Edinburgh.

5

Clonogenic cells and the concept of cell survival

G. Gordon Steel

5.1 Concept of clonogenic cells

The preceding chapter has indicated that the maintenance of tissue size and therefore of tissue function in the normal renewal tissues of the body depends upon the existence of a small number of primitive 'stem cells':

Stem Cells – cells that have the capacity to maintain their numbers whilst at the same time producing cells that can differentiate and proliferate to replace the rest of the functional cell population. Stem cells are at the base of the hierarchy of cells that make up the epithelial and haemopoietic tissues.

Carcinomas are derived from such hierarchical tissues, and our ability to recognise this in histological sections derives from the fact that these tumours often maintain many of the features of differentiation of the tissue within which they arose. Well-differentiated tumours do this to a greater extent than anaplastic tumours. It follows that not all the cells in a tumour are neoplastic stem cells: some have embarked on an irreversible process of differentiation. In addition, carcinomas contain many cells that make up the stroma (fibroblasts, endothelial cells, macrophages, etc.). Stem cells thus may comprise only a small proportion of the cells within a tumour.

When a tumour regrows after non-curative treatment it does so because some neoplastic stem cells were not killed. Radiobiologists have therefore recognised that the key to understanding tumour response is to ask: How many stem cells are left? It is almost impossible to recognise tumour stem cells *in situ*, and therefore assays have been developed that allow them to be detected after removal from the tumour. These assays generally detect stem cells by their ability to form a colony within some growth environment. We therefore call these 'clonogenic' or 'colony-forming' cells:

Clonogenic Cells - cells that form colonies exceeding about 50 cells within a defined growth environment. The number 50 represents 5 - 6 generations of proliferation. It is chosen in order to exclude cells that have a limited growth potential as a result of having embarked on differentiation, or having been sublethally damaged by therapeutic treatment.

After exposure to a therapeutic dose of radiation, damaged cells do not die immediately and they may produce a modest family of descendants. This is illustrated in Figure 5.1 (Trott, 1972). The growth of single mouse L-cells was observed under the microscope and one selected colony was irradiated with 200 roentgens of x-rays at the 4-cell stage. Subsequent growth was carefully recorded and in the figure each vertical line indicates the time from birth at mitosis to subsequent division of a daughter cell. The two irradiated cells on the left and the right of this figure produced continuously expanding colonies, although some daughter cells had a long intermitotic time. The other two irradiated cells fared badly: they underwent a number of irregular divisions including a tripolar mitosis.

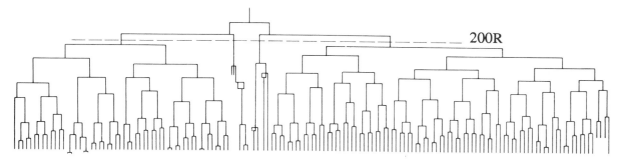

Figure 5.1   Pedigree of a clone of mouse L-cells irradiated with a dose of 200R at the 4-cell stage, illustrating the concept of surviving and non-surviving clonogenic cells. From Trott (1972), with permission.

But note that at the end of the experiment, cells are present from each of the original four cells: the difference is that two produced expanding colonies and the other two did not. The first two were 'surviving clonogenic cells' and the other two are usually described as 'killed' by radiation, since their regrowth is probably unimportant for clinical outcome. It would be more precise to say that two of the cells lost their proliferative ability as a result of irradiation.

5.2 Clonogenic assays

Clonogenic assays have formed the basis of cellular response studies in tumours, also in some normal tissues. The basic idea is to remove cells from the tumour, place them in a defined growth environment and to test for their ability to produce a defined colony of descendants. Many types of assay have been described; we illustrate the principle by a simple assay in tissue-culture that is analogous to a microbiological assay.

A single-cell suspension of tumour cells is prepared and divided into two parts. One is irradiated, the other kept as an unirradiated *control*. The two suspensions are then plated out in tissue culture under identical conditions, except that since we anticipate that irradiation has killed some cells we will have to plate a larger number of the irradiated cells. We here envisage plating 100 control cells and 400 irradiated cells. After a suitable period of incubation the colonies are scored (Figure 5.2). There are 20 control colonies, and we therefore say that the *plating efficiency* was 20/100

= 0.2. The plating efficiency of the treated cells is lower: 8/400 = 0.02.

We calculate a *surviving fraction* as the ratio of these plating efficiencies:

$$\text{Surviving fraction} = \frac{\text{PE}_{\text{treated}}}{\text{PE}_{\text{control}}} = \frac{0.02}{0.2} = 0.1$$

thus correcting for the efficiency with which undamaged clonogenic cells are detected and for the different numbers of cells plated. Surviving fraction is often given as a percentage (10% in this case).

The above description started with a suspension of tumour cells. In order to measure *in vivo* cell survival we take two groups of experimental tumours, irradiate one and keep the other as a control, then at some time after irradiation make cell suspensions from both groups (treated identically) and plate them as before. The difference here is that the cells are irradiated under *in vivo* conditions.

The colonies in Figure 5.2 have been drawn also to illustrate a feature of colony assays that was mentioned in the previous Section. Irradiation not only reduces the colony numbers; it also increases the *number of small colonies*. Some of these small colonies may represent clones that eventually die out; others may arise from cells that have suffered non-lethal injury that reduces colony growth rate. Unless they reach the usual cut-off of 50 cells they will not be counted, although their implications for the evaluation of radiation effects on tumours may be worthy of greater attention (Seymour and Mothersill, 1989).

CONTROL   TREATED

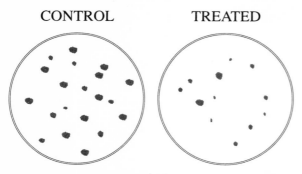

Figure 5.2   Illustrating the principle of measuring a surviving fraction.

5.3 Cell survival curves

A cell survival curve is a plot of surviving fraction against dose (of radiation, cytotoxic drug, or other cell killing agent). Figure 5.3A shows that when plotted on *linear* scales the survival curve for cells irradiated in tissue-culture is often sigmoid: there is a shoulder followed by a curve that asymptotically approaches zero survival. To indicate the sensitivity of the cells to radiation we could just read off the ED_{50} or ED_{90} values (ED_{90} is the dose to kill 90% of the cells) and to do this we need make no assumptions about the shape of the curve.

There are two reasons why survival curves are always plotted on a *logarithmic* scale of survival:

(i)   if cell killing is random then survival will be an exponential function of dose, and this will be a straight line on a semi-log plot;

(ii) a logarithmic scale more easily allows us to see and compare effects at very low survivals.

Such a plot is illustrated in Figure 5.3B. The shapes of radiation survival curves and ways of describing their steepness are dealt with in the next chapter.

Note that for the data shown in Figure 5.3, radiation doses above 5 Gy reduce the survival of clonogenic cells to below 10%. Measurement of radiosensitivity in terms of the parameter D_0 (Section 6.3) is made on the exponential part of the survival curve, which in this case is above 5 Gy. These measurements are therefore made in a dose range where the surviving fraction is very low. Such D_0 values are probably relevant to the problem of exterminating the last few clonogenic cells, but they may not be typical of the radiosensitivity of the bulk of the tumour cell population.

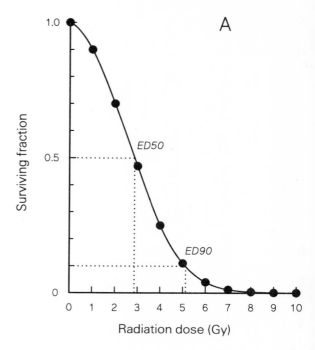

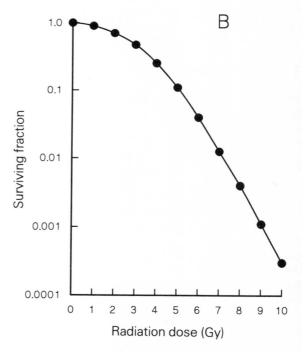

Figure 5.3   A typical cell survival curve for cells irradiated in tissue culture, plotted (**A**) on a linear survival scale. (**B**) shows the same data plotted on a logarithmic scale.

5.4 Assays for the survival of clonogenic cells

Many techniques have been described for detecting colony formation by tumour cells and thus for measuring cell survival. They almost all require first the production of single-cell suspensions. This is not a simple matter, for tumour tissues differ widely in the ease with which they can be disaggregated. Enzymes such as trypsin, collagenase, pronase are often used and some tissues can be disaggregated mechanically.

Such assays can also be used for the assay of colony-forming cells in normal tissues, especially the haemopoietic tissues that can easily be sampled and made into cell suspensions. In addition a variety of *in situ* assays for normal-tissue stem cells have been described (Section 13.3).

The following are some of the principal assays that have been used on tumour cells:

In Vitro Colony Assays

Some tumour cells grow well attached to plastic tissue culture dishes. Others can be encouraged to do so by first laying down a *feeder layer* of lethally irradiated connective-tissue or tumour cells. For cells that have been established as an *in vitro* cell line this often works well but for studies on tissue samples taken directly from patients or animals it is commonly observed that fibroblasts grow better than the tumour cells and overgrow the cultures.

An alternative is therefore to thicken the growth medium with agar or methyl-cellulose. This inhibits the growth of anchorage-requiring cell types, but many epithelial cells will still grow. A widely used assay of this type is the Courtenay-Mills assay for human tumour cells (Courtenay and Mills, 1978). Agar cultures are grown in 15 ml plastic tubes overlaid with liquid medium that can regularly be replenished. The addition of rat red blood cells to the agar has been found to promote the growth of a number of human tumour cell types. An important feature of the Courtenay-Mills assay is the use of a low oxygen tension (a gas phase of 90% nitrogen, 5% oxygen and 5% carbon dioxide) which enhances the plating efficiency of human tumour cells.

Spleen Colony Assay

Till and McCulloch (1961) showed that when mouse bone marrow cells were injected intravenously into syngeneic recipients that had received sufficient whole-body irradiation to suppress endogenous haemopoiesis, colonies were produced in the spleen which derived from the stem cells in the graft. The colonies varied in morphology (erythroid, granulocyte, or mixed) and these stem cells are therefore termed *pluripotent*. Their precise identity was not known and they are often called *colony-forming units (CFU-S)*, where the suffix indicates detection in the spleen. Using this assay, Till and McCulloch obtained the first survival curve for bone marrow cells and found it to be very steep. The spleen colony assay has also been used for some types of mouse lymphoma cells.

Lung Colony Assay

This is analogous to the spleen colony assay and is applicable to any transplanted mouse tumour that readily forms colonies in the lung following intravenous injection of a single-cell suspension. The cloning efficiency can often be increased by mixing the test cells with an excess ($\approx 10^6$) of lethally irradiated tumour cells or plastic microspheres. Not all the tumour cells grow: a few colonies per thousand tumour cells injected would be regarded as satisfactory. Although colonies are formed throughout the lung, they are usually scored only on the lung surface. The method was used by Hill and Stanley (1975) on two experimental tumours and they give further experimental details. *See also* Steel (1977).

Limiting-dilution Assay

This is a non-cloning assay that was used in early radiation cell survival studies and which for some experimental tumours has the advantage of high sensitivity (*see* Steel, 1977, for detailed description). The principle of the method is to prepare a suspension of tumour cells and to make a large number of subcutaneous implants covering a range of inoculum sizes, hopefully spanning the level of 50% tumour takes. The animals, usually mice, are then observed for a long enough period to record nearly every tumour that can grow from a single-cell implant. Take-rate is then plotted against inoculum size and the point of 50% takes is interpolated; this is usually called the 'TD$_{50}$' cell number. The experiment is performed simultaneously on treated cells and control cells and the surviving fraction is given by the ratio of the TD$_{50}$ values. The addition of an excess of lethally irradiated cells improves the take-rate; using this manoeuvre Steel and Adams (1975) found a TD$_{50}$ of 1-3 cells for the Lewis lung tumour and were thus able to measure survival down to 10^{-6}. The method only works well in the absence of an immune response against the tumour grafts.

Short-term In Vitro Assays

The need to develop *in vitro* assays that yield a quicker result than a true clonogenic assay arises from the current interest in prediction of tumour response to treatment (Section 23.3). A variety of assays have been proposed but their reliability has yet to be fully established. The failure of the Salmon-Hamburger 'Human Tumour Stem Cell Assay' that was widely publicised 10 years ago may serve as a warning, both to the developers and users of new assays. There are three pitfalls that must be avoided:

(i) biopsy samples of human tumours contain both tumour cells and normal connective tissue cells; both may grow under the assay conditions and it may be difficult to distinguish colony formation by tumour cells;

(ii) if the method requires the production of single-cell suspensions, great care must be taken to exclude cell clumps, for these may preferentially give rise to scorable colonies;

(iii) radiation-killed cells take time to die and in a short-term assay they may be confused with surviving tumour cells; if this is not done, the method may not distinguish between *radiosensitive* cells and cells that *die rapidly* after irradiation.

Many aspects of the prediction of tumour response are dealt with in the book edited by Chapman, Peters and Withers (1989). Non-clonogenic assays for tumour cells have been reviewed by Mitchell (1988) and they include the following:

The Micronucleus Test. Tumour cells are cultured in the presence of cytochalasin-B which blocks cytokinesis, creates binucleate cells, and thus allows nuclei that have undergone one post-treatment division to be identified. Micronuclei can be scored as small extranuclear bodies. Their frequency is linearly related to radiation dose and gives a measure of radiation sensitivity (Streffer *et al*, 1986). The reliability of the method is limited by the fact that diploid, polyploid and aneuploid cells may differ in their tolerance of genetic loss and therefore of fragment formation.

The Adhesive Tumour Cell Culture System. Human tumour biopsy specimens are disaggregated into a single-cell suspension and plated out in 24-well culture plates that have been coated with a commercially patented adhesive coating (Baker *et al*, 1986). The medium is supplemented with added growth factors. Two weeks after irradiation or drug treatment the cultures are stained with crystal violet and the absorbance is measured using an image analyser.

Growth Assays. A variety of methods have been used to measure the growth of cultures derived from treated and control tumour specimens, thus to derive a measure of radiosensitivity. Incorporation of radioisotopes such as ^{3}H-thymidine has been widely used. MTT is a tetrazolium salt that can be used to stain cell cultures and thus by a colorimetric assay to estimate the extent of growth (Carmichael *et al*, 1987; Wasserman and Twentyman, 1988). It can be used to evaluate growth in microtitre plates and with careful attention to technical factors it can yield a measure of radiosensitivity. Such methods are vulnerable to the variable growth of fibroblasts and for studies on leukaemic cells it may be preferable to differentially stain the cells and analyse the cultures microscopically (Bosanquet, 1991).

5.5 Comparison of assays

Intercomparison of the results of assays of cell survival provides an important check on their validity, yet it has seldom been done. The information can be valuable both at a practical and a fundamental level. At the practical level, it is logical to check a rapid short-term assay against the results of a more laborious but more reliable clonogenic assay.

The more general question is whether assay of cell survival in two different growth environments does actually identify the same population of surviving tumour cells. It is cell survival *in situ* in the patient that we seek to determine, and to subject tumour cells to additional stresses and to artificial growth environments might well produce artefacts. It is therefore reassuring that some careful comparisons between clonogenic assays, *in vitro*, in the mouse lung, and by subcutaneous transplantation, have demonstrated good agreement (Steel and Stephens, 1983).

5.6 The relationship between cell survival and gross tumour response

The objective of studies of clonogenic cell survival is to be able to understand, or to make predictions about, the main features of tumour response to therapy: growth delay and tumour cure.

Tumour Growth Delay

Incomplete treatment of a tumour leads to a temporary phase of tumour regression that is subsequently followed by tumour recurrence. This pattern is illustrated in Figure 2.8. Regression is due to the death and disappearance of cells killed by radiation, also to the loss of those differentiated cells of limited life-span that would have been produced by the killed stem cells. The rate of tumour regression differs widely from one tumour to another, as illustrated in Figure 2.7.

The regrowth component in Figure 2.8 is due to repopulation by surviving clonogenic cells. The speed of regrowth probably varies considerably from one tumour to another, and the broken lines in the figure illustrate the possibilities of a lag period before repopulation gets fully under way, or repopulation at the speed of a small untreated tumour. Fowler (1991) has expressed the view that rapid repopulation may be the norm. He has postulated that irradiation will arrest the proliferation of tumour cells and that if this is the driving force behind the loss of cells to necrosis (Section 11.2) then this loss will temporarily be interrupted. The result will be a period of tumour cell repopulation at a rate that is close to the potential doubling time (Section 3.2) and faster than would have been the case in the absence of treatment. Fowler describes this as the 'unmasking' of rapid tumour cell proliferation.

Growth delay is defined as the difference in time for treated and untreated tumours to reach a fixed multiple of the size at the time of treatment. This has been widely used as a measure of tumour response in transplanted animal tumours (Section 14.3).

What is the relationship between growth delay and cell survival following treatment? For a particular radiation dose, Figure 14.5 shows that the colony-forming ability of tumour cells is depressed immediately after irradiation but that the tumour volume response takes time to appear. In that study, a radiation dose that reduced survival to 0.01 gave only partial remission of tumour growth. Greater cell kill would be expected to lead to longer growth delay and the results of a representative dose-response study (for chemotherapy) are shown in Figure 5.4. Transplanted B16 mouse melanomas were treated either with cyclophosphamide or the nitrosourea CCNU and both parameters were measured over a range of drug doses. Following cyclophosphamide treatment there was an almost linear relationship between the time the tumours took to reach four times the treatment size and the log(survival). The curve for CCNU was much flatter: reducing survival to 10^{-2} gave a growth delay of roughly 4 days, as compared with around 14 days for cyclophosphamide. The explanation appeared to lie in a reduced *rate of repopulation* after cyclophosphamide. The conclusion is that growth delay is a function both of the level of clonogenic cell survival and of the rate of regrowth.

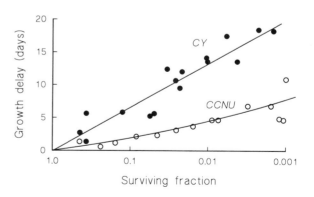

Figure 5.4 Relationship between tumour growth delay and surviving fraction, for B16 mouse melanomas treated either with cyclophosphamide (CY) or CCNU. For a particular level of cell killing, greater growth delay was observed after CY than CCNU. From Steel and Stephens (1983), with permission.

Local Tumour Control

The eradication of every clonogenic tumour cell must lead to tumour cure; this is, however, a daunting objective. Every gram of tumour may contain 10^9 cells of which perhaps 1% might be clonogenic. A human tumour at presentation could weigh some tens or hundreds of grams and the total number of clonogenic cells might therefore exceed 10^9. Cell kill by radiotherapy or chemotherapy is roughly exponential with dose. Thus when treatment has reduced survival to 10^{-2} (which could lead to complete disappearance of all visible tumour) we would expect that four or five times this dose will be needed to reach a curative level. This is illustrated in Figure 2.1.

Whether it is always necessary to eradicate the last clonogenic tumour cell in order to achieve local tumour control has been a matter of intense debate. During the 1970s there was a widespread belief that the immune responses of patients against their tumours may be strong and this gave rise to many attempts at immunotherapy. Unfortunately, it has subsequently been realised that the animal tumours used to support the optimistic claims for immunotherapy were not truly syngeneic and were misleading (Alexander, 1977; Hewitt, 1979). Thus, whilst it is possible that weak tumour-directed immune responses may exist within cancer patients, sufficient perhaps to eradicate the last decade or so of surviving tumour cells, this cannot be relied upon.

5.7 Repair and recovery

The majority of damage induced in cells by radiation is satisfactorily repaired. Evidence for this comes from studies of strand breaks in DNA, most of which disappear during the few hours after irradiation (Section 24.2). Further evidence for repair comes from the wide variety of recovery experiments that have been done, both on *in vitro* cell lines and on normal and tumour tissues *in vivo*. It is useful to draw a distinction between these two sources of evidence:

Repair   refers to the process by which the function of macromolecules is restored. *Rejoining* of DNA strand breaks provides some evidence for this, although the rejoining of a break does not necessarily mean that gene function is restored. *Repair fidelity* is a significant additional factor. 'Repair' has often loosely been used for cellular or tissue recovery.

Recovery   refers to an increase in cell survival or a reduction in the extent of radiation damage to a tissue when time is allowed for this to occur.

There are a number of experimental sources of evidence for recovery, including the following:

Split-dose Experiments. The effect of a given dose of radiation is less if it is split into two fractions, delivered a few hours apart. This effect has been termed recovery from *sublethal damage (SLD)*, or *Elkind recovery* (Elkind and Sutton, 1960). SLD recovery can be observed using various experimental end-points: for instance using cell survival (Figure 5.5A), tumour growth delay (Figure 5.5C), or mouse lethality after irradiating a vital normal tissue (Figure 5.5D). The typical timing of split-dose recovery is shown in Figure 5.5A. Considerable recovery occurs within 15 min - 1 hour, and recovery often seems to be complete by roughly 4 hours. When the split-dose technique is applied to cycling cells there is usually a wave in the data caused by cell-cycle progression effects (Section 5.8).

Delayed-plating Experiments. If cells are irradiated in a non-growing state and left for increasing periods of time before assaying for survival, an increase in survival is often observed (Figure 5.5B). This has been termed recovery from *potentially lethal damage (PLD)*. The kinetics of PLD recovery and SLD recovery are similar.

Dose-rate Effect. The sparing of radiation damage as dose rate is reduced to around 1 Gy/h is primarily due to cellular recovery (Sections 15.1, 15.2).

Fractionation. The sparing effect of fractionating radiation treatment within a relatively short overall time is primarily due to recovery. This is therefore the main reason why iso-effect curves slope upwards as the fraction number is increased (Sections 7.1, 7.2).

What is the relationship between these various ways of detecting recovery? The damage induced in cells by ionizing radiation is complex, as are the enzymatic processes that immediately begin to repair it. The various types of 'recovery experiment' listed above *evaluate* this complex repair process in slightly different ways. For instance, the evaluation based on giving a second dose (i.e.

SLD recovery) is different from that obtained by asking irradiated non-dividing cells to divide (i.e. PLD recovery). There is only one complex entity, but a variety of ways of detecting it.

5.8 Variation of cell killing through the cell cycle

The radiosensitivity of cells varies considerably as they pass through the cell cycle. Although this has not been studied in a large number of cell lines, there seems to be a general tendency for cells in the S-phase (in particular the latter part of the S-phase) to be the most resistant and for cells in G_2 and mitosis to be the most sensitive. The reason for the resistance in S may be related to the conformation of DNA at that time; the sensitivity in G_2 probably results from the fact that those cells have little time to repair radiation damage before the cell is called upon to divide.

The classic results of Sinclair and Morton (1965) are illustrated in Figure 5.6. They synchronised Chinese hamster cells at 5 different points in the cell cycle and performed cell survival experiments. The survival curves showed that it was mainly the *shoulder* of the curve that changed: there was little shoulder for cells in G_2 or mitosis and the shoulder was greatest for cells in S. The right-hand panel shows the profile of variation in cell killing through the cell cycle, constructed from these data.

The effect of this phenomenon is that it must create a degree of synchrony in the cells that survive irradiation. Immediately after a dose of x-rays, all the cells will still be at precisely the same point in the cell cycle as they were before irradiation; but some will have *lost their reproductive integrity* and it is the number that retain this which will tend to be greatest in the S-phase.

The phenomena of induced cell synchrony and *cell-cycle progression* are illustrated in Figure 5.7 for cells treated with an S-phase specific cytotoxic drug. Untreated cells in exponential growth have a distribution through the cell cycle shown by *(a)*. Immediately after treatment the distribution of *surviving clonogenic cells* will be as shown by *(b)*. S-phase killing agents also tend to temporarily block the movement of cells into the S-phase, and a few hours later there may be a pile-up of survivors in the latter part of the G_1 phase *(c)*. Later, these cells will move on in a semi-synchronous wave through the S-phase *(d)*, when the effect of a second dose of the drug would be greatest.

5.9 The 5 Rs of radiotherapy

The biological factors that influence the response of normal and neoplastic tissues to fractionated radiotherapy were summarized by Withers (1975) in the *4 Rs of Radiotherapy*:

Repair As evidenced by cellular recovery during the few hours after exposure (Section 5.7).

Reassortment Cell-cycle progression effects, otherwise known as 'redistribution'. Cells that survive a first dose of radiation will tend to be in a resistant phase of the cell cycle and within a few hours they may progress into a more sensitive phase (Section 5.8).

Repopulation During say a 5–7 week course of radiotherapy, cells that survive irradiation may proliferate and thus increase the number of cells that must be killed (Sections 9.3, 9.4).

Reoxygenation In a tumour, cells that survive a first dose of radiation will tend to be hypoxic but thereafter their oxygen supply may improve, leading to an increase in radiosensitivity (Sections 11.4, 14.4).

Note that two of these processes (repair and repopulation) will tend to make the tissue *more resistant* to a second dose of radiation; the other two (reassortment and reoxygenation) tend to make it *more sensitive*. These 4 factors modify the response of a tissue to repeated doses of radiation and are responsible for the slope of an iso-effect curve (Chapter 7). The overall radiosensitivity of the tissue (i.e. the height of the iso-effect curve on the page) depends on a fifth 'R': *Radiosensitivity*. Thus for a given fractionation course (or for single-dose irradiation) the haemopoietic system shows a greater response than the kidney, even allowing for the different timing of response. Similarly, some tumours are more radioresponsive than others, and this is largely due to differences in *radiosensitivity* (Steel *et al*, 1989).

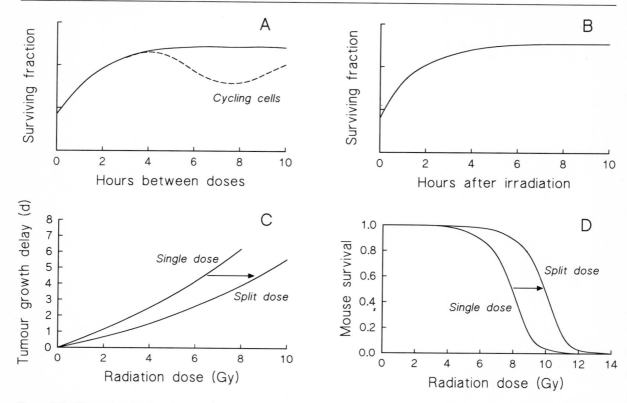

Figure 5.5 Illustrating 4 ways of measuring recovery from radiation damage (see text). Panels A, C and D show three types of split-dose experiment; panel B shows the results of a 'delayed-plating experiment'. The arrows in panels C and D indicate the measurement of $(D_2 - D_1)$ values.

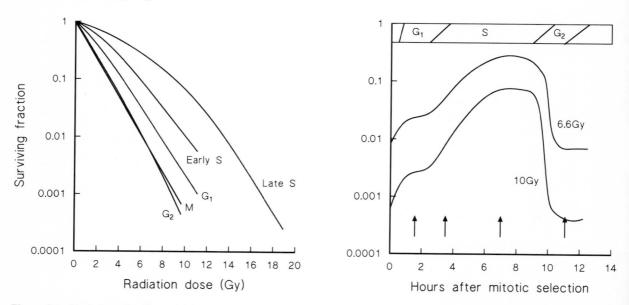

Figure 5.6 Variation of radiosensitivity through the cell cycle of Chinese hamster cells. Adapted from Sinclair and Morton (1965), with permission.

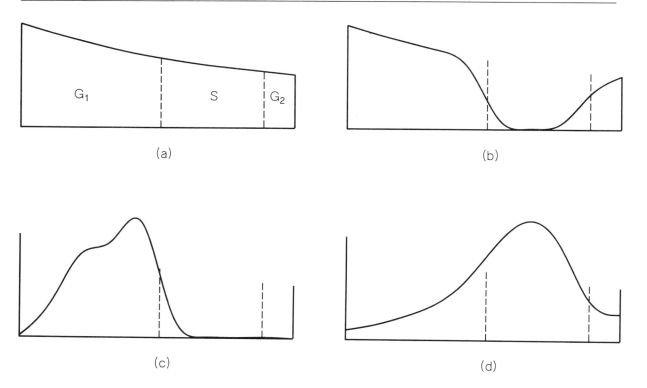

Figure 5.7 Cell-cycle progression (i.e. reassortment) induced in an exponentially growing cell population by an S-phase specific cytotoxic agent. From Steel (1977), with permission.

Key points

1. Tumour recurrence after treatment depends upon the survival of clonogenic cells, which may comprise only a small proportion of the total cells within the tumour.
2. Evaluation of the survival of clonogenic cells following treatment is an important aspect of experimental cancer therapy. In experimental situations this is relatively simple to perform, but for cells removed directly from human tumours great care is necessary in the selection and performance of the assays.
3. In tumour therapy, as with tumour growth, it is important to *think logarithmically*. Partial or complete tumour remission may involve only perhaps two decades of clonogenic cell reduction, yet over nine decades of cell kill may be necessary before long-term tumour control can be assured.
4. Repair of radiation damage is an important feature of irradiated tissues. It can be assessed by a variety of experimental tests.
5. Variation of cell killing through the cell cycle is considerable, and may give rise to cell-cycle progression phenomena.
6. The 5 Rs of radiotherapy: radiosensitivity, repair, reassortment, reoxygenation, repopulation.

Bibliography

Alexander P (1977). Back to the drawing board - the need for more realistic model systems for immunotherapy. *Cancer* 40:467-470.

Baker FL, Spitzer G, Ajani JA *et al* (1986). Drug and radiation sensitivity measurements of successful primary monolayer culturing of human tumour cells using cell-adhesive matrix and supplemented medium. *Cancer Research* 46:1263-1274.

Bosanquet A (1991). Correlations between therapeutic response of leukaemias and *in vitro* drug-sensitivity assay. *Lancet* 337:711-714.

Carmichael J, DeGraff WG, Gazdar AF *et al* (1987). Evaluation of a tetrazolium-based semiautomated colorimetric assay: assessment of radiosensitivity. *Cancer Research* 47:943-946.

Chapman JD, Peters LJ and Withers HR (1989). *Prediction of Tumour Response to Treatment.* Pergamon; New York.

Courtenay VD and Mills J (1978). An *in vitro* colony assay for human tumours grown in immune-suppressed mice and treated in vivo with cytotoxic agents. *Brit J Cancer* 37:261-268.

Elkind MM and Sutton H (1960). Radiation response of mammalian cells grown in culture: I. Repair of X-ray damage in surviving Chinese hamster cells. *Radiat Res* 13:566-593.

Fowler JF (1991). The phantom of tumour treatment - continually rapid proliferation unmasked. *Radiother Oncol* 22:156-158.

Hewitt HB (1979). A critical examination of the foundations of immunotherapy for cancer. *Clin Radiol* 30:361-369.

Hill RP and Stanley JA (1975). The lung colony assay: extension to the Lewis lung tumour and the B16 melanoma. *Int Radiat Biol* 27:377-387.

Mitchell JB (1988). Potential applicability of nonclonogenic assays to clinical oncology. *Radiat Res* 114:401-414.

Steel GG and Adams K (1975). Stem-cell survival and tumour control in the Lewis lung carcinoma. *Cancer Research* 35:1530-1535.

Steel GG, McMillan TJ and Peacock JH (1989). The 5 Rs of radiobiology. *Int J Radiat Biol* 56:1045-1048.

Steel GG and Stephens TC (1983). Stem cells in tumours. In: *Stem Cells* (Ed) Potten CS, Churchill Livingstone; Edinburgh.

Streffer C, van Beunigen D, Gross E *et al* (1986). Predictive assays for the therapy of rectum carcinoma. *Radiother Oncol* 5:303-310.

Seymour CB and Mothersill C (1989). Lethal mutations, the survival curve shoulder and split-dose recovery. *Int J Radiat Biol* 56:999-1010.

Sinclair WK and Morton RA (1965). X-ray and ultraviolet sensitivity of synchronised Chinese hamster cells at various stages of the cell cycle. *Biophys J* 5:1-25.

Till JE and McCulloch EA (1961). A direct measurement of the radiation sensitivity of normal mouse bone marrow. *Radiat Res* 14:213-222.

Trott KR (1972). Relation between division delay and damage expressed in later generations. *Curr Topics Radiat Res* 7:336-337.

Wasserman TH and Twentyman P (1988). Use of a colorimetric microtiter (MTT) assay in determining the radiosensitivity of cells from murine tumours. *Int J Radiat Oncol* 15:699-702.

Withers HR (1975). The four R's of radiotherapy. *Adv Radiat Biol* 5:241-247.

Further reading

Elkind MM and Whitmore GF (1967). *The Radiobiology of Cultured Mammalian Cells.* Gordon and Breach, New York.

Potten CS (Ed) (1983). *Stem Cells, their Identification and Characterisation.* Churchill Livingstone, Edinburgh.

Steel GG (1977). *The Growth Kinetics of Tumours*. Oxford University Press; Oxford.

Tannock IF and Hill RP (1992). *The Basic Science of Oncology*. second edition. Pergamon; New York.

6

Models of radiation cell killing

Michael C. Joiner _____

6.1 Introduction

Research in experimental radiobiology covers studies at the cell, animal and human levels. It deals at the fundamental level with the molecular, biochemical and biophysical nature of radiation damage. Models are a necessary part of radiobiology research, to provide a framework in which to analyze and compare data and ultimately to assist in building up a consistent theory of radiation action both *in vitro* and *in vivo*. Models and mathematics are also sometimes necessary to relate experimental studies to clinical cancer treatment with the aim of improving therapy. This chapter describes some models that are used to analyze the relationship between cell survival and radiation dose.

6.2 Molecular targets

Radiation kills cells by producing secondary charged particles and free radicals in the nucleus which in turn produce a variety of types of damage in DNA. Evidence that damage to DNA is the primary cause of radiation cell killing and mutation is set out in Section 24.2. Each 1 gray dose of low-LET radiation produces about 2000 initial single-strand breaks and 40 initial double-strand breaks. Some lesions are more important than others and radiation lethality correlates most significantly with the number of residual, unrepaired double-strand breaks (DSB) several hours after irradiation. Table 24.2 shows that for a fixed radiation dose, if cell kill is modified by changing LET, oxygen level, thiol concentration or temperature, only the number of DSB follows the change in cell kill. Single-strand breaks, base damage and DNA-protein crosslinks do not reflect the change in cell kill for all of these modifiers. The DNA double-strand break is therefore thought to be the most important type of cellular damage. Just one residual DSB in a vital section of DNA may be sufficient to produce a significant chromosome aberration and to sterilize the cell.

6.3 Target theory

One way of explaining the shape of cell survival curves is the idea that there may be regions of the DNA that are crucial to maintain the reproductive ability of cells. These sensitive regions could be thought of as specific *targets* for radiation damage so that the survival of a cell after radiation exposure will be related to the number of targets inactivated. There are two versions of this idea that have been used commonly. The first version of the theory proposes that just one hit by radiation on a single sensitive target leads to death of the cell. This is called *single-target single-hit inactivation*, and it leads to the form of survival curve shown in Figure 6.1A. The survival curve is exponential (i.e. linear in the semi-logarithmic plot against dose). To derive an equation for this survival curve, Poisson statistics can be applied, as during irradiation there are a very large number of hits on different cells taking place, but the probability (p) of the next hit occurring in a given cell is very small. Thus for each cell,

$$p(\text{survival}) = p(0 \text{ hits}) = e^{-D/D_0}$$

where D_0 is the dose that gives an average of one hit per target. A dose of D_0 Gy reduces survival from 1 to 0.37 (i.e. to e^{-1}), or from 0.1 to 0.037, etc. D/D_0 is the average number of hits per target (and in this case per cell). This is the reason why (as in Figure 6.4) a scale of cell survival is some-

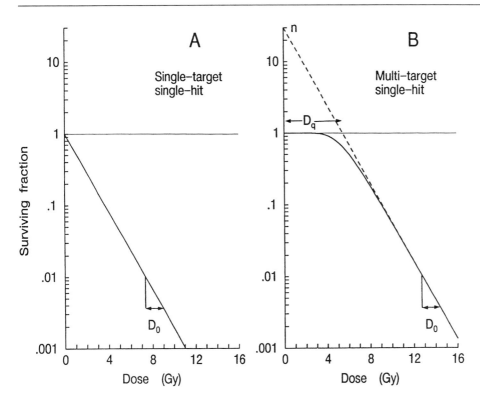

Figure 6.1 The two most common types of target theory. A: single-target inactivation; B: multi-target inactivation.

times labelled -ln(SF): this is a scale of the natural logarithm of surviving fraction and it is also the *equivalent* number of lethal lesions per cell.

In this example (Figure 6.1A) D_0 = 1.6 Gy. These simple straight survival curves are usually found for the inactivation of viruses and bacteria. They may also be useful in describing the radiation response of some very sensitive human cells (normal and malignant), also the radiation response at very low dose rates (Section 15.2) and the response to high LET radiations (Section 16.3).

A more general version of target theory is called *multi-target single-hit inactivation*. This proposes that just one hit by radiation on each of n sensitive targets in the cell is required for death of the cell. The shape of this survival curve is shown in Figure 6.1B. Again, using Poisson statistics,

$$p(\text{0 hits on a specific target}) = e^{-D/D_0}$$

Thus
$$p(\text{specific target inactivated}) = 1 - e^{-D/D_0}$$

As there are n targets in the cell,

$$p(\text{all } n \text{ targets inactivated}) = (1 - e^{-D/D_0})^n$$

Thus $p(\text{survival})$
$$= p(\text{not all targets inactivated})$$
$$= 1 - (1 - e^{-D/D_0})^n \qquad \text{(Eqn 6.1)}$$

Figure 6.1B shows that multi-target single-hit survival curves have a shoulder whose size can be indicated by the *quasi-threshold dose* (D_q). This is related to n and D_0 by the relation:

$$D_q = D_0 \log_e n \qquad \text{(Eqn 6.2)}$$

For the example in Figure 6.1B we have chosen n = 30 and D_0 = 1.6 Gy, giving D_q = 5.4 Gy. Such multi-target survival curves have proved useful for describing the radiation response of mammalian cells at high doses, 'off the shoulder'. They do not describe the survival response well at lower more clinically-relevant doses.

6.4 More complex models

The main shortcoming of the multi-target model is that, as shown in Figure 6.1B, it predicts a response that is flat for very low radiation doses. On the contrary, much experimental cell survival data show evidence for a finite initial slope. To take account of this, the multi-target model can be modified by adding a single-hit component. The resulting equation for the survival curve is called the *two-component model*:

$$p(\text{survival}) = e^{-D/D_1}(1 - (- e^{-D(1/D_0 - 1/D_1)})^n) \quad \text{(Eqn6.3)}$$

This type of survival curve is illustrated in Figure 6.2A. In addition to the parameters n, D_0 and D_q, this curve also has a parameter D_1 which fixes the initial slope, i.e. the dose required in the low-dose region to reduce survival from 1 to 0.37. In this example, $n = 30$ and $D_0 = 1.6$ Gy, and $D_1 = 4.6$ Gy. This type of curve does predict finite cell killing in the low-dose region but it has the drawback that the change in cell survival over the range $0 - D_q$ occurs almost linearly. This implies that no sparing of damage should occur as dose per fraction is reduced below ≈ 2 Gy, which is usually not found to be the case either experimentally or in clinical radiotherapy (Section 9.2).

6.5 The linear-quadratic model

A better description of radiation response in the low-dose region $(0 - 3$ Gy$)$ is given by the Linear-Quadratic (LQ) model shown in Figure 6.2B:

$$p(\text{survival}) = \exp(-\alpha D - \beta D^2) \quad \text{(Eqn 6.4)}$$

This is a continuously-bending survival curve with no straight portion at high radiation doses. Its shape (or 'bendiness') is determined by the ratio α/β. Since the dimensions of the parameters are α Gy^{-1} and β Gy^{-2}, the dimensions of α/β are Gy: as shown in Figure 6.2B, this is the dose at which the *linear* contribution to damage (αD on the logarithmic scale) equals the quadratic contribution (βD^2).

The response of cells to densely-ionizing radiations like neutrons or α-particles is usually a steep and almost exponential survival curve (Section 16.3). As shown in Figure 6.2, this would

be explained in the two-component model by the ratio D_1/D_0 being near to 1.0, or in the LQ model by a high α/β ratio.

The LQ model is in widespread use in radiobiology and generally works well in describing responses to radiation *in vitro* and also *in vivo* (Section 8.4). Is there a mechanistic justification for the LQ model? One simple idea is that the linear component $[\exp(-\alpha D)]$ might be due to *single-track* events while the quadratic component $[\exp(-\beta D^2)]$ might arise from *two-track* events. This interpretation is supported by studies of the dose-rate effect (Section 15.2) which show that as dose rate is reduced, cell survival curves become straight and tend to extrapolate the initial slope of the high dose-rate curve: the quadratic component of cell killing disappears, leaving only the linear component. This would be expected, for at low dose rate single-track events will occur far apart in time and the probability of interaction between them will be low. Although this interpretation of the LQ equation seems reasonable, the nature of the interactions between separate tracks is still a matter of considerable debate. Chadwick and Leenhouts (1973) postulated that separate tracks might hit opposite strands of the DNA double helix and thus form a double-strand break; this now seems an unlikely mechanism in view of the very low probability of such a close interaction at a dose of a few gray. Interaction between more widely-spaced regions of the complex DNA structure, or between DNA in different chromosomes, may be a more plausible mechanism.

6.6 The lethal, potentially lethal damage (LPL) model

Curtis (1986) proposed this model as a 'unified repair model' of cell killing. Ionizing radiation is considered to produce two different types of lesion: repairable (potentially lethal) lesions and non-repairable (lethal) lesions. The non-repairable lesions produce single-hit lethal effects and therefore give rise to a linear component of cell killing $[= \exp(-\alpha D)]$. The eventual effect of the repairable lesions depends on competing processes of repair and *binary misrepair*. It is this latter process that leads to a quadratic component in cell killing. As shown in Figure 6.3, the model has two sensitivity parameters (η_L determines the number of non-repairable lesions produced per

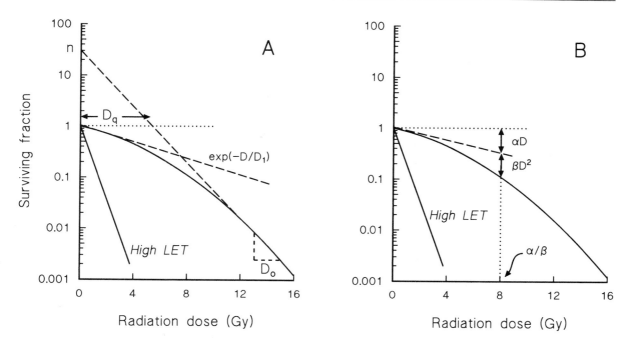

Figure 6.2 Models with non-exponential cell killing but a finite initial slope. A: the two-component model and B: the linear-quadratic model. From Hall (1988), with permission.

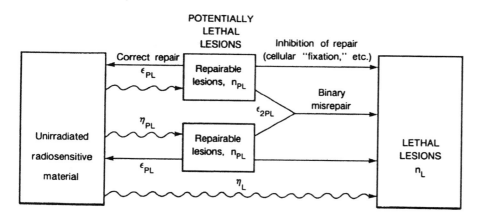

Figure 6.3 The Lethal, Potentially Lethal (LPL) damage model of radiation action. From Curtis (1986), with permission.

unit dose, and η_{PL} the number of repairable lesions). There are also two rate constants (ϵ_{PL} determines the rate of repair of repairable lesions, and ϵ_{2PL} the rate at which they undergo interaction and thus misrepair).

This model produces almost identical cell survival curves to the LQ model, down to a survival level of perhaps 10^{-2}. It can therefore be taken to provide one possible mechanistic model for the LQ equation. It predicts that as dose rate is reduced the probability of binary interaction of potentially lethal lesions will fall and parameter values can be found that allow the model to accurately simulate cell survival data on human and animal cells irradiated at various dose rates (Section 15.2).

Curtis' LPL model is an example of a lesion-interaction model, which additionally incorporates repair processes. Figure 6.4A shows how this produces the downward-bending cell survival curve: the dashed curve indicates the component of cell killing that is due to single-track non-repairable lesions. It is the extra lethal lesions produced by the binary interaction of potentially lethal lesions which give the downward-bending curve.

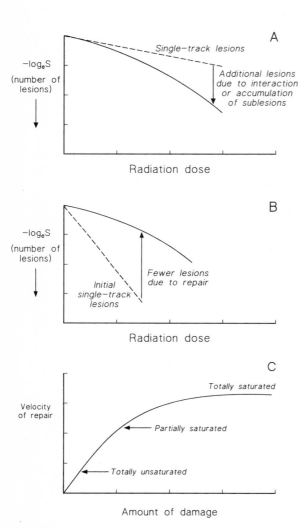

Figure 6.4 The contrast between lesion-interaction models and repair saturation models. A: the LPL model; B: the effect of repair becoming less effective at higher radiation doses; C: the basic concept of repair saturation. Adapted from Goodhead (1985), with permission.

6.7 Repair-saturation models

Another class of model are the *repair-saturation models*, which propose that the shape of the survival curve depends *only* on a dose-dependent rate of repair. Figures 6.4B and 6.4C demonstrate this idea. Only one type of lesion and single-hit killing are postulated, and in the absence of any repair these lesions produce the steep dashed survival curve in Figure 6.4B. The final survival curve (solid line) results from repair of some of these lesions but if the repair enzymes become saturated (Figure 6.4C), there is not enough repair enzyme to bind to all damaged sites simultaneously and so the reaction velocity of repair no longer increases with increasing damage. Therefore at higher doses (more lesions), there is proportionally less repair during the time available before damage becomes fixed; this will lead to more residual damage and to greater cell kill. The mechanisms of fixation of non-repaired damage are not understood but they may be associated with the entry of cells carrying such damage into DNA synthesis or mitosis. It should be noted that an alternative 'saturation' hypothesis, leading to the same consequence, is that the pool of repair enzymes is used up during repair, so that at higher doses the repair system is depleted and is less able to repair all the induced damage.

Table 6.1 illustrates how the basic conceptual difference between the lesion accumulation/interaction models such as Curtis' LPL and the dose-dependent repair models affects the interpretation of some radiobiological phenomena (Goodhead, 1985). Both types of model predict linear-quadratic cell-survival curves in the clinically relevant dose region. They also provide good explanations of split-dose recovery (Section 5.7), changing effectiveness with LET (Section 16.3) and the dose-rate effect (Section 15.2). At present, radiation scientists are uncertain whether lesion interaction or repair saturation really exist in cells but it may well be that molecular and microdosimetric studies will eventually determine which explanation (maybe both!) is correct.

Table 6.1 Different interpretations of radiobiological phenomena by lesion-interaction and saturable-repair models.

Observation	Explanation	
	Lesion-interaction	*Repair Saturation*
Curved dose-effect relationship	Interaction of sub-lesions	Saturation of capacity to repair sublesions
Split-dose recovery	Repair of sublesions (sublethal damage repair)	Recovery of capacity to repair sublesions
RBE increase with LET	More non-repairable lesions at high LET	High-LET lesions are less repairable
Low dose rate is less effective	Repair of sublesions during irradiation	Repair system not saturating

Adapted from Goodhead (1985).

Key points

1. A number of different mathematical models adequately simulate the shape of cell-survival curves for mammalian cells. So far it has not been possible to strongly prefer one model to others.
2. Target theory proposes that a specific number of targets or DNA sites must be inactivated or damaged to kill the cell. This approach is only satisfactory if a component of single-hit killing is also introduced. So far it has not been possible to identify the location of these vital 'targets' within the cell nucleus.
3. Lesion-interaction models explain downward-bending cell-survival curves by postulating two classes of lesion. One class is directly lethal, but the other type is only *potentially* lethal and may be repaired enzymatically or may interact with other potentially-lethal lesions to form lethal lesions.
4. Repair-saturation models assume that potentially lethal lesions are either repaired successfully or fixed as the cell goes through some critical stage in its cycle (e.g. mitosis). Downward-bending survival curves occur because higher doses produce too much damage for the repair system to handle and it saturates; proportionally less damage can be therefore be repaired in the time available before fixation than at lower doses where the system is unsaturated.

Bibliography

Chadwick KH and Leenhouts HP (1973). A molecular theory of cell survival. *Phys Med Biol* 13:78-87.

Curtis SB (1986). Lethal and potentially lethal lesions induced by radiation: A unified repair model. *Radiat Res* 106:252-270.

Frankenberg-Schwager M (1989). Review of repair kinetics for DNA damage induced in eukaryotic cells *in vitro* by ionizing radiation. *Radiother Oncol* 14:307-320.

Goodhead DT (1985). Saturable repair models of radiation action in mammalian cells. *Radiat Res* 104:S58-S67.

Further reading

Alpen EL (1990). *Radiation Biophysics*. Prentice-Hall, London.

Chapman JD (1980). Biophysical models of mammalian cell inactivation by radiation. In: *Radiation Biology in Cancer Research*, pp.21-32. (Eds) Meyn RE and Withers HR. Raven Press; New York.

Douglas BG and Fowler JF (1976). The effect of multiple small doses of X-rays on skin reactions in the mouse and a basic interpretation. *Radiat Res* 66:401-426.

Elkind MM and Sutton H (1960). Radiation response of mammalian cells grown in culture:

I. Repair of X-ray damage in surviving Chinese hamster cells. *Radiat Res* 13:556-593.

Hall EJ (1988). *Radiobiology for the Radiologist*, Chapter 2: Cell-survival curves. Lippincott; Philadelphia.

Ward JF (1990). The yield of DNA double-strand breaks produced intracellularly by ionizing radiation: a review. *Int J Radiat Biol* 57:1141-1150.

7

Time-dose relationships in radiotherapy

Søren M. Bentzen and Jens Overgaard _____

7.1 From Strandqvist to Ellis

Early in the history of radiotherapy it became evident that the biological effect of a dose given as 'fraktioniert-protrahiert' irradiation was less than the effect of the same total dose given as a single treatment. However, in the first half of this century treatments were given daily and there was no clear distinction between the effect of overall treatment time and the number or size of dose fractions. The monograph by Strandqvist (1944) presented the first attempt to establish a mathematical relationship between overall treatment time and response to radiotherapy. Strandqvist plotted recurrences and complications in patients treated for basal and squamous cell carcinomas of the skin and lip as a function of total dose and treatment time. He documented the complications of delayed wound healing and skin necrosis. In 91 patients treated between 1933 and 1937 there were 15 recurrences and 14 complications. Strandqvist's idea was to establish in a dose-time scattergram an exclusion line that would lie below most of the complications and above most of the recurrences. When dose and overall time were plotted on double-logarithmic co-ordinates the exclusion line was drawn as a straight line with an exponent of 0.22 (Figure 7.1). Mathematically, the total dose (D) is related to overall treatment time (T) as:

$$D = k \times T^{0.22} \qquad \text{(Eqn 7.1)}$$

where **k** is a constant.

Strandqvist tested this relationship for other data sets as well and concluded that the formula described 'biologisch äquivaleute Gesamtdosen',

or using modern terminology, isoeffective doses. Note that practically all treatments were single doses or fractionated courses lasting less than 15 days.

Strandqvist defined overall treatment time as the time between the first and the last fraction. With this convention, one problem with the use of logarithmic axes was the representation of single-dose treatments. Strandqvist used 0.35 days as the time for a single treatment (not shown in Figure 7.1) but was fully aware of the fact that this choice substantially influences the steepness of the exclusion lines.

Cohen (1949) elaborated on Strandqvist's work and analyzed three different sets of skin damage data using the type of representation shown in Figure 7.1. The endpoints were weak or strong erythema and *skin tolerance*. Cohen found a *recovery exponent* for skin of 0.33, and concluded that the difference between this value and the 0.22 estimated for squamous cell carcinomas by Strandqvist was 'real and significant'. However, Cohen defined the time for a treatment to be numerically equal to the number of fractions. This meant that the single-dose treatments were plotted at time 1 day instead of the 0.35 days used by Strandqvist. If the same convention had been used for tumour and skin data, there would have been no significant difference between the two exponents. In other words, the alleged difference was an artefact (Liversage, 1971).

7.2 The Ellis NSD formula

In 1969 Frank Ellis published a paper with the title *Dose, time and fractionation. A clinical*

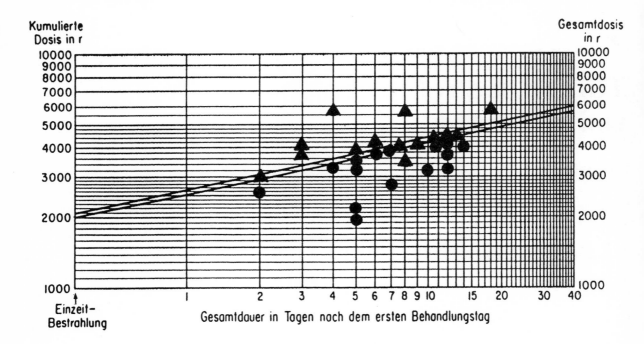

Figure 7.1   The classic data of Strandqvist (1944) on the radiotherapy of skin tumours. The ordinate shows the total radiation dose in roentgens (exposure units); the abscissa gives the overall treatment time in days after the first treatment (Einzeit-Bestrahlung = single dose). Both axes are logarithmic. The circles show recurrences and the triangles show skin complications. Adapted, with permission.

hypothesis. Ellis was inspired by the difference in recovery exponent observed by Cohen, also by the experimental studies by Fowler on pig skin which showed that the number of fractions (N) was more important than the overall treatment time (T), at least when T was under 28 days. This led Ellis to the important realization that the 'time factor' was actually a composite effect of N and T. This is in accordance with our present knowledge, although current models emphasize the importance of dose per fraction rather than number of fractions. Ellis based his derivation of an isoeffect relationship on 3 assumptions, derived from his own earlier work:

(i)   the healing of skin epithelium depends on the condition of the underlying connective-tissue stroma;

(ii)   apart from bone and brain, connective tissues throughout the body are similar;

(iii)   within and around a malignant tumour normal connective-tissue elements make up the stroma.

'Therefore', he wrote, 'apart from bone and brain, the tumour dose limited by the normal tissue tolerance dose, could be based on skin tolerance.' This is essentially a two-tissue-type model, distinguishing only between *normal tissues* (excepting brain and bone) and *tumours*. Furthermore, Ellis assumed from (ii) and (iii) above, that the N exponent was the same for tumours and normal tissues and that the overall treatment time was of no importance for tumour control by radiotherapy. His argument for the latter was based on the idea that it was homeostatic control in normal tissues that gave rise to the time factor. His further reasoning is remarkable: 'Malignant cells are not susceptible to homeostatic control as are normal cells. . . . We know that some tumours are hormone sensitive to some extent. In so far as they are sensitive to hormones they are not behaving like malignant cells.'

So the recovery exponent from Strandqvist's work (0.22) was interpreted as the number-of-fractions exponent, and the difference between this value and the 0.33 observed for skin by Cohen was interpreted as a T exponent of 0.11 (remember that T was numerically equivalent to N in Cohen's work). Therefore Ellis suggested the following formula for the total dose, D, at normal-tissue tolerance:

$$D = NSD \times N^{0.22} \times T^{0.11} \qquad \text{(Eqn 7.2)}$$

where NSD, the *Nominal Standard Dose*, is a constant. Later versions of the formula had a number-of-fractions exponent of 0.24 rather than 0.22 to adjust for schedules treating in 5 rather than 6 days per week. The NSD was expressed in units of rad-equivalent-therapy, i.e. in *rets*. A similar formula was proposed for tumours, with the same number-of-fractions exponent but omitting the time factor. An unfortunate side-effect of the general acceptance of the NSD formula was that many subsequent papers did not present dose-fractionation details in terms of dose, number of fractions, and overall treatment time, but only as the nominal standard dose in rets.

7.3 Variants of the NSD formula

A number of extensions and modifications of the NSD formula have been developed. The *Cumulative Radiation Effect* (CRE) of Kirk *et al* (1971) was mathematically a simple rearrangement of the NSD formula, but more importantly it incorporated the notion of isoeffect at subtolerance doses. Ellis introduced the concept of *partial tolerance,* which has the advantage of being additive for two or more schedules. The disadvantage was that the partial effect value was calculated from clinical experience in each specific institution and therefore could not readily be compared. Orton and Ellis (1973) introduced the TDF (*Time-Dose-Fractionation*) factors, mainly for computational convenience.

It is important to realize that all of these formulae are derived from the basic NSD formula, therefore the criticisms of the NSD apply to these variations as well.

During the 1970s, the NSD formula and its variants came into widespread use and at the time of writing they continue to be used in many institutions throughout the world. As early as 1971, Liversage pointed to the dangers of a formula in which the therapeutic ratio is independent of the number of fractions so long as they are given in

a constant overall time. The social and economic advantages of treating patients in fewer, larger, fractions thus became a temptation in many institutions. It is fair to note that Ellis actually regarded his contribution as an *hypothesis* which he encouraged others to test in the clinic.

7.4 Critique of the NSD formula

Liversage (1971) published a critical analysis of the NSD formula. He started by considering the general case of a power-law model:

$$D = k \times N^m \times T^\tau \qquad \text{(Eqn 7.3)}$$

where **m** and τ are constants that have to be determined from clinical data. Ellis' two fundamental assumptions were that **m** is the same for tumours and normal tissues and that τ is zero for tumours. Liversage's basic criticisms were:

(i) Isoeffect curves in the Strandqvist plots are curved, not linear as expected from Eqn 7.3 (*see* Figure 8.1). Thus the mathematical form of the power-law model cannot be correct, no matter what the actual values of **m** and τ.

(ii) The difference in recovery exponents is, as indicated above, an artefact of the different time-scale conventions for single-fraction data.

(iii) **m** varies from one set of tumour data to another.

(iv) The values of τ vary from one data set to another. For example, Strandqvist's data yields $\tau = 0$.

(v) Two experimental animal studies, known to Liversage, gave substantially different values of τ.

These arguments led Liversage to the conclusion that the NSD formula could not be a valid description for all tumours and normal tissues; he also doubted its validity for squamous cell carcinoma and skin reactions. In hindsight, Liversage's criticism appears to be crucial, but it had a limited penetration at the time. The following 20 years have produced even stronger evidence from the laboratory and the clinic that the basic biology of the NSD formula is wrong for tumours, for early-responding, and for late-responding normal tissues and that power-law models have a mathematical form that is inconsistent with basic radiobiological observations.

The shortcomings of the NSD formula may be listed as follows:

(i) The NSD formula underestimates the incidence of late sequelae after large dose fractions.

Table 7.1 shows the clinical experience of Singh (1978) with intracavitary plus external-beam radiotherapy for carcinoma of the uterine cervix. The intracavitary schedules were identical, delivering 40 Gy to point A of the Manchester system. The two external-beam schedules had an equivalent TDF value. Changing the number of fractions (and therefore the dose per fraction) had no effect on early reactions (33% in each case) but radiotherapy with fewer larger fractions gave a

significant increase in late sequelae (33% → 83%, p = 0.001).

Figure 7.2 shows one example of evidence for dissociation between *early* and *late* tissue responses as a result of altered dose per fraction (Overgaard *et al*, 1987). It shows the relationship between acute skin reaction (erythema) and late subcutaneous fibrosis in 73 patients treated with 12 fractions, and 66 with 22 fractions. Each dot represents data for an individual patient. The total doses were equivalent on the basis of the NSD formula. The incidence of grade 3 erythema was similar (35% compared with 31%) but the incidence of marked subcutaneous fibrosis (grade ≥ 2) was much higher in the 12-fraction schedule (68% compared with 5%). Note that some patients developed late complications without a preceding

Table 7.1 Incidence of early and late reactions following an increase in fraction size. Cervix carcinomas treated with combined intracavitary and external-beam radiotherapy

Regimen*	No. of patients	Early reactions	Late sequelae
40/20/26 + IC+10/5/5	24	8 (33%)	8 (33%)
29/5/28 + IC + 6.7/1/1	24	8 (33%)	20 (83%)

* Dose in Gy / number of fractions / overall time in days.
IC = intracavitary radiotherapy
From Singh (1978)

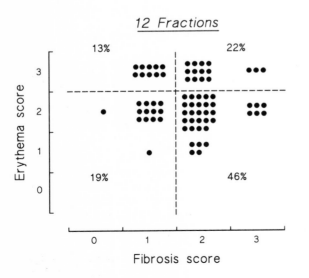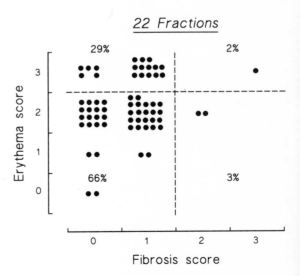

Figure 7.2 Relationship between acute skin reaction (erythema) and late subcutaneous fibrosis in breast cancer patients treated with an equivalent total dose according to the NSD formula but with very different fraction numbers. From M. Overgaard *et al* (1987), with permission.

early complication. Results of this type revealed shortcomings in the NSD approach and led to the more recent preference for the linear-quadratic model. These data represent a breakdown in the first two of Ellis' assumptions listed in Section 7.2. But once again it should be stressed that even if the exponents of the power-law model are allowed to vary from one tissue to another, this type of model has a mathematical form that is inconsistent with biological knowledge.

(ii) There is no appreciable treatment-time factor for late sequelae.

Table 7.2 shows isoeffect doses for late normal-tissue injury in patients treated with continuous or split-course radiotherapy for laryngeal carcinoma (Overgaard et al, 1988). The overall treatment times were 6 and 10 weeks. The isoeffect doses in the two schedules are statistically indistinguishable, from which it can be concluded that no recovery was observed in the 4 weeks gap of the split-course schedule.

(iii) Prolonged overall treatment time gives poorer local tumour control in squamous cell carcinoma.

One clinical example in support of this conclusion is shown in Table 7.3. It summarizes the results of three studies in head and neck cancer where split-course radiotherapy was instituted as a treatment policy for a period of time. The estimated loss of local tumour control was 7 – 10%. Other estimates of the effect of prolonged treatment are found in the literature but in most of these bias cannot be ruled out in the sense that patients with poor prognosis tended to have prolonged treatment. More extensive data are shown in Figure 9.4.

(iv) The number-of-fractions exponent (m) is not constant, even for a specific endpoint.

Support for this conclusion comes mainly from radiobiological data on experimental animals. Figure 7.3 (Fowler, 1984) shows isoeffect curves for radiation damage to mouse kidney, skin (i.e. desquamation) and lung (i.e. pneumonitis). The NSD formula predicts the relationship to be a straight line with slope 0.24 (the dashed line). In each case the data define a bending curve. Local values of the number-of-fractions exponent (m) are shown underneath the curves. The linear-quadratic model predicts that m increases with dose per fraction (and decreases with increasing fraction number) to a limiting value of 0.5.

The dependence of the isoeffective total dose on number of fractions has been found in a very large collection of normal-tissue data to correspond with the predictions of the L-Q model (Thames

Table 7.2 Isoeffect doses for late normal-tissue injury in patients treated with continuous or split-course radiotherapy for laryngeal carcinoma

Endpoint	Continuous RT*	Split-course RT*	Recovery ratio§
5% late oedema	59.3 (57.1–61.6)	62.6 (56.4–69.5)	1.06 (0.95–1.17)
35% late oedema	66.9 (55.8–80.2)	69.6 (67.9–71.4)	1.04 (0.88–1.23)
22.5% fistula	57–60	61.4 (44.2–85.2)	1.02–1.07

* Isoeffect doses in grays, with 95% confidence limits.
§ Ratio of split-course to continuous doses.
Adapted from Overgaard et al (1988)

Table 7.3 The estimated fall in tumour control probability for 1 week extra overall treatment time in squamous cell carcinoma of the head and neck

Tumour site	Authors	Estimated loss per week (%)
Larynx	Overgaard et al (1988)	10
Oropharynx	Bentzen et al (1991)	7
Various head and neck cancers	Parsons et al (1980)	7

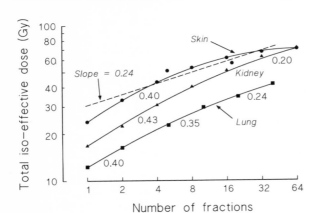

Figure 7.3 Isoeffect curves for radiation damage to mouse kidney, skin and lung. Local values of the number-of-fractions exponent (m) are shown underneath the curves. From Fowler (1984), with permission.

and Hendry, 1987). Turesson and Notter (1975) have made a similar observation for telangiectasia after clinical postoperative radiotherapy. A correction was needed for the isoeffective dose estimated from the NSD formula. This again can be interpreted as an increasing value of *m* with increasing dose per fraction. Thus, a power-law model cannot describe the outcome of radiotherapy for late radiation reactions, no matter what value is assigned to *m*.

(v) A power-law model for the effect of overall treatment time has the wrong mathematical form.
A power-law relationship of the form T^τ (with $\tau < 1$) predicts a *decreasing* dose compensation for proliferation as the duration of treatment increases. This is contrary to biological data for both early-responding tissues and tumours (Withers and Peters, 1980).

7.5 The cell population kinetics (CPK) Model of Cohen

The CPK model of Cohen (1971) represented a new point of view, completely different from the empirical Strandqvist-NSD approach. Many of the ideas incorporated in the CPK model still play a role in more recent approaches to time-dose relationships. Cohen's biological starting point was the target-cell hypothesis: that radiation reactions in human tissues depend on the depletion of some critical cell population below a certain

threshold level. Cell survival was assumed to be described by the two-component model (Section 6.4) but Cohen subsequently substituted the linear-quadratic model. Cohen also included the kinetics of cellular renewal in his model. In its basic formulation the CPK model employed 7 parameters, and a brief list of these provides a feeling for the biological effects that Cohen attempted to model. The two-component model contained 3 parameters (D_0, D_1, and n). The other 4 parameters were the growth rate of the target-cell population, the number of available cell cycles in the tissue (a factor limiting repopulation), the critical threshold for cell depletion, and a field-size correction for both tumours and normal tissues. The field-size effect was intended as a correction for the number of target cells in the tumour and as a representation of the (possibly) reduced normal-tissue tolerance for larger field sizes.

The model parameters were to be estimated from clinical dose-response data and were assumed to be specific for the different normal tissues or tumour types. Cohen took full advantage of the computers that became generally available in the 1960s. He and his collaborators wrote a number of computer programs for obtaining best-fit values of the parameters in the model and

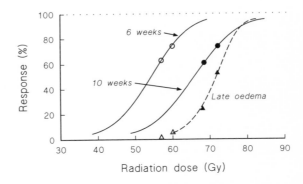

Figure 7.4 The influence of overall treatment time on the dose-response relationship for local control of squamous cell carcinoma of the larynx (circles) and late oedema (triangles). Open symbols show data for continuous-course radiotherapy (nominal duration 6 weeks); closed symbols show data for split-course radiotherapy (nominal duration 10 weeks). Proliferation during the additional 4 weeks shifted the dose-response curve for local control towards higher doses. In contrast, the data for late oedema fit a single dose-response curve independently of treatment time, implying that the split had no effect. Adapted from Overgaard et al (1988), with permission.

for predicting response to radiotherapy for a given treatment and tissue characteristics.

Some aspects of Cohen's model are inconsistent with biological observations, for example that no delay occurs before the onset of regeneration in normal tissues. But more seriously, and Cohen himself was aware of this, very few clinical data sets can provide sufficient information to allow the parameters of the CPK model to be estimated. A considerable variation in treatment characteristics is required, also sufficiently accurate clinical observations of response to radiotherapy. For ethical reasons it is doubtful whether this kind of data can be obtained from current radiotherapy practices.

Cohen's model provided arguments in favour of split-course radiotherapy, i.e. fractionation schedules including typically a 2–4 week treatment-free interval. The basic rationale was that proliferation during the treatment gap would improve normal-tissue tolerance and thereby allow the tumour dose to be escalated. At the Department of Oncology in Aarhus, a 3–week split was introduced and the total dose was raised by 10–12 Gy. The expectation from the CPK model was that tumour control would improve and that the incidence of early and late normal-tissue complications would decrease. The clinical observation was that tumour cell proliferation during the gap completely offset the gain in tumour control expected from the higher dose, and late sequelae increased (Figure 7.4).

In the early 1980s, the linear-quadratic model came into widespread use for calculating isoeffect relationships. This model was deliberately kept simple in order to describe quantitatively the clinically important effect of dose per fraction. The relative simplicity of this model matched the biological resolution of clinical and experimental animal studies. That is the subject of the next chapter.

Key points

1. The NSD formula and its derivations may underestimate the incidence of late normal-tissue sequelae after radiotherapy.
2. Even if the exponents of the NSD formula are determined for each specific normal tissue and tumour type, the model incorrectly describes the effect of number of fractions or treatment duration.
3. Overall treatment time is important for tumour control after radiotherapy, at least for squamous cell carcinomas.
4. There is no appreciable proliferation in *late-responding* normal tissues during a standard 6–10 week course of radiotherapy.
5. The sensitivity to large fraction sizes is much higher for late-responding than for early-responding normal tissues.
6. It is possible to construct models of response to radiotherapy that contain many known biological processes but these inevitably become too complex to be defined by the available clinical data; hence the attraction of the linear-quadratic approach.

Bibliography

Bentzen SM, Johansen LV, Overgaard J and Thames HD (1991). Clinical radiobiology of squamous cell carcinoma of the oropharynx. *Int J Radiat Oncol Biol Phys* 20:1197-1206.

Cohen L (1949). Clinical radiation dosage, Pt.II. *Br J Radiol* 22:706-713.

Cohen L (1971). A cell population kinetic model for fractionated radiation therapy. I. Normal tissues. *Radiology* 101:419-427.

Ellis F (1969). Dose, time and fractionation: a clinical hypothesis. *Clin Radiol* 20:1-7.

Fowler JF (1984). Review: Total doses in fractionated radiotherapy - implications of new radiobiological data. *Int J Radiat Biol* 46:103-120.

Kirk J, Gray WM and Watson ER (1971). Cumulative radiation effect. Part I. Fractionated treatment regimes. *Clin Radiol* 22:145-155.

Liversage WE (1971). A critical look at the ret. *Br J Radiol* 44:91-100.

Orton CG and Ellis F (1973). A simplification in the use of the NSD concept in practical radiotherapy. *Br J Radiol* 46:529-537.

Overgaard M, Bentzen SM, Christensen JJ and Hjøllund Madsen E (1987). The value of the NSD formula in equation of acute and late radiation complications in normal tissue following 2 and 5 fractions per week in breast cancer patients treated with postmastectomy radiotherapy. *Radiother Oncol* 9:1-12.

Overgaard J, Hjelm-Hansen M, Johansen LV and Andersen AP (1988). Comparison of conventional and split-course radiotherapy as primary treatment in carcinoma of the larynx. *Acta Oncol* 27:147-152.

Parsons JT, Bova FJ and Million RR (1980). A re-evaluation of split-course technique for squamous cell carcinoma of the head and neck. *Int J Radiat Oncol Biol Phys* 6:1645-1652.

Singh K (1978). Two regimes with the same TDF but differing morbidity used in the treatment of stage III carcinoma of the cervix. *Br J Radiol* 51:357-362.

Strandqvist M (1944). Studien über die kumulative Wirkung der Röntgenstrahlen bei Fraktionierung. *Acta Radiol* 55(Suppl.):1-300.

Turesson I and Notter G (1975). Skin reactions after different fractionation schedules giving the same cumulative radiation effect. *Acta Radiologica Therap* 14:475-484.

Further reading

Thames HD and Hendry JH (1987). *Fractionation in Radiotherapy*, Taylor & Francis Ltd.; London.

Withers HR and Peters LJ (1980). Biological aspects of radiation therapy. In: *Textbook of Radiotherapy*. (Ed) Fletcher GH. Lea & Febiger; Philadelphia.

8

The linear-quadratic approach to fractionation

Michael C. Joiner

8.1 Introduction

The linear-quadratic (LQ) cell-survival model, introduced in Chapter 6, can also be used to describe the relationship between total isoeffective dose and the dose per fraction in fractionated radiotherapy *in vivo*. This is one of the most important recent developments in radiobiology applied to therapy. This chapter describes the theoretical background and the animal data which have led to the adoption of the LQ approach; specific calculations using the model are described in detail in Chapter 10.

8.2 Linear-quadratic versus NSD

Experiments using animal models carried out over many years have shown that if isoeffective total dose (or tolerance dose) is measured as a function of decreasing dose per fraction or increasing number of fractions, then this relationship is steeper for late-responding tissues than for acutely-responding tissues. Figure 8.1 illustrates this for some studies on mice: skin is an early-responding tissue and kidney a late-responding tissue. The charts are isoeffect plots (the total radiation dose to give a fixed level of damage is plotted against dose per fraction and fraction number). Note that the curve for kidney is steeper than that for skin.

The solid lines in Figure 8.1 are calculated by an equation based on the LQ model:

$$\text{Total dose} = \frac{\text{constant}}{1 + d/(\alpha/\beta)} \qquad \text{(Eqn 8.1)}$$

where d is the dose per fraction. See Section 8.4 for the derivation of this equation. The steepness and curvature of these lines are both determined by one parameter, the α/β ratio. For the skin data (Figure 8.1A) α/β is about 10. The units of α/β are grays, so the α/β ratio in this case is 10 Gy. For the kidney data α/β is about 2 Gy.

The LQ model fits these data very well. Also shown in Figure 8.1A is the fit of Ellis' Nominal Standard Dose model to the skin data. The equation is:

$$\text{Total dose} = NSD \, N^{0.24} \, T^{0.11}$$

where T is constant in this case. This gives a straight line in this type of plot (Sections 7.2, 7.3). The NSD equation can be made to fit the data well from 4 to 32 fractions but is not as accurate as the LQ model for large doses per fraction or, more importantly, for doses per fraction of 1–2 Gy that are of current interest in hyperfraction (Chapter 9). As illustrated by the kidney data (Figure 8.1B), for late reactions the NSD formula again does not fit as well as the LQ formula and overestimates tolerance doses when the dose per fraction is below 2 Gy. In addition, the N exponent needs to be raised from 0.24 to 0.35 for kidney. A similar modification, but not necessarily by the same amount, must be made for all late-responding tissues if the NSD formulation is to be even approximately correct. The conclusion is that it is always better to use the linear-quadratic model, with correctly chosen α/β ratio, to describe isoeffect dose relationships, especially when considering doses per fraction below 2 Gy.

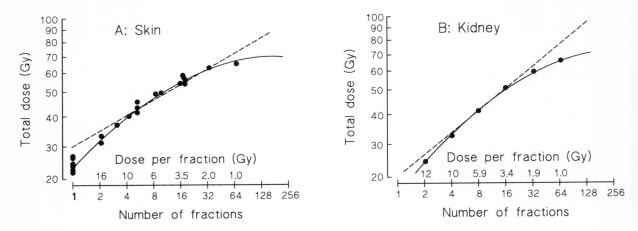

Figure 8.1. Relationship between total dose to achieve an isoeffect and fractionation. **A**: for acute reactions in mouse skin (Douglas and Fowler, 1976) and **B**: for late injury in mouse kidney (Stewart *et al*, 1984). Note that the curve for kidney is steeper than that for skin. The broken lines are NSD relationships fitted to the central part of each data set. Reproduced with permission.

8.3 Cell-survival basis of the LQ model

What is the explanation for the difference between the fractionation response of early- and late-responding tissues? Figure 8.2 shows hypothetical single-dose (1 fraction) survival curves for the target cells in early- and late-responding tissues, drawn according to the LQ equation (see Figure 6.2B). E represents the reduction in cell survival equivalent to tissue tolerance. The total doses

that would need to be given in 2 fractions are obtained by drawing a straight line from the origin through the survival curve at E/2 and measuring the intersection of this line with the dose axis. The total dose for 3 fractions is obtained in the same way by drawing a line through E/3 on the survival curve, and similarly for the other fraction numbers. Because the late-responding survival curve (Figure 8.2B) is more 'bendy' (it has a lower α/β ratio), there is a *larger* change in total dose with increasing number of fractions

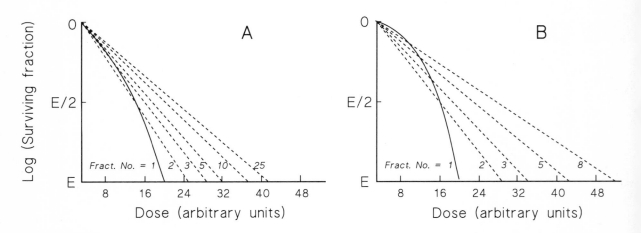

Figure 8.2. Schematic survival curves for target cells in **A**: acutely responding and **B**: late-responding normal tissues. The abscissa is radiation dose on an arbitrary scale. From Thames and Hendry (1987), with permission.

compared with the early-responding tissue where the survival curve bends less.

8.4 The LQ model in detail

The surviving fraction (SF_d) of target cells after a dose per fraction d is given in Chapter 6 as:

$$SF_d = \exp(-\alpha d - \beta d^2)$$

Radiobiological studies have shown that each successive fraction in a series is equally effective, so the effect (E) of n fractions can be expressed as:

$$E = -\log_e (SF_d)^n = -n \log_e(SF_d)$$
$$= n(\alpha d + \beta d^2) = \alpha D + \beta dD$$

where the total radiation dose $D = nd$. This equation may be rearranged into the following forms:

$$1/D = (\alpha/E) + (\beta/E)d \qquad \text{(Eqn 8.2)}$$
$$1/n = (\alpha/E)d + (\beta/E)d^2 \qquad \text{(Eqn 8.3)}$$
$$D = (E/\alpha)/[1 + d/(\alpha/\beta)] \qquad \text{(Eqn 8.4)}$$
$$D_2 / D_1 = (d_1 + \alpha/\beta)/(d_2 + \alpha/\beta) \qquad \text{(Eqn 8.5)}$$

Figure 8.3 shows the results of an experiment in which a measure of functional damage in the kidney is plotted against the total dose given in fractionated schedules of 1–64 fractions. To apply the LQ model to this example, first we measure off from the graph the total doses at a fixed level of effect (arrowed) and then plot the reciprocal of these total doses against the corresponding dose per fraction. Eqn 8.2 shows that this should give a straight line whose slope is β/E and whose

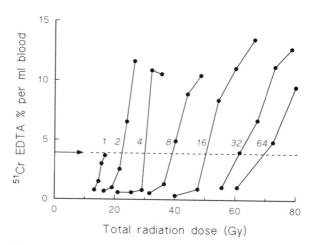

Figure 8.3. Dose-response curves for late damage to the mouse kidney with fractionated radiation exposure. Damage is indicated by EDTA clearance, curves determined for 1 to 64 dose fractions, illustrating the sparing effect of increased fractionation. From Stewart *et al* (1984), with permission.

intercept on the vertical axis is α/E. This plot is shown in Figure 8.4A. The points fit well to a straight line. This line cuts the x-axis at -3 Gy; it can be seen from Eqn 8.2 that this is equal to $-\alpha/\beta$, thus providing a measure of the α/β ratio for these data. The relative contributions of α and β to the α/β ratio can be judged by comparing the reciprocal total dose intercept (α/E) and the slope of the line β/E.

Figure 8.4. The data of Figure 8.3 after two different transformations. **A**: a reciprocal-dose plot according to Eqn 8.2. **B**: transformation according to Eqn 8.3 with the same data plotted as a proportion of full effect.

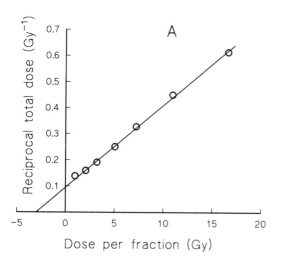

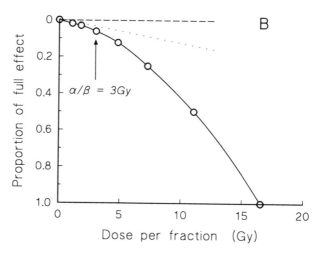

An alternative way of deriving parameter values from these data is to plot the reciprocal of the number of fractions against the dose per fraction as suggested by Eqn 8.3. Figure 8.4B shows that this gives the shape of the target-cell survival curve with the y-axis proportional to $-\log_e (SF_d)$. [Statistical note: This method combined with non-linear least-squares curve fitting is preferred over the linear-regression method shown in Figure 8.4A for determining α/β, because the $1/n$ and dose per fraction axes are independent.]

Eqns 8.4 and 8.5 are further ways of expressing the linear-quadratic model. Eqn 8.4 shows the LQ model in the form used already to describe the relationship between total dose and dose per fraction (Figure 8.1). Eqn 8.5 shows what change in total dose ($D_1 \rightarrow D_2$) is required when the dose per fraction is changed from $d_1 \rightarrow d_2$ in a fractionated schedule (Section 10.1).

8.5 The value of α/β

Many detailed fractionation studies of the type shown in Figures 8.1 and 8.3 have been made in animals over the last fifteen years. Table 8.1 summarises the α/β values obtained from these experiments. For acutely responding tissues which express their damage within a period of days to weeks after irradiation, the α/β ratio is in the range 7-20 Gy while, for late-responding tissues which express their damage months to years after irradiation, α/β generally ranges from 0.5–6 Gy. *The α/β ratio is not constant and its value should be chosen carefully to match the specific tissue under consideration.*

Table 8.1   Values for the α/β ratio for a variety of acute- and late-responding normal tissues in experimental animals

Early reactions			Late reactions		
	α/β	References		α/β	References
Skin			Spinal cord		
Desquamation	9.1–12.5	Douglas and Fowler (1976)	Cervical	1.8–2.7	van der Kogel (1979)
	8.6–10.6	Joiner *et al* (1983)	Cervical	1.6–1.9	White and Hornsey (1978)
	9–12	Moulder and Fischer (1976)	Cervical	1.5–2.0	Ang *et al* (1983)
Jejunum			Cervical	2.2–3.0	Thames *et al* (1988)
Clones	6.0–8.3	Withers *et al* (1976)	Lumbar	3.7–4.5	van der Kogel (1979)
	6.6–10.7	Thames *et al* (1981)	Lumbar	4.1–4.9	White and Hornsey (1978)
Colon				3.8–4.1	Leith *et al* (1981)
Clones	8–9	Tucker *et al* (1983)		2.3–2.9	Amols, Yuhas (quoted by
Weight loss	9–13	Terry and Denekamp (1984)			Leith *et al*, 1981)
Testis			Colon		
Clones	12–13	Thames and Withers (1980)	Weight loss	3.1–5.0	Terry and Denekamp (1984)
Mouse lethality			Kidney		
30d	7–10	Kaplan and Brown (1952)	Rabbit	1.7–2.0	Caldwell (1975)
30d	13–17	Mole (1957)	Pig	1.7–2.0	Hopewell and Wiernik (1977)
30d	11–26	Paterson *et al* (1952)	Rats	0.5–3.8	van Rongen *et al* (1988)
Tumour bed			Mouse	1.0–3.5	Williams and Denekamp
45d	5.6–6.8	Begg and Terry (1984)			(1984 a,b)
			Mouse	0.9–1.8	Stewart *et al* (1984 a)
			Mouse	1.4–4.3	Thames *et al* (1988)
			Lung		
			LD_{50}	4.4–6.3	Wara *et al* (1973)
			LD_{50}	2.8–4.8	Field *et al* (1976)
			LD_{50}	2.0–4.2	Travis *et al* (1983)
			Breathing rate	1.9–3.1	Parkins and Fowler (1985)
			Bladder		
			Frequency, capacity	5–10	Stewart *et al* (1984 b)

α/β values are in grays.
From Fowler (1989); for references, see the original.

The fractionation response of well-oxygenated tumours is thought to be similar to acutely responding normal tissues, sometimes with an even higher α/β ratio. The values shown in Figure 8.5 were compiled by Williams *et al* (1985) from a review of the literature. Values calculated from data obtained in experiments under fully radiosensitized conditions (marked 'Miso' and 'Oxic' in the figure) are plotted directly, and values calculated from fractionation responses under hypoxic conditions (marked 'Clamp', 'Anoxic' and 'Hypoxic') are plotted after dividing by an assumed Oxygen Enhancement Ratio (OER) of 2.7, because the α/β ratios for a tissue under anoxic and oxic conditions are in the same proportion as the OER. Error bars are estimates of the 95% confidence range on each value. Such experiments can assay the effect of radiation either *in situ* by regrowth delay or local tumour control, or by excising the tumour from the animal and measuring the survival of cells *in vitro* (Section 5.4).

Table 8.2 α/β values for human tissues and tumours

	Analysis	α/β (Gy)	Reference
Early reactions			
Skin (erythema)	D	7.5(5.4–10.9)	Turesson and Thames (1989)
(Desquamation) (T>29 days)	D	11.2(7.8–18.6)	
(T<29 days)	D	18–35	
Lung (acute)	TR	<8.8	Cox (1987)
Late reactions			
Supraglottic larynx			
(Late sequelae)	D	3.8(0.8–14)	Maciejewski *et al* (1986)
Larynx	TR	≈3.4	Henk and James (1978)
(Cartilage necrosis)	TR	<4.4	Horiot *et al* (1972)
	TR	<4.2	Stell and Morrison (1973); Fletcher *et al* (1974)
Oropharynx (Late sequelae)	TR	≈4.5	Horiot *et al* (1988)
Skin (Telangiectasia)	D	3.9(2.7–4.8)	Turesson and Thames (1989)
	D	3.7(0.2–47)	Bentzen *et al* (1989 b)
Skin (Subcutaneous fibrosis)	D	1.9(0.8–3)	
Shoulder (Impaired movement)	D	3.5(0.7–6.2)	Bentzen *et al* (1989 a)
Nipple (Retraction)	TR	≈2.5	van Limbergen *et al* (1989)
Lung (Pneumonitis)	TR	<3.8	Cox (1987)
Cord (Myelopathy)	TR	<3.3	Dische *et al* (1981)
Bowel (Stricture/perforation)	TR	2.2<α/β<8	Bennet (1978) Edsmyr *et al* (1985)
Tumours			
Vocal cord	TR	<9.9	Harrison *et al* (1988)
Oral cavity/oropharynx	TR	<6.5–10.3	Byhardt *et al* (1977)
	TR	<7	Hands *et al* (1980)
Lung (Squamous cell, large cell, adenoca.)	D	≈50–90	Cox (1987)
Cervix	TR	<13.9	Watson *et al* (1978)
Skin	D	8.5(4.5–11.3)	Trott *et al* (1984)
Melanoma	D	0.6(-1.1–2.5)	Bentzen *et al* (1989 c)
Liposarcoma	D	0.4(-1.4–5.4)	Thames and Suit (1986)

D: Direct analysis; TR: two-regimen analysis.
Parentheses enclose 95 per cent confidence interval.
From Thames *et al* (1989); for references, see the original.

Analysis of data from human tissues and tumours to determine α/β ratios has been made by Thames *et al* (1989) and the results are shown in Table 8.2. Estimates from these data are much less precise than the animal values because 'experiments' using a wide range of fraction numbers cannot be performed on human patients for obvious ethical reasons. However, the agreement between human and animal data is generally good and confirms that animal tissues are good models for comparing the effects of different fractionation schemes that might be used clinically.

8.6 Incomplete repair

The simple LQ model described by Eqns 8.1 to 8.5 assumes that sufficient time is allowed between fractions for complete repair of sublethal damage to take place after each dose. This *full-repair* interval is at least 6 hours but in some cases (e.g. spinal cord) may be as long as 1 day. If the interfraction interval is reduced below this value, the overall damage from the whole treatment is increased because then there is interaction between residual unrepaired damage from one fraction and the damage from the next fraction. As an example of this phenomenon, Figure 8.6 shows data from mouse jejunum irradiated with 5 x-ray fractions in which the number of surviving crypts per gut circumference is plotted against total dose. Much less dose is needed to produce the same effects when the interfraction interval is reduced from 6h to 1h or 0.5h. This phenomenon is called *incomplete repair*.

Modification of the LQ model to take incomplete repair into account is described in Section 10.1. Figure 8.7 demonstrates the fit of such an incomplete-repair LQ model to data for pneumonitis in mice following fractionated thoracic irradiation with intervals of 3h between doses (Thames *et al*, 1984). The end-point was mortality, expressed as the LD_{50}. On these reciprocal-dose plots, incomplete repair makes the data bow upwards away from the straight line (dashed) which shows the pure linear-quadratic relationship obtained when there is complete repair between successive doses, as will be the case with long time intervals between fractions. Chapter 10 describes calculations using the incomplete-repair model.

The influence of incomplete repair is determined by the repair half-time ($T_{1/2}$) in the tissue. This is the time required between fractions, or during low dose-rate treatment, for half the maximum possible repair to take place. The half-time can be found by fitting the incomplete repair model (Section 10.1) to data like those shown in Figures 8.6 and 8.7. For

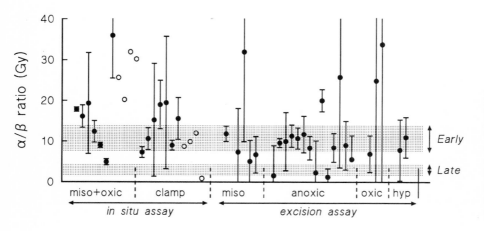

Figure 8.5. Values of α/β for experimental tumours, determined under a variety of conditions of oxygenation (see text). The stippled areas indicate the range of values for early- and late-responding normal tissues. From Williams *et al* (1985), with permission.

Table 8.3 Half-times for recovery from radiation damage in various normal tissues

Tissue	Species	Dose delivery†	T₁/₂/(hours)	Source
Haemopoietic	mouse	CLDR	0.3	Thames *et al* (1984)
Spermatogonia	mouse	CLDR	0.3–0.4	Delic *et al* (1987)
Jejunum	mouse	F	0.45	Thames *et al* (1984)
Lip mucosa	mouse	F	0.8	Ang *et al* (1985)
Skin (acute injury)	mouse	F	1.5	Rojas *et al* (1991)
Skin (acute injury)	mouse	CLDR	1.0	Joiner *et al* (unpublished)
Skin (acute injury)	pig	F	0.4 + 1.2*	Aardweg and Hopewell (1992)
Skin (acute injury)	human	F	0.35–1.2	Turesson and Thames (1989)
Skin (late injury)	human	F	0.4 + 3.5*	"
Lung	mouse		0.5–1.2	Travis *et al* (1987)
				Parkins *et al* (1988)
				Fowler *et al* (1989)
Lung	mouse	CLDR	0.85	Down *et al* (1986)
Lung	rat	FLDR	1.0	van Rongen (1989)
Spinal cord	rat	F	0.7 + 3.8*	Ang *et al* (1992)
Lung	rat	CLDR	1.4	Scalliet *et al* (1989)
Kidney	rat	F	1.6–2.1	van Rongen *et al* (1990)
Kidney	mouse	F	1.0	Joiner *et al* (1993)
Colon (acute)	mouse	F	0.8	Thames *et al* (1984)
Kidney	rat	F	1.15	Sassy *et al* (1988)
Rectum (late)	rat	CLDR	1.15	Kiszel *et al* (1985)

† F = acute dose fractions, FLDR = fractionated low dose rate, CLDR = continuous low dose rate.
* Two components of repair with different half-times.

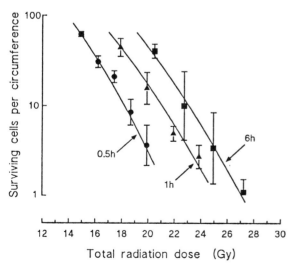

Figure 8.6. Effect of inter-fraction interval on intestinal radiation damage in mice. The total dose required in 5 fractions for a given level of effect is less for short intervals, illustrating incomplete repair between fractions. From Thames, Withers and Peters (1984), with permission.

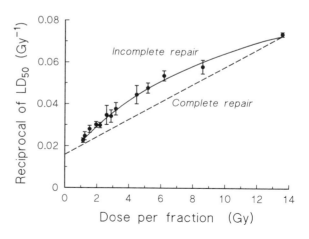

Figure 8.7. Reciprocal dose plot (compare Figure 8.4A) of data for pneumonitis in mice produced by fractionated irradiation; the points derive from experiments with different dose per fraction (and therefore different fraction numbers), always with 3 h between doses. The upward bend in the data illustrates lack of sparing due to incomplete repair. From Thames, Withers and Peters (1984), with permission.

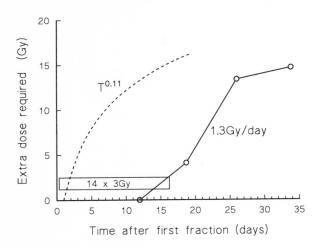

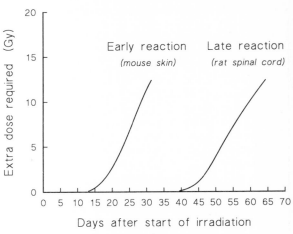

Figure 8.8. Extra dose required to counteract proliferation in mouse skin. Test doses of radiation were given at various intervals after a priming treatment with fractionated radiation. The slope of the line through the data corresponds to an extra dose of 1.3 Gy/day. The broken line shows the prediction of the NSD equation. Adapted from Denekamp (1973), with permission.

Figure 8.9. The extra dose required to counteract proliferation does not become significant until much later for late-responding normal tissues such as spinal cord, beyond the 6-week duration of conventional radiotherapy. From Fowler (1984), with permission.

isoeffect calculations it is important to select the appropriate $t_{1/2}$ for the tissue in question. Table 8.3 lists some values.

8.7 The time factor

So far, we have not discussed the change in total dose necessary to compensate for changes in the overall duration of treatment. Overall time is included in the NSD model (Eqn 7.2) but not in the basic LQ approach described above. The reason is because the time factor in radiotherapy is now perceived to be more complex than has previously been supposed. For example, Figure 8.8 shows that the extra dose needed to counteract proliferation in mouse skin does not become significant until about 2 weeks after the start of daily fractionation. For this situation the time factor in the NSD formula (broken line; total dose $\propto T^{0.11}$) gives a false picture because it predicts a large amount of sparing if overall time were increased from 1 to 12 days. These wrong time factors have not led to major clinical disasters because they have little effect over the 6 weeks of

conventional radiotherapy, corresponding at most to about one-third of the total increase in dose as the number of fractions increases. Thus the $T^{0.11}$ factor in the NSD model predicts only an 8% increase in total dose for a doubling of overall time.

Nevertheless, the $T^{0.11}$ factor is clearly misleading and should **not** be used (see Chapter 7). The use of the LQ model in clinical practice with **no** time factor at all is probably the best strategy for late-reacting tissues because any extra dose needed to counteract proliferation does not become significant until beyond the overall time of treatment even up to 6 weeks. This is illustrated in Figure 8.9 which diagrammatically shows the different effects of overall time in early- and late-responding tissues. Attempts are now being made to include time factors in the LQ model for acutely responding normal tissues and tumours but such factors depend in a complex way on the dose per fraction and interfraction interval as well as on the tissue type, and will need to take account of any delay in onset of proliferation which will probably depend in some way on these factors also.

Key points

1. The linear-quadratic model satisfactorily describes the relationship between total isoeffective dose and dose per fraction over the range of dose per fraction from 1 Gy up to large single doses. In contrast, the NSD formulation can only be made to fit data over a limited range of dose per fraction.
2. The α/β ratio describes the *shape* of the fractionation response: a low α/β (0.5–6 Gy) is characteristic of late-responding normal tissues and indicates a rapid increase of total dose with decreasing dose per fraction and a survival curve for the putative target cells that is significantly curved.
3. A higher α/β ratio (7–20 Gy) is characteristic of acutely responding normal tissues and tumours; it indicates a less rapid increase in total dose with decreasing dose per fraction and a less curved survival response for the target cells.
4. The basic LQ model is appropriate for calculating the change in total dose for an altered dose per fraction, assuming that fractions are given with *long intervals* between (typically one day). For shorter interfraction intervals, a correction may be necessary for incomplete repair.
5. The basic LQ model is appropriate for calculating the change in total dose for an altered dose per fraction, assuming the new and old treatments are given in the *same overall time*. Total dose probably does not need to be modified according to changes in overall time for late reactions, but for acute reactions (and tumour response) there will be a *time factor*. It is recommended that this be considered separately from the LQ calculation.

Bibliography

Dale RG (1985). The application of the linear quadratic dose effect equation to fractionated and protracted radiotherapy. *Br J Radiol* 58:515-528.

Denekamp J (1973). Changes in the rate of repopulation during multifraction irradiation of mouse skin. *Br J Radiol* 46:381-387.

Douglas BG and Fowler JF (1976). The effect of multiple small doses of x-rays on skin reactions in the mouse and a basic interpretation. *Radiat Res* 66:401–426.

Fowler JF (1984). What next in fractionated radiotherapy? *Br J Cancer* 49, Suppl.VI:285-300.

Michael BD (1985). A simple graphical determination of α/β from reciprocal dose plots. *Int J Radiat Biol* 47:119-120.

Stewart FA, Soranson JA, Alpen EL *et al* (1984). Radiation-induced renal damage: the effects of hyperfractionation. *Radiat Res* 98:407-420.

Thames HD, Bentzen SM, Turesson I *et al* (1989). Fractionation parameters for human tissues and tumors. *Int J Radiat Biol* 56:701-710.

Thames HD, Withers HR and Peters LJ (1984). Tissue repair capacity and repair kinetics deduced from multifractionated or continuous irradiation regimens with incomplete repair. *Br J Cancer* 49, Suppl.VI:263-269.

Thames HD, Withers HR, Peters LJ and Fletcher GH (1982). Changes in early and late radiation responses with altered dose fractionation: implications for dose survival relationships. *Int J Radiat Oncol Biol Phys* 8:219-226.

Williams MV, Denekamp J and Fowler JF (1985). A review of α/β ratios for experimental tumors: implications for clinical studies of altered fractionation. *Int J Radiat Oncol Biol Phys* 11:87-96.

Further reading

Fowler JF (1989). The linear-quadratic formula and progress in fractionated radiotherapy. *Br J Radiol* 62:679-694.

Joiner MC (1989). The dependence of radiation response on the dose per fraction In: *The Scientific Basis for Modern Radiotherapy* (BIR Report 19), pp.20-26. (Ed) McNally NJ. British Institute of Radiology; London.

Thames HD and Hendry JH (1987). *Fractionation in Radiotherapy*. Taylor & Francis; London.

9

Hyperfractionation and accelerated radiotherapy

Michael C. Joiner

9.1 Introduction

The relationships between total dose and dose per fraction for late-responding tissues, acutely responding tissues, and tumours, provide the basic information required to optimize radiotherapy according to the dose per fraction and number of fractions. Much work still needs to be done to determine the time of onset and rate of repopulation in normal tissues and tumours during and after radiotherapy, but enough is now known about this proliferative response to support the view that reduction in the overall duration of fractionated radiotherapy should be considered. This chapter discusses changes in clinical practice that are being made to take account of these two issues.

9.2 Hyperfractionation

The dependence of isoeffective total dose on dose per fraction is addressed in Chapter 8 in terms of the linear-quadratic model. Figure 9.1 shows a collection of isoeffect curves for acutely responding tissues (dashed lines) and late-responding tissues (full lines) in experimental animals exposed to fractionated x- or γ-irradiation (Thames *et al* 1982). The data that have been selected were for short treatment times, thus excluding any influence of proliferation on the total dose during these multifraction experiments. This summary thus represents purely the influence of dose per fraction on response and excludes the influence of overall treatment time. The data show that isoeffective total doses increase more rapidly with decreasing dose per fraction for late effects than

for acute effects. A reminder from Chapter 8 is that, in consequence, late effects have low α/β ratios (0.5 to 6 Gy) and acute effects have high α/β ratios (7 to 20 Gy). The vertical axis can be regarded as tissue tolerance dose and it can be seen that for low dose per fraction (right-hand end of the horizontal scale) late reactions tend to require a higher dose and are therefore spared. It was indicated in Section 8.5 that the available data on tumours suggest that in terms of fractionation

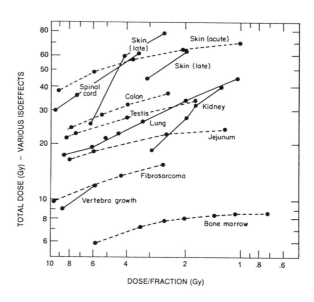

Figure 9.1 Relationship between total dose and dose per fraction for a variety of normal tissues in experimental animals. The results on late-responding tissues (full lines) are systematically steeper than those on early-responding tissues (broken lines). Chart from Hall (1988) quoting the data of Thames *et al* (1982), with permission.

response they may tend to behave like acutely responding normal tissues; thus, provided that late reactions are dose-limiting, small doses per fraction should give the best therapeutic index.

It is possible to summarize data of the type shown in Figure 9.1 by plotting the ratio of total dose for each dose per fraction to total dose for a reference treatment (usually 2 Gy per fraction). This is done in Figure 9.2A using calculations on the basis of the LQ equation. The shaded areas enclose the range of these ratios, for α/β values of 1 to 4 Gy and 8 to 15 Gy, which apply to most late- and acute-responding tissues respectively. The change in total dose is greater for the lower α/β values, as is the potential for error if the wrong α/β value is used. α/β values should therefore be selected carefully and always conservatively when doing calculations involving changing dose per fraction.

An increase in dose per fraction relative to 2 Gy is termed *hypofractionation* and a decrease is *hyperfractionation*. We can calculate a therapeutic gain factor (TGF) for a new dose per fraction from the ratio of the relative isoeffect doses for tumour and normal tissue. An example is shown in Figure 9.2B. Remember that we are assuming here that the new regimen is given in the same overall time as the 2 Gy regimen and that treatment is always limited by the late reactions. TGF curves are shown for a range of (late-responding) α/β values from 1.5 to 4 Gy.

Hyperfractionation using a larger number of dose fractions below 2 Gy is predicted to give a therapeutic gain, and hypofractionation a therapeutic loss. Note, however, that this situation would be nullified, or even reversed, for specific tumours that have low α/β ratios (e.g. some melanomas). TGF values for hyperfractionation would also be less than those shown if an unacceptable increase in acute normal-tissue reactions prevented the total dose from being increased to the full tolerance of the late-responding tissues.

Hyperfractionation has now been tested in a randomized clinical trial of oropharyngeal cancer (EORTC No. 22791) and the results are shown in Figure 9.3. A hyperfractionated treatment with 70 fractions of 1.15 Gy (2 fractions per day with a 4–6 h interval, total dose 80.5 Gy) produced a similar incidence of late tissue damage as a conventional schedule of 35 fractions of 2 Gy (70 Gy given in the same overall time of 7 weeks). However, the larger total dose in the hyperfractionated treatment produced a substantial increase of

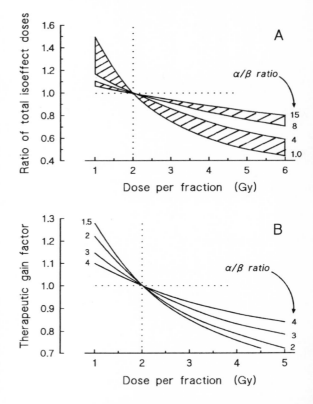

Figure 9.2 A: Theoretical isoeffect curves based on the LQ model for various α/β ratios. The hatched areas enclose curves corresponding to early-responding and late-responding normal tissues. B: Therapeutic gain factors for various α/β ratios of normal tissue, assuming an α/β ratio of 10 Gy for tumours. From Withers, Maciejewski and Taylor *et al.* (1989) with permission.

about 19% in long-term local tumour control. The results of this study are in good agreement with the linear-quadratic model and support hyperfractionation as a way of increasing the therapeutic benefit in radiotherapy.

9.3 The effect of tumour cell proliferation during radiotherapy

It is possible that tumour cell proliferation during treatment may reduce the effectiveness of radiotherapy. Withers *et al* (1988) drew attention to this and their results are shown in Figure 23.4. A more recent analysis of these data by Bentzen and Thames (1991) is shown in Figure 9.4. The data

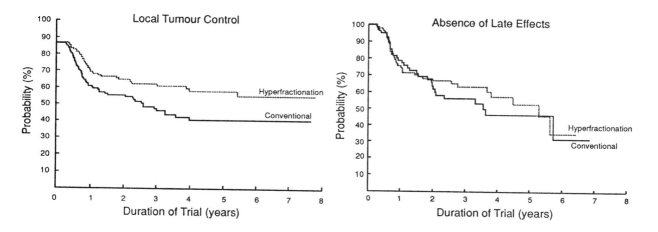

Figure 9.3 Results of the EORTC (22791) trial of clinical hyperfractionation. A: local tumour control (logrank p = 0.02); B: patients free of late radiation effects, grade 2 or worse (logrank p = 0.72). From Horiot *et al* (1992), with permission.

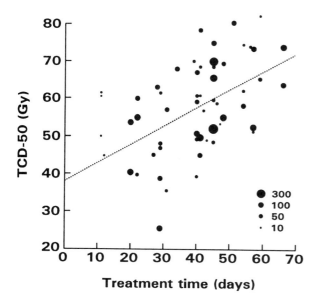

Figure 9.4 Tumour control dose (TCD$_{50}$) in head and neck cancer as a function of the overall treatment time. Each point indicates the result of a particular trial, the size of the symbol indicating the size of the trial. There is a trend for the curative radiation dose to increase with overall treatment time. From Bentzen and Thames (1991); *see also* Figure 23.4.

show doses to achieve tumour control in 50% of cases (i.e. TCD$_{50}$ values) plotted against overall treatment time, for squamous-cell carcinomas of the head and neck. Since a variety of doses per

fraction were used in the various studies, the LQ model was used with an α/β ratio of 25 Gy to convert from the actual doses per fraction used into equivalent doses with 2 Gy per fraction. The various studies achieved different tumour control rates and it was also necessary to extrapolate to the 50% control level. This required an assumed value for the steepness of the dose-control relationship for the tumours; Bentzen and Thames assumed that the dose to increase control from 40% to 60% was 10.5 Gy.

The slope of the line through the data in Figure 9.4 is 0.48 Gy per day. From reasonable estimates of tumour cell radiosensitivity, this would correspond to clonogen doubling times of less than 1 week, similar to the values of pretreatment potential doubling time measured in human tumours (Figure 9.6). Thus *accelerated fractionation*, which uses a reduced overall treatment time below the conventional 6 to 7 weeks, should increase tumour cure rates by restricting the time available for tumour cell proliferation. From Figure 9.4, for example, the dose in a 5-week schedule would be effectively larger than that in a 7-week schedule by a factor $0.48 \times (7-5) \times 7 = 6.7$ Gy, or nearly 10% of a 70 Gy treatment.

Figure 9.4 is a retrospective analysis and therefore is not ideal. From a particular clinical study Figure 7.4 shows more clearly the loss in tumour response that resulted from the introduction of a split of 4 weeks during treatment so that overall time was 10–10.5 weeks compared with 6 weeks.

It showed that the extra 4 weeks gap was worth about 11–12 Gy in total dose and, using reasonable estimates of tumour cell radiosensitivity, this would correspond to clonogen doubling times of about 4 to 5 days.

Various calculations have been made of the efficacy of short schedules in radiotherapy. As an example, Figure 9.5 shows calculations made by J.F. Fowler comparing schedules with 5, 10 and 15 fractions per working week, i.e. 1, 2 and 3 fractions per day. Log(tumour cell kill) was determined using the linear-quadratic cell survival equation with $\alpha = 0.35$ Gy^{-1} and $\alpha/\beta = 10$ Gy (*see* Section 8.4). As overall time increases (and thus the number of fractions) the dose per fraction has been continually adjusted to keep the same late effects as a reference schedule with 30 fractions of 2 Gy, using the LQ model with $\alpha/\beta = 3$ Gy. Tumour cell proliferation is assumed to occur after each fraction, with the clonogen doubling times shown against each curve. The star symbols show the maximum cell kill and hence the optimum overall time for each tumour-cell doubling time and number of fractions per week. The horizontal dotted line shows the expected log cell kill needed to sterilize a 1 gram tumour that is assumed to contain 10^9 cells. The following points should be noted:

1. For clonogen doubling times below 7 days, the optimum overall time is always less than 6 weeks and for such tumours accelerated

radiotherapy should be better than conventional 6–7 week radiotherapy.

2. Whatever the value of the clonogen doubling time, it should always be better to use more than one treatment per day, to take advantage of the hyperfractionation effect (Figure 9.2) unless tumours have low α/β ratios.

9.4 Predicting the influence of proliferation

The potential doubling time (T_{pot}, Section 3.2) is a cell-kinetic parameter that indicates the rate at which cells are proliferating in an untreated tumour. Although there is much uncertainty about this, it has been suggested that *during* treatment the rate at which clonogenic cells within the tumour repopulate may also resemble the T_{pot} value. It could be therefore that the T_{pot} value for a tumour (measured before the start of treatment) will indicate whether it will benefit from accelerated radiotherapy.

Figure 9.6 shows measurements of T_{pot} using flow cytometry on tumour biopsies from patients at Mount Vernon Hospital and the Gray Laboratory in the UK (Wilson *et al*, 1988). Most tumours (62%) had T_{pot} less than 7 days, and so might benefit from accelerated fractionation. However, the other 38% of tumours had T_{pot} greater than 7 days. Figure 9.5 suggests that acceleration would

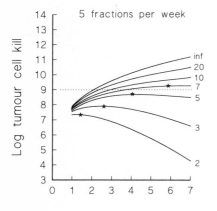
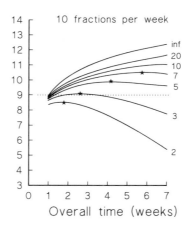
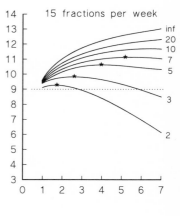

Figure 9.5 Calculations of the anti-tumour effect of accelerated fractionation over overall times up to 7 weeks. The ordinate shows the log cell kill for constant late normal-tissue reactions. Assumptions: $\alpha/\beta = 3$ Gy for late-responding normal tissues, 10 Gy for tumour; reference schedule is 30 fractions of 2 Gy. Lines are calculated for different assumed repopulation doubling times in days; the stars show the optimum schedule for each line. From Fowler (1990), with permission.

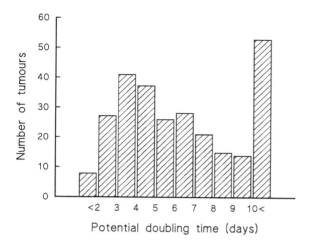

Figure 9.6 Distribution of T_{pot} values in 269 human tumours of various histological types. Personal communication from G.D. Wilson.

from differences between tumours and of course from experimental errors. In parentheses is the percentage of tumours of each type with $T_{pot} \leq 5$ days. There is a trend towards cervix and head and neck tumours proliferating the fastest, with lung tumours and melanomas proliferating more slowly. However, this diagram emphasizes the danger of making generalizations, as a significant proportion of tumours in *all* groups are proliferating quickly.

It seems unlikely that accelerated radiotherapy will be appropriate for all patients in any given histopathological category. As indicated in Chapter 23, it will probably be necessary to employ a predictive test for tumour cell repopulation, on the basis of which to identify those patients who are likely to benefit. The future pattern of radiotherapy may well be to individualize treatments, using information such as the T_{pot} value.

be of little or no benefit in these cases and if T_{pot} is longer than about 10 days, then accelerated therapy could actually be detrimental if it means reducing the total dose. This demonstrates the importance of predicting repopulation rate as accurately as possible in each tumour prior to therapy in order to determine which treatment schedule would maximize the response.

Figure 9.7 shows T_{pot} values according to tumour type. The columns indicate the median T_{pot} and the range of values is also indicated; remember that scatter in such data results both

9.5 Accelerated radiotherapy

There are now a number of trials of accelerated radiotherapy taking place and this could prove to be one of the most significant advances in cancer treatment during the last 20 years. Of particular interest is the EORTC trial # 22851 (Section 23.4). It has been found that within the whole trial, patients with slowly proliferating tumours (defined by $T_{pot} > 4$ days) responded significantly better than patients with rapidly proliferating tumours ($T_{pot} \leq 4$ days). If these patients are stratified into those receiving a conventional (7.5 weeks) and an accelerated (5 weeks) treatment, then patients with rapidly proliferating tumours responded significantly better if they received accelerated treatment; for those with slowly proliferating tumours it made no difference. A feature of this particular trial is that the same total dose (72 Gy) was used in both arms.

A different strategy has been developed at the Mount Vernon Hospital in the UK under the supervision of Dr. M. Saunders and Prof. S. Dische (Saunders *et al*, 1989; Saunders and Dische, 1989). It is called *Continuous Hyperfractionated Accelerated Radiotherapy* (CHART) and it is now over 5 years since the first group of patients began receiving this treatment. The protocol is 36 fractions given over 12 consecutive days (including weekends), using 3 fractions per day with an interval of 6 h between the fractions within each day. Dose per fraction

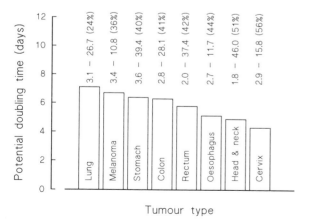

Figure 9.7 T_{pot} values according to tumour type. Numbers in parentheses indicate the proportion of tumours with T_{pot} below 5 days. Personal communication from G.D. Wilson.

is now 1.5 Gy to a total of 54 Gy. Total dose is therefore *reduced* compared with conventional therapy, in order to remain within the tolerance of acutely-responding epithelial tissues. In 99 cases with advanced squamous cell cancer of the head and neck, complete regression has been seen in 95%. The left-hand panel of Figure 9.8 compares these results with 84 cases from the same sites and T and N stages treated conventionally with curative intent during the period 1980–85. 74% of these patients achieved complete regression of their primary disease. There has remained a significant benefit from using CHART compared with conventional therapy.

In addition, 76 cases with locally-advanced carcinoma of the bronchus have been treated with CHART and compared with a previously treated group of 62 patients with similar disease who had been included in a study with the radiosensitizer misonidazole. With CHART, complete radiologi-

cal disappearance of tumour was obtained in 42% of cases compared with 15% treated in the sensitizer study (Figure 9.8, right). This difference has remained significant, and a significant increase in 5-year survival has also been obtained in this site. A phase III multi-centre randomized trial of CHART *versus* conventional therapy in head and neck and bronchial carcinomas is now in progress in the UK.

Although it could be that accelerated radiotherapy as in the CHART regime is an improved treatment for certain categories of cancer, the future may (as indicated above) lie with its use in subgroups of patients that are selected on the basis of a predictive assay for tumour-cell repopulation (Section 23.4). This is because slowly growing tumours might be expected to do worse as a result of the reduced total dose compared with conventional radiotherapy.

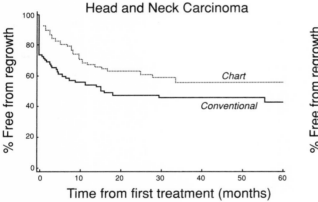 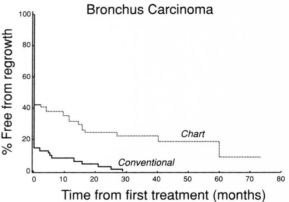

Figure 9.8. Results of a phase II CHART trial of accelerated radiotherapy in head and neck and bronchial cancer, as of February 1992. In each case there is a significant difference in local control: head and neck, p = 0.005; bronchus, p < 0.001. Personal communication from M.I. Saunders and S Dische.

Key points

1. *Hyperfractionation* is the use of a reduced dose per fraction over a conventional overall treatment time, employing multiple fractions per day. The therapeutic advantage is thought to derive from a more rapid increase in tolerance with decreasing dose per fraction for late-responding normal tissues than for tumours.
2. *Accelerated radiotherapy* is the use of a reduced overall treatment time with a conventional dose per fraction, achieved using multiple fractions per day. The aim is to reduce the protective effect of tumour-cell repopulation during radiotherapy.

Bibliography

Bentzen SM and Thames HD (1991). Clinical evidence for tumor clonogen regeneration: interpretations of the data. *Radiother Oncol* 22:161-166.

Fowler JF (1990). How worthwhile are short schedules in radiotherapy?: A series of exploratory calculations. *Radiother Oncol* 18:165-181.

Hall EJ (1988). *Radiobiology for the Radiologist*. Lippincott; Philadelphia.

Horiot J-C, Le Fur R, N'Guyen T *et al* (1992). Hyperfractionation *versus* conventional fractionation in oropharyngeal carcinoma: final analysis of a randomized trial of the EORTC cooperative group of radiotherapy. *Radiother Oncol* 25:231-241.

Saunders MI, Dische S, Hong A *et al* (1989). Continuous hyperfractionated accelerated radiotherapy in locally advanced carcinoma of the head and neck region. *Int J Radiat Oncol Biol Phys* 17:1287-1293.

Thames HD, Withers HR, Peters LJ *et al* (1982). Changes in early and late radiation responses with altered dose fractionation: implications for dose-survival relationships. *Int J Radiat Oncol Biol Phys* 8:219-226.

Wilson GD, McNally NJ, Dische S *et al* (1988). Measurement of cell kinetics in human tumours *in vivo* using bromodeoxyuridine incorporation and flow cytometry. *Br J Cancer* 58:423-431.

Withers HR, Taylor JMG and Maciejewski B (1988). The hazard of accelerated tumor clonogen repopulation during radiotherapy. *Acta Oncol* 27:131-146.

Further reading

Begg AC, Hofland I, van Glabekke M *et al* (1992). Predictive value of potential doubling time for radiotherapy of head and neck tumor patients: Results from the EORTC cooperative trial 22851. *Sem Radiat Oncol* 2:22-25.

Saunders MI and Dische S (1989). Continuous hyperfractionated accelerated radiotherapy in non-small-cell carcinoma of the bronchus. In: *The Scientific Basis of Modern Radiotherapy (BIR Report 19)*, pp. 47-51. (Ed) McNally NJ. British Institute of Radiology; London.

Thames HD, Peters LJ, Withers HR and Fletcher G. (1983). Accelerated fractionation vs hyperfractionation: rationales for several treatments per day. *Int J Radiat Oncol Biol Phys* 9:127-138.

Withers HR, Maciejewski B and Taylor JMG (1989). Biology of options in dose fractionation. In: *The Scientific Basis of Modern Radiotherapy*, pp. 27-36. (Ed) McNally NJ. British Institute of Radiology; London.

10

Calculation of isoeffect relationships

Albert J. van der Kogel and Arnout C.C. Ruifrok _____

10.1 Derivation of LQ-based isoeffect formulae

The isoeffect or tolerance calculations in this chapter are based on the linear-quadratic (LQ) formulae introduced in Chapter 8. The linear-quadratic approach has led to various ways of calculating isoeffect relationships for radiotherapy, all based on similar underlying assumptions. Two principal formulations are the concept of Extrapolated Tolerance Dose (ETD) introduced by Barendsen (1982) and Total Effect (TE) by Thames and Hendry (1987). Fowler (1989) has preferred the term Biologically Effective Dose (BED), which is mathematically identical to ETD. BED has the advantage that it can logically be calculated for levels of effect that are below normal-tissue tolerance, whereas ETD implies the full tolerance effect. Throughout this book we are using the BED terminology.

These formulae seek to describe a range of fractionation schedules that are *isoeffective*. First, we must define a particular effect, or *endpoint*. Although the validity of the LQ approach to fractionation depends principally on its ability to predict isoeffective schedules successfully, there is an implicit assumption that the isoeffect has a direct relationship with a certain level of cell inactivation (or cell survival, *SF*). Generally, the fraction of surviving cells associated with an isoeffect is unknown and it is customary to work in terms of a level of tissue effect, which we denote *E*. As shown in Section 8.4:

$$\text{Effect } (E) = -\log_e(SF)$$
$$= D\,(\alpha + \beta d)$$

Dividing both sides of this equation by α, we get

$$E/\alpha = D\,[1 + d/(\alpha/\beta)]$$
$$= \text{Biologically Effective Dose (BED)}$$

BED is a measure of the effect (E) of a course of fractionated or continuous irradiation; it has the units of *dose* and is usually expressed in grays. Note that as the dose per fraction (d) is reduced towards zero, BED becomes D, i.e. the total radiation dose. BED thus has a simple conceptual significance: it is the theoretical total dose that would be required to produce the isoeffect E using a large number of very small dose fractions. It is also the total dose required for a *single* exposure at very low dose rate (Section 15.4). As will be illustrated below, values of BED from separate parts of a course of treatment may be added in order to calculate the overall BED value.

The TE formulation is conceptually similar and is also used in the literature. In this case we divide E by β rather than α to get

$$\text{TE} = E/\beta = D(\alpha/\beta + d).$$

The units of TE are (grays)^2, which makes it less convenient than BED. But note the simple conversion: $\text{TE} = (\alpha/\beta) \times \text{BED}$.

Incomplete Repair

When multiple fractions per day are used, the repair (or more correctly, recovery) of damage due to one radiation dose may not be complete before the next fraction is given, especially if the half-time for repair ($T_{1/2}$) is relatively long in relation to the time interval between fractions. Incomplete repair will tend to reduce the isoeffective dose and corrections have to be made for the consequent loss of tolerance. This can be accomplished by the use of the *incomplete repair model* as introduced by Thames (Section 8.6; Thames and Hendry, 1987). In this model, the amount of unrepaired damage is expressed by a function H_m which depends upon the number of equally-spaced fractions (m), the time interval between them, and the repair half-time. For the purpose of tolerance calculations, an extra term is added to the basic BED formula:

$$BED = D\,[1 + d/(\alpha/\beta) + H_m.d/(\alpha/\beta)]$$
(for fractionated radiotherapy)

Once again, d is the dose per fraction and D the total dose. Since repair from one day to the next is assumed to be complete, m is the *number of fractions per day*. Values of H_m are given in the Appendix (Table 10.3) for repair half-times up to 4 hours and for 2 or 3 fractions per day given with interfraction intervals down to 3 hours. Other values can be calculated using the spreadsheet computer program described in Section 10.3

Another common situation in which incomplete repair occurs in clinical radiotherapy is during continuous irradiation. As described in Chapter 15, irradiation must be given at a very low dose rate (below about 5 cGy/h) for full repair to occur during irradiation. At the other extreme, a single irradiation at a high dose rate may allow no significant repair to occur during exposure. As the dose rate is reduced below the range used in external-beam radiotherapy, the duration of irradiation becomes longer and the induction of damage is counteracted by repair, leading to an increase in the isoeffective dose. The corresponding BED formula for continuous irradiation incorporates the factor g to allow for incomplete repair:

$$BED = D\,[1 + D.g/(\alpha/\beta)]$$
(for continuous low dose rate radiotherapy)

where D is the total dose (= dose rate × time). Table 10.4 gives values of the g-factor for exposure times between 1 hour and 4 days.

Effect on Tolerance of Overall Treatment Duration

Changes in overall treatment time were dealt with in the NSD equation by assuming that tolerance

dose increases as power function (for instance proportional to $T^{0.11}$) of the overall duration of treatment (Section 7.2). Such an approach is now thought to be unsatisfactory, as described in Sections 7.4 and 8.7.

The effect of overall time on normal-tissue tolerance depends very much on the proliferation rate of the *target cells* in the tissue in question. The effect will be large in rapidly proliferating (i.e. early responding) tissues, and it may be absent in tissues in which cell turnover is slow (late responding) tissues). At the present time there is no consensus on how to apply a correction for change in overall time.

10.2 Tolerance calculations using the BED formula

General procedure: changes in fraction size

We deal here with the situation in which fraction size is changed *without change in the overall duration of treatment*.

Formula: $BED = D\,[1 + d/(\alpha/\beta)]$
(D = total dose in n fractions of size d)

First decide what is the dose-limiting normal tissue for this treatment.

1. Select a value for α/β for the specific tissue endpoint in question; examples are given in Tables 8.1 and 8.2.
    Select the reference tolerance dose D_{ref}. This will depend on clinical experience and on the dosage policy of the treatment centre (some examples are given in Table 10.1).
    Select a fraction size for the reference treatment (d_{ref}).

2. Calculate for the reference treatment:
    $BED_{ref} = D_{ref}\,[1 + d_{ref}/(\alpha/\beta)]$

    This value of BED is constant for the chosen α/β and reference treatment.

Assuming conditions of complete repair (high dose rate, one fraction per day), we can calculate as follows:

New fraction size, constant throughout treatment:

3. For new fraction dose d, calculate total dose
    $D = BED_{ref}/\,[1 + d/(\alpha/\beta)]$

Change of fraction size during treatment:

4. For the first part of treatment, calculate the partial BED value (PE_1) from d_1 and D_1 as in #3.

5. The partial tolerance remaining for second part of treatment is: $PE_2 = BED_{ref} - PE_1$.

6. For the new fraction dose d_2, the remaining total dose is given by:
    $$D_2 = PE_2/[1 + d_2/(\alpha/\beta)].$$

A similar procedure can be performed for more than 2 fraction sizes during treatment.
A fundamental aspect of these calculations is that partial BED values (PE) are additive:

$$BED = PE_1 + PE_2 + PE_3 \ldots$$

When fractions of radiotherapy are given so close in time that repair is incomplete, it is necessary to adjust the BED formulae as described in Section 10.1.

What degree of reliability can be placed on these calculations?

It is important to stress that the results of these calculations must only be taken as a *guide* to clinical practice. The LQ approach to fractionation overcomes some of the deficiencies of the older NSD approach (Section 7.4) but it cannot be claimed to be universally correct. Indeed, it would be surprising if such simple equations satisfactorily describe all of the possible effects of changing dose prescriptions in radiotherapy.

The validity of the equations is limited to more or less *standard conditions*. Deviations from the predictions of the incomplete-repair LQ model have become apparent under more extreme conditions, such as a reduced spinal cord tolerance in the CHART regime (3 fractions/day continuous over 12 days). Most of the deviations that have so far been observed from the LQ model may have arisen from incorrect choice of the two basic parameters: α/β and $T_{1/2}$. As experience grows in the application of this method of calculation it may be expected that fewer deviations will be observed. The exploration of new treatment schedules based on extrapolations from standard conditions using the current mathematical models must be done with caution.

Practical Calculations - Example 1

Background: Head and neck cancer. The planned treatment is 70 Gy in 35 fractions (abbreviated 70 Gy/35 fx). Due to a dosimetric error the first 6 fractions were given with 4 Gy/fx instead of 2 Gy/fx. The accumulated dose is thus 24 Gy in 6 fx. Treatment will be continued using 2 Gy/fx.
Question: How many fractions of 2 Gy should be given to maintain an equal probability of late fibrosis?
Assumption: α/β for late fibrosis = 3.5 Gy

Solution:

1.	$BED = 70 \times (1 + 2/3.5) = 110$	*calculate BED*
2.	$PE_1 = 24 \times (1 + 4/3.5) = 51.4$	*PE of first 6 fractions*
3.	$PE_2 = BED - PE_1 = 58.6$	*remaining PE*
4.	$PE_2 = D_2 \times (1 + 2/3.5) = 58.6$	*D_2 at 2 Gy/fraction*
5.	$D_2 = 58.6/1.57 = 37.3$ Gy	*remaining total dose*
6.	At 2 Gy/fx: 37.3 / 2 = 18 or 19 fractions	*remaining no. of fractions*

Practical Calculations - Example 2

Background: Cancer of the oral tongue, stage T_2 (3.5 cm). The planned treatment is in two parts: external beam 50 Gy in 25 fractions (part 1) followed by an interstitial implant giving 30 Gy in 3 days (part 2).

Question: If the total treatment were to be given in 2 Gy fractions, what would be the total biologically equivalent dose for late fibrosis?
Assumptions: $\alpha/\beta = 3.5$ Gy; $T_{1/2} = 1.0$ h ; *g*-factor (3 days) = 0.04 (Table 10.4).

Solution:

1. $PE_1 = 50 \times (1 + 2/3.5) = 78.6$	*PE for part 1 – external beam*
2. $PE_2 = 30 \times (1 + (0.04 \times 30 \div 3.5)\,) = 40.3$	*PE for part 2 = interstitial irrad.*
3. $BED = 78.6 + 40.3 = 118.9$	$BED = PE_1 + PE_2$
4. $BED = D \times (1 + 2/3.5\,) = 118.9$	*total dose D given in 2 Gy/fx*
5. $D = 118.9 / 1.57 = 75.7$ Gy in 2 Gy/fx	

Caution: because of the smaller volume and different dose distribution for the interstitial irradiation, the calculated biologically equivalent fractionated dose may be too high for an external beam irradiation.

Practical Calculations - Example 3

Background: Melanoma, selective radiotherapy of nodal area. The planned treatment is 5 fractions of 6 Gy (2 fx/week). After the first fraction it was discovered that by mistake a single dose of 12 Gy had been given. It was decided to complete the treatment with the same total number of 5 fractions.

Question: What fraction size should be used for the remaining 4 treatments? Is there a risk of radiation damage to the spinal cord? *Assumptions*: α/β for late fibrosis = 3.5 Gy ; α/β for damage to the spinal cord = 2 Gy. *Solution:*

Solution, late fibrosis:

1. $BED = 30 \times (1 + 6/3.5) = 81.4$	*BED of planned treatment*
2. $PE_1 = 12 \times (1 + 12/3.5\,) = 53.1$	*partial BED for first fraction*
3. $PE_2 = 81.4 - 53.1 = 28.3$	*partial BED for remaining 4 fx*
4. $PE_2 = D_2 \times (1 + D_2/(4 \times 3.5))$	
5. $28.3 = D_2 + (D_2)^2/14$	*filling in the known values*
6. $0.714\,(D_2)^2 + D_2 - 28.3 = 0$	*quadratic equation:* $D = \{-b + \sqrt{(b^2 - 4\,a\,c)}\} / 2a$
7. $D_2 = 14$ Gy $d_2 = 3.5$ Gy	

Solution, spinal cord tolerance:

1. $BED_{ref} = 50 \times (1 + 2/2\,) = 100$	*reference BED for the cord; 2Gy/fx*
2. $BED_{plan} = 30 \times (1 + 6/2\,) = 120$	*planned treatment: 5 × 6 Gy*
3. $BED_{plan} / BED_{ref} = 1.2$	*cord tolerance exceeded by 20%*
4. $100 = D_{max} \times (1 + 6/2\,)$	D_{max} *(cord) for 6 Gy fractions*
5. $D_{max} = 100 / 4 = 25$ Gy	*maximum 4 fractions of 6 Gy*

Additional Question: The actual treatment was: 1 × 12 Gy + 4 × 3.5 Gy. Calculate how this dose compares with the spinal cord reference dose of 50 Gy in 2 Gy fractions.

Note: it is much safer to use small doses per fraction for spinal cord tolerance; it is therefore better to reduce the dose for all fractions, rather than shielding after 4 large fractions of 6 Gy.

10.3 Advanced calculations with a computer spreadsheet

The calculations performed in the previous section are designed to identify schedules that have an equivalent probability of normal-tissue injury (i.e. for which the BED is the same). A much more difficult assignment is to calculate the relative tissue effects of two schedules that are *not* isoeffective. As illustrated in Chapters 13 and 14, dose-response relationships for radiation damage to normal tissues and tumours are never linear; in most cases they tend to be sigmoidal. Tissue effects are thus not proportional to BED and in order to calculate a difference in effect it is necessary to have information or to make assumptions about the shape of the dose-response relationship.

This is illustrated by Example 3 above. The BED_{ref} for spinal cord tolerance was calculated to be 100 Gy (50 Gy in 2 Gy/fx) and BED_{plan} was 120 Gy for the schedule of 5×6 Gy. Although the BED of the latter schedule was 20% higher than the reference schedule, we do not know how the risk for induction of myelopathy compares.

To address this problem we have developed a simple spreadsheet program that will run on a personal computer and which incorporates many aspects of the linear-quadratic model, including multiple daily fractionation, fractionated low dose rate, pulsed dose rate, estimates of proliferation, etc. (Thames, 1985; Fowler, 1989; Nilsson *et al*, 1990; Guttenberger *et al*, 1992). It allows the calculation and comparison of BED values and, in order to deal with the problems raised in the last paragraph, dose-response curves are constructed based on the double-log transformation of a Poisson model for cell inactivation (Gilbert, quoted in Thames and Hendry, 1987). This model assumes that the probability of tissue failure P is a function of the number of surviving Tissue Rescuing Units (TRU). If K is the initial number of TRU, then the probability function is:

$$P = \exp\left[-\exp\left(\log_e K - E\right)\right]$$

where E is the (negative) logarithm of the fraction of *surviving* TRU. The position and steepness of the sigmoid dose-incidence curve is determined by the parameters of the LQ-survival equation (α, β) and the value of $\log_e K$. With sufficient data these values can be derived by a direct analysis (e.g. Turesson and Thames, 1989, for human

skin) or estimated in the spreadsheet if two treatments with different levels of effect are entered.

The greatest advantage of the spreadsheet approach is to obtain insight into the meaning and impact of the various parameters of the LQ model. A change in any parameter is immediately reflected in a change in all the dependent variables, together with an estimate of the probability of normal-tissue complications or tumour cure.

Description and Use of the Spreadsheet
A simplified layout of the spreadsheet is shown in Table 10.2. The spreadsheet has two main parts, *the upper part* deals with the calculation of new (or combined) schedules and BED values based on a reference treatment. For an estimate of the therapeutic ratio of a particular schedule, α/β and repair $T_{\frac{1}{2}}$ values can be entered for both normal tissue and tumour. In *the lower part*, two dose-incidence curves (normal-tissue and tumour) can be estimated and compared in the accompanying chart. The most reliable curves are those for which the values of α, β, and $\log_e K$ are obtained by a direct analysis. For such cases the values can be entered directly, and curves are plotted for the conditions as specified for the reference treatment (fraction size, number of fractions per day, time intervals between fractions). As an alternative, approximate values can be derived if the α/β ratio is known, together with two dose-levels with different effects.

Other options available in the more extensive versions of the software are: 2 repair components, continuous low dose rate (also fractionated or pulsed), and correction for proliferation.

The use of the spreadsheet is demonstrated for Example 3 of the practical calculations, in particular for the second part dealing with spinal cord tolerance. As a first step, the parameters for the reference tolerance of the spinal cord, 50 Gy in 2 Gy/fx, 1 fx/day, are entered in the upper left quadrant. Next, the components of the actually given treatment are entered in the upper right quadrant: one fraction of 12 Gy in part 1, and 14 Gy in 3.5 Gy fractions in part 2. The BED estimates at the bottom of this quadrant immediately show that the cord dose is 22.5% higher than the reference tolerance dose.

To obtain an estimate of the probability of spinal cord injury at this increased BED, two dose-levels are entered in the bottom left quadrant: 5% incidence of myelopathy at 60 Gy (2 Gy/fx) and 50% incidence at 70 Gy, both schedules given as 1

Table 10.1 Tolerance doses and LQ parameter estimates for some normal tissues

Organ/tissue	Endpoint	TD$_5$* (2Gy/fx)	TD$_{50}$* (2Gy/fx)	α/β (Gy)	T$_{1/2}$ (hour)
CNS	necrosis	60	70	2	1.5–2.0
Lung	pneumonitis	18	24	3–4	0.6–1.0
Kidney	nephritis	20	24	2.5	1.0–2.0
Heart	pericarditis	45		55	2.5
Skin	fibrosis	50	65	2–4	
Intestine	ulceration	50	60	7–10	0.5–0.8

* TD$_5$ and TD$_{50}$ are the radiation doses that give 5% or 50% incidence of complications (in each case for a dose per fraction of 2 Gy with complete repair). These values have been compiled from various sources and should only be regarded as a guideline for the tolerance calculations in this chapter. The TD$_5$ and TD$_{50}$ estimates are for *human tissues*, while α/β and T$_{1/2}$ estimates are from *animal and human studies* (*see* also Tables 8.1 to 8.3).

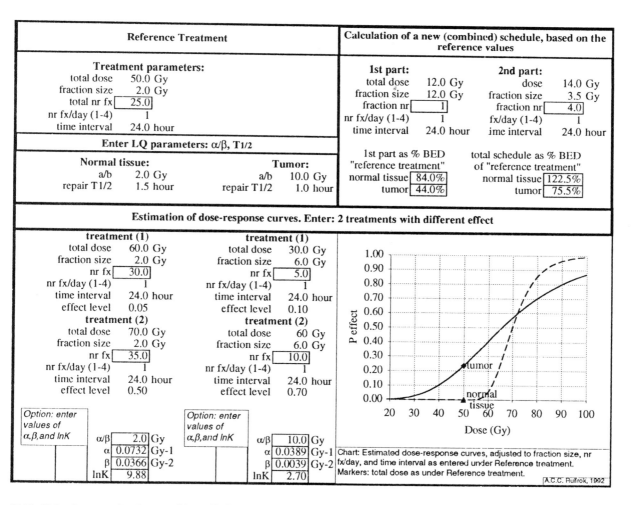

Table 10.2 An example of a spreadsheet display for advanced LQ calculations.

fraction per day with 24 h interval. The associated dose-incidence curve is shown in the chart.

In the previous example, only information about the normal-tissue tolerance is taken into consideration, while in many clinical situations the treatment decision is based on a comparison of the risk of complications and the probability of tumour control. The spreadsheet accommodates two tissues simultaneously, and can thus handle this situation. Dose-response curves for both the normal tissue and the tumour are displayed in the chart if the appropriate information is entered.

Table 10.3   Incomplete repair factors: fractionated irradiation (H_m factors)

Repair half-time (h)	Interval (h)				
	3	4	5	6	8
0.5	0.0156	0.0039	0.0010	0.0002	–
	0.0210	0.0052	0.0013	0.0003	–
0.75	0.0625	0.0248	0.0098	0.0039	0.0006
	0.0859	0.0335	0.0132	0.0052	0.0008
1.0	0.1250	0.0625	0.0312	0.0156	0.0039
	0.1771	0.0859	0.0423	0.0210	0.0052
1.25	0.1895	0.1088	0.0625	0.0359	0.0118
	0.2766	0.1530	0.0859	0.0487	0.0159
1.5	0.2500	0.1575	0.0992	0.0625	0.0248
	0.3750	0.2265	0.1388	0.0859	0.0335
2.0	0.3536	0.2500	0.1768	0.1250	0.0625
	0.5547	0.3750	0.2565	0.1771	0.0859
2.5	0.4353	0.3299	0.2500	0.1895	0.1088
	0.7067	0.5124	0.3750	0.2766	0.1530
3.0	0.5000	0.3969	0.3150	0.2500	0.1575
	0.8333	0.6341	0.4861	0.3750	0.2265
4.0	0.5946	0.5000	0.4204	0.3536	0.2500
	1.0285	0.8333	0.6784	0.5547	0.3750

m = number of treatments per day; the table applies for m values of 2 or 3.
From Thames and Hendry (1987), with permission.

Table 10.4   Incomplete repair factors: continuous irradiation (g factors)

Repair half-time (h)	Exposure time (h)						Exposure time (days)						
	1	2	3	4	8	12	1	1.5	2	2.5	3	3.5	4
0.5	0.6622	0.4774	0.3671	0.2959	0.1641	0.1130	0.0583	0.0393	0.0296	0.0238	0.0198	0.0170	0.0149
0.75	0.7517	0.5888	0.4774	0.3983	0.2339	0.1641	0.0861	0.0583	0.0441	0.0354	0.0296	0.0254	0.0223
1	0.8040	0.6622	0.5571	0.4774	0.2959	0.2115	0.1130	0.0769	0.0583	0.0469	0.0393	0.0338	0.0296
1.25	0.8382	0.7137	0.6165	0.5394	0.3504	0.2555	0.1390	0.0952	0.0723	0.0583	0.0488	0.0420	0.0369
1.5	0.8622	0.7517	0.6622	0.5888	0.3983	0.2959	0.1641	0.1130	0.0861	0.0695	0.0583	0.0502	0.0441
2	0.8938	0.8040	0.7276	0.6622	0.4774	0.3671	0.2115	0.1475	0.1130	0.0916	0.0769	0.0663	0.0583
2.5	0.9136	0.8382	0.7720	0.7137	0.5394	0.4269	0.2555	0.1803	0.1390	0.1130	0.0952	0.0822	0.0723
3	0.9272	0.8622	0.8040	0.7517	0.5888	0.4774	0.2959	0.2115	0.1641	0.1339	0.1130	0.0977	0.0861
4	0.9447	0.8938	0.8471	0.8040	0.6622	0.5571	0.3671	0.2693	0.2115	0.1739	0.1475	0.1280	0.1130

From Thames and Hendry (1987), with permission.

Key points

1. The BED formulae provide a simple and convenient way of calculating isoeffective radiotherapy schedules.
2. Tolerance calculations require: a reference tolerance dose and an estimate of the α/β ratio; for schedules with multiple fractions per day or continuous (low) dose rate an estimate of the repair half-time is also needed.
3. With the help of a simple spreadsheet computer program, more advanced calculations based on the incomplete repair model can be performed, allowing BED values to be calculated, also the probability of tissue damage, both for normal tissue and tumour response.

Bibliography

Barendsen GW (1982). Dose fractionation, dose rate, and isoeffect relationships for normal tissue responses. *Int J Radiat Oncol Biol Phys* 8:1981-1997.

Fowler JF (1989). The linear-quadratic formula and progress in fractionated radiotherapy. *Br J Radiol* 62:679-694.

Guttenberger R, Thames HD and Ang KK (1992). Is the experience with CHART compatible with experimental data? A new model of repair kinetics and computer simulations. *Radiother Oncol* 25:280-286.

Nilsson P, Thames HD and Joiner MC (1990). A generalized formulation of the 'incomplete-repair' model for cell survival and tissue response to fractionated low dose-rate irradiation. *Int J Radiat Biol* 57:127-142.

Thames HD and Hendry JH (1987). *Fractionation in Radiotherapy*. Taylor & Francis; London.

Turesson I and Thames HD (1989). Repair capacity and kinetics of human skin during fractionated radiotherapy: erythema, desquamation, and telangiectasia after 3 and 5 years' follow-up. *Radiother Oncol* 15:169-188.

Appendix: summary of formulae

Basic Equations:

$$E \quad = n\,(\alpha d + \beta d^2) = D\,(\alpha + \beta d)$$

$d = dose\ per\ fraction$
$D = total\ dose$
$n = fraction\ number$

$$SF \quad = \exp(-E) = \exp[-(\alpha + \beta d)\,D]$$

$$BED \quad = E/\alpha = D\,[1 + d/(\alpha/\beta)]$$

$$\frac{D}{D_{ref}} = \frac{\alpha/\beta + D_{ref}}{\alpha/\beta + d}$$

$$P \quad = \exp[-\exp(\log_e K - E)]$$

$K = probability\ constant$

$$\quad = \exp\{-\exp[\log_e K - (\alpha + \beta d)\,D]\}$$

Low Dose-rate:

$$\mu \quad = \log_e 2\,/\,T_{\frac{1}{2}}$$

$T_{\frac{1}{2}} = repair\ half\text{-}time$

$$\mathbf{g} \quad = 2\,[\mu t - 1 + \exp(-\mu t)]\,/\,(\mu t)^2$$

$t = exposure\ duration$

$$BED \quad = D\,[1 + g.d/(\alpha/\beta)]$$

Incomplete Repair Correction:

$$\Phi \quad = \exp(-\mu\,\Delta T)$$

$\Delta T = interval\ between\ fractions$

$$H_m = \frac{2}{m}\ \frac{\Phi}{1-\Phi}\,[m - \frac{1-\Phi_m}{1-\Phi}]$$

$m = number\ of\ fractions\ per\ day$

$$BED = D\,[1 + (1 + H_m).d/(\alpha/\beta)]$$

11

The oxygen effect

Michael R. Horsman and Jens Overgaard

11.1 Importance of oxygen

The response of cells to ionizing radiation is strongly dependent upon oxygen (Gray *et al*, 1953; Wright and Howard-Flanders, 1957). This is illustrated in Figure 11.1 for mammalian cells irradiated in culture. Cell surviving fraction is shown as a function of radiation dose administered either under normal aerated conditions or under

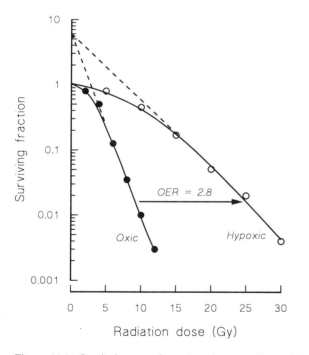

Figure 11.1 Survival curves for cultured mammalian cells exposed to x-rays under oxic or hypoxic conditions (diagrammatic), illustrating the radiation dose-modifying effect of oxygen. Note that the broken lines extrapolate back to the same point on the survival axis (n = 5.5).

hypoxia, generally achieved by flowing nitrogen gas over the surface of the cell suspensions for a period of 30 minutes or more. The enhancement of radiation damage by oxygen is *dose-modifying*, i.e. the radiation dose that gives a particular level of survival is reduced by the same factor at all levels of survival. This allows us to calculate an *oxygen enhancement ratio (OER)* which is simply the ratio of radiation dose in hypoxia to the dose in air needed to achieve the same biological effect. For most cells the OER for x-rays is around 3.0. However, recent studies suggest that at radiation doses of 3 Gy or less the OER is actually reduced (Palcic and Skarsgard, 1984). This is an important finding because this is the dose range for clinical fractionation treatments.

It has been demonstrated from rapid-mix studies that the oxygen effect only occurs if oxygen is present either during irradiation or within a few milliseconds thereafter (Howard-Flanders and Moore, 1958; Michael *et al*, 1973). The dependence of the degree of sensitization on oxygen tension is shown in Figure 11.2. By definition, the OER under anoxic conditions is 1.0. As the oxygen level increases there is a steep increase in radiosensitivity (and thus in the OER). The greatest change occurs from 0 to about 20 mm Hg; further increase in oxygen concentration, up to that seen in air (155 mm Hg) or even to 100% oxygen (760 mm Hg), produce a small though definite increase in radiosensitivity. Also shown in Figure 11.2 are the oxygen partial pressures typically found in arterial and venous blood. Thus from a radiobiological standpoint most normal tissues can be considered to be well-oxygenated, although it is now recognized that moderate hypoxia is a feature of some normal tissues such as cartilage and skin.

The mechanism responsible for the enhancement of radiation damage by oxygen is generally

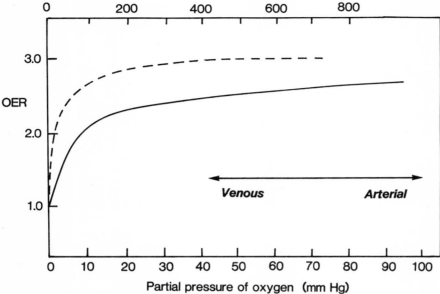

Figure 11.2 Variation of oxygen enhancement ratio (OER) with oxygen tension. The dashed curve shows the same curve plotted on the upper scale. The range of blood oxygen tensions is indicated. Adapted from Denekamp (1989), with permission.

referred to as the oxygen-fixation hypothesis and is illustrated in Figure 11.3 (*see also* Section 24.1). When radiation is absorbed in a biological material, free radicals are produced. These radicals are highly reactive molecules and it is these which break chemical bonds, produce chemical changes, and initiate the chain of events that result in biological damage. They can be produced either directly in the target molecule (usually DNA) or indirectly in other cellular molecules and diffuse far enough to reach and damage critical targets. Most of the indirect effects occur by free radicals produced in water, since this makes up 70-80% of mammalian cells. A free radical, designated $R^\bullet$, has several fates. If oxygen is present then it can react with $R^\bullet$ to produce $RO_2^\bullet$ which then undergoes further reaction ultimately to yield ROOH in the target molecule. Thus we have a change in the chemical composition of the target and the damage is chemically fixed. Subsequently this damage can be processed enzymatically and perhaps repaired (Section 24.5). In the absence of oxygen, or in the presence of reducing species, $R^\bullet$ can react with H, thus restoring its original form.

11.2 Hypoxia in tumours

Oxygen plays an important role in the radiation response of tumours. The growth of solid tumours

requires the induction of a blood supply, a process which is referred to as angiogenesis. This new blood supply is primitive in nature and it may be inadequate for meeting all the needs of the growing tumour. Nutrient-deprived and oxygen-deprived regions may develop, yet the hypoxic cells existing in these areas may still be viable, at least for a time. The first clear indication that hypoxia could exist in tumours was made in 1955 by Thomlinson and Gray from their observations on histological sections of fresh specimens from human carcinoma of the bronchus (Figure 11.4). They observed viable tumour regions surrounded by vascular stroma from which the tumour cells obtained their nutrient and oxygen requirements. As these regions expanded, areas of necrosis appeared at the centre. The thickness of the resulting shell of viable tissue (100–180 μm) was found to be similar to the calculated diffusion distance of oxygen in respiring tissues; it was thus suggested that as oxygen diffused from the stroma it was consumed by the cells and, while those cells beyond the diffusion distance were unable to survive, cells immediately bordering on to necrosis might be viable yet hypoxic.

Tannock (1968) made similar observations in mouse mammary tumours. The extent of necrosis in these tumours was much greater and each patent blood vessel was surrounded by a cord of viable tumour cells outside which

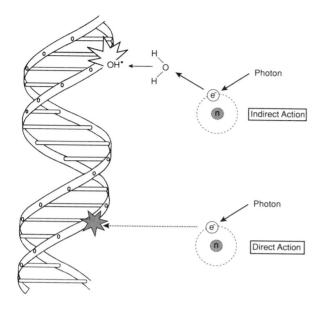

Figure 11.3 The oxygen fixation hypothesis. Free radicals produced in DNA either by a direct or indirect action of radiation can be repaired under hypoxia but fixed in the presence of oxygen. Adapted from Hall (1988), with permission.

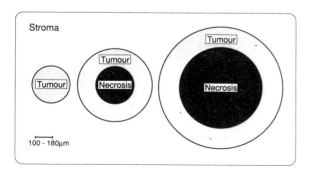

Figure 11.4 Conclusions by Thomlinson and Gray from studies on histological sections of human bronchial carcinoma showing the development of necrosis beyond a limiting distance from the vascular stroma. Adapted from Hall (1988), with permission.

was necrosis (Figure 11.5). Cells at the edge of the cords are thought to be hypoxic and are often called *chronically hypoxic cells*. Tannock showed, however, that since the cell population of the cord is in a dynamic state of cell turnover these hypoxic cells will have a short life-span, being continually replaced as other cells are displaced away from the blood vessel and in turn become hypoxic. More recently it has been suggested that some tumour blood vessels may periodically open and close, leading to *transient or acute hypoxia* (Figure 11.5). The mechanisms responsible for intermittent blood flow in tumours are not entirely clear. They might include the plugging of vessels by blood cells or by circulating tumour cells; collapse of vessels in regions of high tumour interstitial pressure; or spontaneous vasomotion in incorporated host arterioles affecting blood flow in downstream capillaries.

Since hypoxic cells are resistant to radiation, their presence in tumours is critical in determining the response of tumours to treatment with large doses of radiation. The presence of such cells in experimental tumours can easily be demonstrated, as shown in Figure 11.6. This shows the radiation survival response of KHT mouse sarcomas, irradiated *in situ* in air-breathing mice; or in nitrogen-asphyxiated mice (i.e. hypoxic); or as a single-cell suspension *in vitro* under fully oxic conditions. The studies in air-breathing mice were made both under normal and anaemic conditions. Cell survival was estimated immediately after irradiation using a lung-colony assay (Section 5.4). The survival curves for tumours in air-breathing mice are biphasic. At low radiation doses the response is dominated by the aerobic cells and the curves are close to the oxic curve; at larger radiation doses the presence of hypoxic cells begins to influence the response and the survival curve eventually parallels the hypoxic curve. The proportion of hypoxic cells (the *hypoxic fraction*) can be calculated from the vertical separation between the hypoxic and air-breathing tumour survival curves in the region where they are parallel. In this mouse sarcoma the hypoxic fraction was calculated to be 0.06 in mice with a high haemoglobin level ($\approx$16.5 g%) and 0.12 in anaemic mice (Hb level $\approx$9.5 g%). These data thus illustrate not only the presence of hypoxic cells in these tumours but also the influence on them of oxygen transport. Most experimental tumours have been found to contain hypoxic cells and estimates of hypoxic fraction range from below 1% to over 50%.

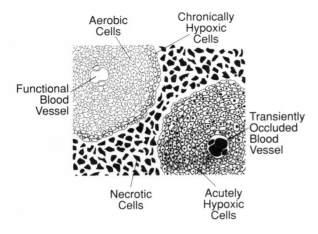

Figure 11.5 Schematic representation of diffusion-limited *chronic* hypoxia and perfusion-limited *acute* hypoxia within tumour cords. From Horsman and Overgaard (1992), with permission.

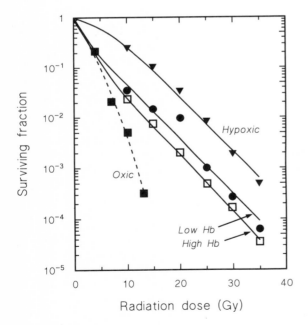

Figure 11.6 Cell survival curves for KHT mouse sarcoma cells irradiated under aerobic or hypoxic conditions. The 'hypoxic' data were obtained by killing the mice shortly before irradiation. Two sets of data for tumours in air-breathing mice are shown, with high and low haemoglobin levels. The dashed curve shows the *in vitro* survival of oxic cells. From Hill *et al* (1971), with permission.

A variety of procedures have been found to reduce or eliminate hypoxic cells in animal tumours. These include:

(i) increasing oxygen availability by allowing animals to breathe oxygen or carbogen (i.e. 95% oxygen + 5% carbon dioxide) under normobaric or hyperbaric conditions; introducing perfluorochemical emulsions into the vascular system to increase the oxygen-carrying capacity of the blood; using drugs that modify the affinity of haemoglobin for oxygen; or by the use of agents that increase tumour blood perfusion;

(ii) chemically radiosensitizing hypoxic cells using drugs such as misonidazole, etanidazole or nimorazole (Section 19.3);

(iii) preferentially killing hypoxic cells by means of bioreductive drugs that are active under hypoxic conditions, or by hyperthermia.

11.3 Hypoxia in human tumours

Although the presence of radiation-resistant hypoxic cells in animal tumours is well established and their impact on response to radiation can be reduced subtantially by the procedures listed above, the improvement of radiation response in human tumours as a result of these approaches has not been so successful. This could be because the phenomenon of reoxygenation (*see* below) is effective in some human tumours. Another possible explanation is that most of these treatments work well against chronically hypoxic cells, but apart from the radiosensitizing/bioreductive drugs, they have little or no influence on cells that are acutely hypoxic. More recent studies have now shown that there are agents that can specifically reduce acute hypoxia and these include nicotinamide, angiotensin II and flunarizine.

The failure to see significant clinical benefit from some manoeuvres designed to reduce the impact of hypoxia has led to questions about the presence and relevance of hypoxia in human tumours. Numerous attempts have been made to estimate hypoxia in human tumours. Unfortunately, the direct procedures that have been used in animal tumours, such as the paired survival curve assay (Figure 11.6) or clamped tumour growth/control assays, are not applicable to the human situation. Clinical estimates of tumour hypoxia have been made indirectly by measurements of tumour vascularization or tumour metabolic activity as well as by the binding of specific radioactive or fluorescent-labelled compounds to hypoxic cells.

Direct measurements of hypoxia in human tumours have been made by determining oxygen partial pressures (pO_2) using microelectrodes. Recent studies in a mouse tumour system have found a direct relationship between microelectrode estimates of tumour oxygenation and the actual percentage of hypoxic clonogenic cells. This is illustrated in Figure 11.7 in which the hypoxic fraction, determined using a clamped tumour-control assay, was altered in a C3H mouse mammary carcinoma by allowing the mice to breathe different gas mixtures. A strong correlation was found between hypoxic fraction and the percentage of measured pO_2 values that were equal to or less than 5 mm Hg.

Results from two clinical studies in which the pO_2 distributions in cervix cancers and tumours of the head and neck were measured by microelectrodes and related to local tumour

response after radiation therapy are shown in Figure 11.8. Good correlations were observed in both tumour types, with the less well oxygenated tumours showing the poorest response.

Several other clinical trials have provided evidence that hypoxia exists in human tumours and can influence radiation response. Significant improvement in local tumour control has been seen, particularly in head and neck cancers, from hyperbaric oxygen, chemical radiation sensitizers, and improved oxygen supply. This is illustrated in Figure 11.9, in which local regional control of tumours is expressed as a function of pretreatment haemoglobin concentration in male or female patients treated with radiotherapy for squamous cell carcinoma of the larynx and pharynx. Local tumour control was lower in those patients with reduced haemoglobin concentrations. Such a reduction in haemoglobin would make less oxygen available to the tumour and thus increase the level of tumour hypoxia.

11.4 Reoxygenation

Following a large single dose of radiation most of the radiosensitive aerobic cells in a tumour will be

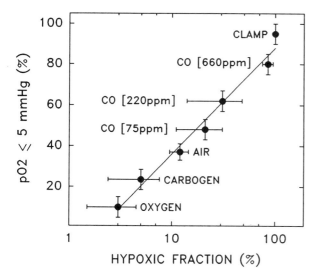

Figure 11.7 Relationship between pO_2 microelectrode measurements and the hypoxic fraction in a C3H mouse mammary carcinoma. Results were obtained from normal air-breathing mice, in clamped tumours, and in mice allowed to breathe oxygen, carbogen, or various concentrations of carbon monoxide (CO). Horsman *et al.* (1993).

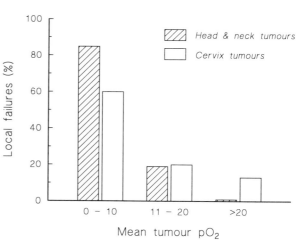

Figure 11.8 Correlation between local failure after radiation therapy and the mean tumour pO_2 measured before treatment using microelectrodes. The hatched columns show results on head and neck cancers (Gatenby *et al*, 1988); open columns are the results of Kolstad (1968) on cervix carcinomas. Data reproduced with permission.

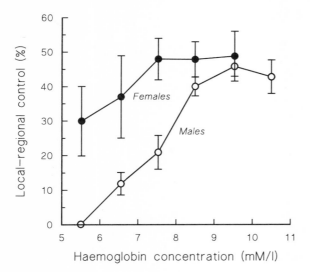

Figure 11.9 Local-regional tumour control as a function of sex and pre-treatment haemoglobin value in 1112 patients treated with radiotherapy for squamous cell carcinoma of the larynx and pharynx. From Overgaard (1988), with permission.

Table 11.1 Possible mechanisms and timescales of tumour reoxygenation

Recirculation through temporarily closed vessels	Minutes
Reduced respiration rate in damaged cells	Minutes to hours
Ischaemic death of cells without replacement	Hours
Mitotic death of irradiated cells	Hours
Cord shrinkage as dead cells are resorbed	Days

killed. The cells that survive will predominantly be hypoxic and therefore the hypoxic fraction immediately after irradiation will be close to 100%. This is illustrated in Figure 14.8. Subsequently, the hypoxic fraction falls and approaches its starting value. This phenomenon is termed *reoxygenation* (Section 14.4). The process of reoxygenation has been reported to occur in a variety of tumour systems. The speed of reoxygenation varies widely, occurring within a few hours in some tumours and taking several days in others. Furthermore, the final level of hypoxia after reoxygenation can also be higher or lower than its value prior to irradiation.

The mechanisms underlying reoxygenation in tumours are not clearly understood. A number of possible processes are listed in Table 11.1. If reoxygenation occurs rapidly then it may be due either to recirculation of blood through vessels that were temporarily closed or to a decreased cellular respiration (which will increase the oxygen diffusion distance). Reoxygenation occurring at longer time intervals is probably the result of cell death leading to tumour shrinkage and a reduction in intercapillary distances, thus allowing oxygen to reach hypoxic cells.

Reoxygenation has important implications in clinical radiotherapy. Figure 11.10 illustrates the hypothetical situation in a tumour following fractionated radiation treatments. In this example, 98% of the tumour cells are considered well-oxygenated and 2% are hypoxic. The responses of oxic and hypoxic cells to 6 large dose fractions are illustrated. If no reoxygenation occurs, then each dose of radiation would be expected to kill only a small number of the hypoxic cells and the resultant curve is therefore shallow. At the end of treatment the tumour response will be dominated by the hypoxic cell population. However, if reoxygenation occurs between fractions then the radiation killing of initially hypoxic cells will be greater and the hypoxic cells then have less impact on response. It has not been possible to detect reoxygenation directly in human tumours, but its existence is supported by the fact that local control can be achieved in a variety of tumours given fractionated radiotherapy with 30 fractions of 2 Gy, consistent with the measured SF_2 values for oxic tumour cells (Section 14.5).

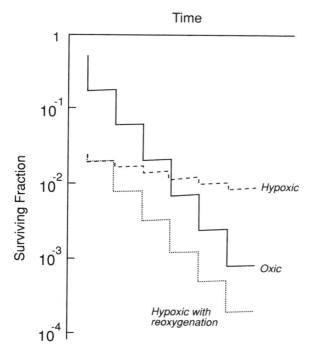

Figure 11.10 Calculated survival curves for a tumour containing 98% well oxygenated cells and 2% hypoxic cells when given 6 fractions of radiotherapy, showing the role of reoxygenation on the influence of hypoxic cells. Adapted from Hall (1988), with permission.

Bibliography

Denekamp J (1989). Physiological hypoxia and its influence on radiotherapy. In: *The Biological Basis of Radiotherapy*, Second Edition. (Eds) Steel GG, Adams GE and Horwich A. Elsevier Science Publishers BV; Amsterdam.

Gray LH, Conger AD, Ebert M *et al* (1953). The concentration of oxygen dissolved in tissues at the time of irradiation as a factor in radiotherapy. *Br J Radiol* 26:638-648.

Gatenby RA, Kessler HB, Rosenblum JS *et al* (1988). Oxygen distribution in squamous cell carcinoma metastases and its relationship to outcome of radiation therapy. *Int J Radiat Oncol Biol Phys* 14:831-838.

Hall EJ (1988). *Radiobiology for the Radiologist.* Lippincott; Philadelphia.

Hill RP, Bush RS and Yeung P (1971). The effect of anaemia on the fraction of hypoxic cells in an experimental tumour. *Br J Radiol* 44:299-304.

Horsman MR, Khalil A, Nordsmark M, Grau C and Overgaard J (1993). Relationship between radiobiological hypoxia in clonogenic tumour cells and direct estimates of tumour oxygenation in a mouse tumour model. *Radiother Oncol* (in press).

Horsman MR and Overgaard J (1992). Overcoming tumour radiation resistance resulting from acute hypoxia. *Eur J Cancer* 28:717-718.

Howard-Flanders P and Moore D (1958). The time interval after pulsed irradiation within which injury in bacteria can be modified by dissolved oxygen. I. A search for an effect of oxygen 0.02 seconds after pulsed irradiation. *Radiat Res* 9:422-437.

Kolstad P (1968) Intercapillary distance, oxygen tension and local recurrence in cervix cancer.

Key points

1. Hypoxic cells are much less sensitive to radiation than well-oxygenated cells.
2. Hypoxic cells probably occur in most animal and human tumours; they are believed to be an important cause of radioresistance to radiotherapy, especially using a small number of large dose fractions.
3. Hypoxia in tumours can be chronic or acute, for which the underlying mechanisms differ. Attempts to eliminate these radioresistant tumour cells require treatments that are effective against each of these types of hypoxia.
4. Reoxygenation has been shown to occur in animal tumours; some tumours reoxygenate rapidly, others more slowly. The evidence for reoxygenation in human tumours is less direct.

Scand J Clin Lab Invest Suppl 106:145-157.

Michael BD, Adams GE, Hewitt HB *et al* (1973). A post-effect of oxygen in irradiated bacteria: a submillisecond fast mixing study. *Radiat Res* 54:239-251.

Overgaard J (1988). The influence of haemoglobin concentration on the response to radiotherapy. *Scand J Clin Lab Invest* 48, Suppl 189:49-53.

Palcic B and Skarsgard LD (1984). Reduced oxygen enhancement ratio at low doses of ionizing radiation. *Radiat Res* 100:328-339.

Tannock IF (1968). The relation between cell proliferation and the vascular system in a transplanted mouse mammary tumour. *Br J Cancer* 22:258-273.

Thomlinson RH and Gray LH (1955). The histological structure of some human lung cancers and the possible implications for radiotherapy. *Br J Cancer* 9:539-549.

Wright EA and Howard-Flanders P (1957). The influence of oxygen on the radiosensitivity of mammalian tissues. *Acta Radiol* 48:26-32.

Further reading

Brown JM (1979). Evidence for acutely hypoxic cells in mouse tumours and a possible mechanism of reoxygenation. *Br J Radiol* 52:650-656.

Chapman JD (1984). The detection and measurement of hypoxic cells in solid tumors. *Cancer* 54:2441-2449.

Chaplin DJ, Durand RE and Olive PL (1986). Acute hypoxia in tumors: implication for modifiers of radiation effects. *Int J Radiat Oncol Biol Phys* 12:1279-1282.

Dische S (1989). The clinical consequences of the oxygen effect. In: *The Biological Basis of Radiotherapy*, Second Edition. (Eds) Steel GG, Adams GE and Horwich A. Elsevier Science Publishers BV; Amsterdam.

Kallman RF and Rockwell S (1977). Effects of radiation on animal tumour models. In: *Cancer* vol 6. (Ed) Becker FF. Plenum Press; New York.

Moulder JE and Rockwell S (1984). Hypoxic fractions of solid tumors: experimental techniques, methods of analysis and a survey of existing data. *Int J Radiat Oncol Biol Phys* 10:695-712.

Overgaard J (1989). Sensitization of hypoxic tumour cells–clinical experience. *Int J Radiat Biol* 56:801-811.

Rasey JS and Evans ML (1991). Detecting hypoxia in tumours. In: *Tumour Blood Supply and Metabolic Microenvironment*. (Eds) Vaupel P and Jain RK. Gustav Fischer Verlag; Stuttgart.

Sutherland RM and Franco AJ (1980). On the nature of the radiobiologically hypoxic fraction in tumours. *Int J Radiat Oncol Biol Phys* 6:117-120.

Urtasun RC (1992). Tumor hypoxia, its clinical detection and relevance. In: *Radiation Research. A Twentieth Century Perspective*, vol 2. (Eds) Dewey WC, Edington M, Michael Fry RJ, Hall EJ and Whitmore GF. Academic Press; San Diego.

Vaupel P, Kallinowski F and Okunieff P (1989). Blood flow, oxygen and nutrient supply, and metabolic micro-environment of human tumors: a review. *Cancer Res* 49:6449-6465.

12

Clinical manifestations of normal-tissue damage

Søren M. Bentzen and Jens Overgaard

12.1 Documentation of normal-tissue injury is an essential component of radiotherapy research

Radiotherapy is associated with a broad spectrum of normal-tissue reactions and no reporting of the outcome of radiotherapy is satisfactory without a thorough description of the treatment-related morbidity. With an increasing number of long-term survivors after cancer treatment, particularly in childhood and adolescence, long-term side-effects are increasingly important. Systems for tumour staging and tumour response evaluation are generally agreed upon, but there is as yet no widely accepted comprehensive system for classification and grading of normal-tissue injury after radiotherapy. Dische *et al* (1989) surveyed the reporting of radiotherapy trials in leading international journals for the years 1985 and 1988. Over half (in 1985) and one-third (in 1988) of the papers gave no or only anecdotal accounts of treatment-related morbidity. Few papers employed a previously published scoring system. Sismondi *et al* (1989) analyzed the reporting of complications of radiotherapy for carcinoma of the uterine cervix in 96 papers published between 1938 and 1986. Only 37 papers used some kind of classification of the complications, and 30 of these employed a grading system. In these 30 papers, 22 different systems were used! This makes a comparison of published complication frequencies virtually impossible.

12.2 Classification of clinical normal-tissue endpoints

There are several ways in which normal-tissue endpoints may be classified in clinical practice. The choice between them is influenced by clinical and/or biological relevance and by the choice of methods of data recording and analysis. The main classifications are as follows.

Subjective v. Objective Endpoints

Objective endpoints are preferable in clinical science in general but they do not provide a complete picture of the patient's situation after therapy. Table 12.1 shows an example where the physician's evaluation of impairment of shoulder movement was compared with the patient's perception of pain. Whether or not a given grade of objective reaction actually limits the patient's ability to live a normal life is of crucial importance in evaluating treatment-related morbidity. For example, the fact that 27% of patients with a 'moderate' (i.e. grade 2) impairment of shoulder movement had pain associated with movement of the shoulder is important information characterising the patient's condition.

The patient's perception of normal-tissue damage is not necessarily well-correlated with any objective clinico-biological changes. How the patient actually copes with treatment sequelae is influenced by a number of cultural and psychosocial factors. The use of questionnaires and such measures as the *visual-analogue-scale* (Till, 1988) may to some extent overcome these problems.

The objective evaluation of normal-tissue damage may depend to a considerable extent on the observer. Physical measurements often have minimal observer or operator dependency and should in general be preferred, but the results of such measurements may not be superior to

Table 12.1   Severity of impaired shoulder movement compared with frequency of subjective symptoms

Grade	Pain at movement	Pain* at rest	Reduced working ability
	%	%	
0	6	6	8
1	9	4	28
2	27†	16‡	62
3	31†	20‡	99

* Defined as moderate or severe (grade 3 only) pain on a scale including no pain and light pain.
† 5% had severe pain.
‡ 1.5% had severe pain.
From Bentzen *et al*, 1989a.

an overall judgement by a physician, taking into account many different aspects of response to radiotherapy.

Cosmetic v. Functional Endpoints

Cosmetic changes may constitute a major problem for the patient and must therefore be a concern of the radiotherapist as well. Serious cosmetic changes after radiotherapy may arise from retardation of the growth of muscle and bone in children and adolescents, or visible skin changes on the face or hands. Changes in body image may also lead to secondary problems like sexual dysfunction. Cosmetic endpoints have an obvious importance when cosmesis is one of the motivations for changing a treatment schedule, for example in the evaluation of combined tumorectomy and radiotherapy for early breast cancer. There are, however, some cosmetic effects that rarely trouble the patient, such as telangiectasia on parts of the body normally covered by clothes. In contrast, functional endpoints of injury almost inevitably influence the patient's quality of life.

Early v. Late Endpoints

A consistent distinction between early responses ('Frühreaktion') and late responses ('Spätwirkungen') is found in the German literature of the 1930s. The irreversibility of the late reactions was recognized in the term 'Dauerveränderungen' and Holthusen (1936) recommended that late reactions be assessed after a minimum observation time of 2 years.

The distinction between early and late responses came to play a key role with the 1982 paper by Thames and colleagues in which the observation was made that early and late reactions could be classified according to the α/β ratio of the linear-quadratic model (Sections 8.5, 9.2). They interpreted this as reflecting a difference in the shape of the survival curves for the (in some cases hypothetical) underlying target cell populations. Biologically, as well as clinically, this classification is of great importance as the reactions of early- and late-responding tissues differ in a number of important respects (Table 12.2). These two types of clinical response are defined operationally: any treatment-related morbidity that occurs within the first 90 days of the end of treatment is usually regarded as an early response. The clinical course of the two types of reactions is different, early reactions tending to be transient whereas late reactions are often irreversible.

Binary v. Graded Responses

Statistically as well as clinically, there is yet another important classification of normal-tissue endpoints (Table 12.3). Binary endpoints are *all-or-nothing* events, and no grading is possible for these. An example is radiation-induced neoplasia, often called a *stochastic response* to radiotherapy because it is the *frequency* that varies with radiation dose rather than the *intensity* of the response. A further example is radiation myelopathy which is a binary-threshold endpoint (Withers *et al*, 1988) where damage beyond a critical limit results in an all-or-nothing response.

In contrast, many functional tests give rise

Table 12.2 Typical clinical and biological characteristics of early and late radiation reactions

	Early reactions	**Late reactions**
Latency	≤90 days, typically 3–9 weeks. No strong dependence on treatment toxicity, but high toxicity may lead to slower healing of injury	>90 days, typical range 0.5–5 years. Shorter latent period with increasing treatment toxicity
Fractionation sensitivity	Low, $\alpha/\beta \approx 10$ Gy	High, $\alpha/\beta \approx 1$ to 5 Gy
Overall treatment time	Shorter time → more injury	No significant influence
Clinical course	Transient, but consequential late reactions may occur	Irreversible, compensatory mechanisms may occur (e.g. saliva production). rehabilitation programs or treatment for complications may relieve

to a *continuum* of responses. In between are the graded response endpoints where different outcomes can be ranked in order of increasing severity. However, no numerical relationship can be assumed between the various grades and the reporting of average scores should be avoided as this practice mixes up the severity and the incidence of reactions.

It is possible by data reduction to move from the bottom to the top of Table 12.3. Continuous responses may be graded, and graded responses may be converted to an all-or-nothing endpoint by defining a binary variable to be severity above or below a specific threshold value (Figure 12.1).

12.3 Systems for reporting normal-tissue injury

Several attempts have been made to devise a comprehensive system for grading and reporting

of normal-tissue complications (Table 12.4). None of them has so far gained general acceptance. The ideal system would be easy to use, clinically relevant, and would ensure that as much information as possible is available for radiobiological analysis. For example, both the RTOG/EORTC system and the French-Italian Glossary are clinically rather than radiobiologically oriented. In the former, the grading of late skin reactions involves hair loss, telangiectasia, and atrophy/ulceration, which biologically are 3 different endpoints, most likely resulting from the depletion of different target-cell populations. In the French-Italian system, only the *maximum* grade of reaction is recorded, and this means that a specific grade of reaction may have been reached during either the early or the late phase of expression of injury. Table 12.4 provides a broad comparison between these 4 systems.

In spite of the problems with these multiple systems, the use of a standard system of reporting

Table 12.3 Classification of radiation reactions according to data type

Type of Tendpoint	Statistical data type	Scoring system	Examples
Binary (quantal)	Categorical; all-or-nothing responses	'Yes/no'	Radiation-induced leukaemia; radiation myelitis
Graded	Ordinal; a ranking of severity is possible	'None/mild/ moderate/severe'	Telangiectasia; subcutaneous fibrosis
Continuous	Continuous; a continuum of responses is obtained	'Laboratory value'	Kidney ^{51}Cr-EDTA clearance; computed tomography density of pulmonary fibrosis

is strongly encouraged. It is to be hoped that a comprehensive system, widely acceptable both to radiotherapists and biologists, will in future be realised. An example of part of a system that has proven feasible in practice is given in Table 12.5; it has been incorporated into the European system (Dische *et al*, 1989).

12.4 Latent period

Late radiation responses in humans occur after latent periods of between 3 months and many years. To obtain a reliable estimate of the incidence of late complications therefore requires an extended period of follow-up (Figure 12.2).

Table 12.4 Some comprehensive systems for reporting and grading of treatment-related morbidity after radiotherapy

System	Basic features	Separates early and late reactions?	Limitations	Reference
RTOG/ EORTC	Very comprehensive: scoring available for virtually all major organs that may be injured by radiotherapy.	Yes	Mixes various endpoints for the same organ. Requires judgement by an experienced radiotherapist.	Perez and Brady (1992)
WHO	Derived from a system for use in medical oncology.	Focuses on early reactions	Focuses on early reactions and is therefore not very well suited for radiotherapy.	Miller *et al* (1981)
French/ Italian	Aimed at treatments for gynaecological cancer. Suited for surgical complications as well.	No	Mixes various endpoints for the same organ. Requires judgement by an experienced radiotherapist/ gynaecologist.	Chassagne *et al* (1993)
European	Focuses on endpoints rather than organs. Attempts to break down scores in specific symptoms thus allowing retrospective re-scoring of grades. Easy to use.	Yes	Based on previously published systems but has only been used in a limited number of studies so far. Still under evaluation.	Dische *et al* (1989)

Table 12.5 Definition of early and late cutaneous and subcutaneous reactions

Endpoint	Grade 0	Grade 1	Grade 2	Grade 3
Moist desquamation	none	< 10% of field	10–49% of field	≥50% of field.
Erythema	none	mild	moderate	severe with dry desquamation.
Telangiectasia	none	< 1/cm^2	1–4/cm^2	> 4/cm^2
Subcutaneous fibrosis	none	mild (just palpably increased firmness)	moderate (definitely increased firmness)	severe (very marked firmness, retraction and fixation)

From M. Overgaard *et al*, 1987.

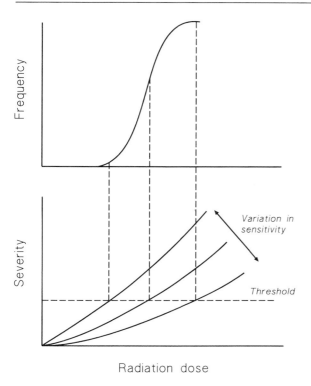

Figure 12.1 The *incidence* of a binary endpoint increases with increasing dose. No grading of severity is possible (top panel). Graded and continuous endpoints increase in *severity* as well as in incidence with increasing dose (bottom panel). The proportion of patients with a reaction above a certain threshold may be treated as a binary endpoint. From Field and Upton (1985), with permission.

Typically a 5-year follow-up is preferable. Patients who die from their disease or from an unrelated cause early after therapy are clearly less likely to have developed late normal-tissue damage than patients who live longer. Similarly, some patients may have incomplete follow-up because they were entered late into the study and only a short period before the data analysis. Such data are said to be *censored*, because the status of the patients after a certain time is unknown. To restrict the analysis to patients who have completed a specified minimum observation time, say 2 years or 5 years, may involve a considerable loss of information. But even more seriously, such a procedure may lead to selection bias, as it is not necessarily a random subset of all patients who would be included in this analysis. In statistical terminology, this type of data is called *failure-time data*: for each patient we record the time of reaching the endpoint or, for patients who were alive without complications when last seen, the time of their last follow-up.

There is an extensive statistical literature on the analysis of failure-time data. Popularly, these methods are often referred to as *survival statistics*, analyzed by *actuarial* methods. It is far beyond the scope of this chapter to provide a full description of this field but a few key methods should be mentioned. Estimates of the complication rate at a given time may be obtained by the life-table

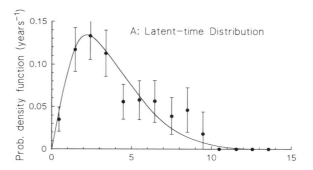

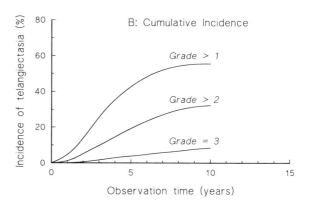

Figure 12.2 A: The latent-time distribution for any grade of telangiectasia as observed in 174 treatment fields with an intermediate probability of developing this reaction (grade ≥ 1). The probability density function may be interpreted as the fraction of patients who express the radiation reaction within a specific year after treatment. Even 9 years after treatment, about 2% of the patients showed the mildest grade of telangiectasia for the first time. **B:** The cumulative incidence of telangiectasia as a function of time for various grades of reaction following 44.4 Gy in 25 fractions. Model calculation based on observation in a total of 401 treatment fields. From Bentzen *et al* (1990), with permission.

method or the Kaplan-Meier estimate (Machin and Gardner, 1989). In statistical literature the latter is called the product-limit estimate. From these estimates the median latent time can be estimated (Bentzen *et al*, 1990).

To test for a statistically significant difference between the time-course of complications in two groups may be done by one of the versions of the log-rank test. Finally, multivariate methods have been used for analyzing failure-time data in radiobiology: the Cox Proportional Hazards Model (Taylor *et al*, 1987) and the Mixture Model (Bentzen *et al*, 1989). The former has become very popular in the analysis of survival data and is readily available in many standard statistical computer programs. There are, however, reasons to prefer the latter in the analysis of complication and tumour control data. For an (admittedly technical!) discussion see Bentzen *et al* (1989 c).

Biologically, it has been established that higher grades of reactions are on average seen at later times than lower grades, and that increased treatment toxicity may considerably shorten the latent period. Thus, in general, a follow-up at a fixed time interval after treatment is not sufficient. A complete description of the latent-time distribution is required.

12.5 Additional factors influencing normal-tissue damage

Apart from the details of dose fractionation, a number of other factors can influence the incidence and severity of normal-tissue reactions. These include concomitant treatment with other modalities.

Interaction with other Treatment Modalities

Figure 12.3 illustrates the influence of adjuvant chemotherapy on the development of subcutaneous fibrosis following post-mastectomy radiotherapy. The data have been corrected for latency, and error bars indicate binomial standard errors on the frequency of responders. Radiotherapy and the first cycles of chemotherapy were given concomitantly. After 44 Gy in 22 fractions the risk of ultimately developing marked subcutaneous fibrosis increased from 19% to 50% when the CMF combination (cyclophosphamide, methotrexate and 5-fluorouracil) was given as an adjuvant to radiotherapy. No such change was seen with cyclophosphamide as a single agent (data not shown). Figure 18.7 illustrates the time-dependence of gastro-intestinal damage in testicular teratoma patients treated with radiotherapy and combination chemotherapy.

An example of the influence of laparotomy on radiation-induced gastro-intestinal damage is shown in Figure 12.4 (Cosset *et al*, 1988). 345 patients with supra-diaphragmatic stage I or II Hodgkin's disease were entered into two EORTC trials. All patients received 39–41 Gy in less than 35 days. Due to the work-load in one of the participating institutions, other fractionation schedules than the standard 5 × 2 Gy per week were tried. No dose reduction was implemented to correct for the increase in biological effect from the larger dose fractions. There was a highly significant increase in late gastro-intestinal injury with increasing dose per fraction (p < 0.001). Also patients having a previous laparotomy had a significantly increased risk of intestinal damage, whatever the dose per fraction (p < 0.001).

Figure 12.5. shows the incidence of arm oedema after postmastectomy radiotherapy as a function of the number of lymph nodes excised from the axilla. Oedema was defined as more than 2 cm difference in the circumferences of the ipsilateral (relative to the treatment field) and

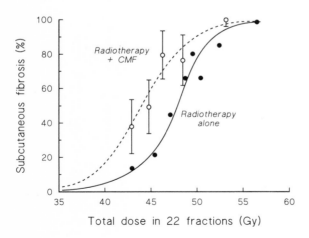

Figure 12.3 Effect of adjuvant chemotherapy on the incidence of radiation-induced subcutaneous fibrosis. (●) post-mastectomy radiotherapy alone; (○) radiotherapy plus adjuvant CMF (cyclophosphamide + methotrexate + 5-fluorouracil). From Bentzen *et al* (1989b), with permission.

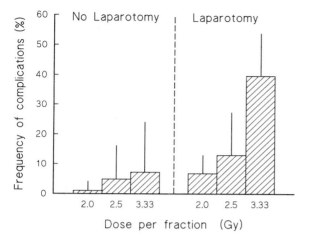

Figure 12.4 The risk of late gastro-intestinal injury in patients with supra-diaphragmatic stage I or II Hodgkin's disease is increased by previous laparotomy. From Cosset *et al* (1988), with permission.

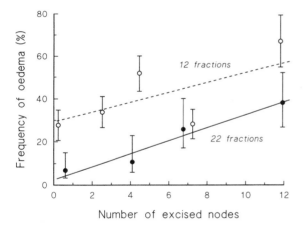

Figure 12.5 The frequency of arm oedema following postmastectomy radiotherapy increases in relation to the number of lymph nodes previously excised from the axilla. Adapted from Bentzen *et al* (1989a), with permission.

the contralateral arms. The total doses in the 12 and the 22 fraction groups were presumed to be equivalent according to the NSD formula (Chapter 7). In spite of this, large dose fractions considerably increased the incidence of late oedema of the arm. However, the extent of surgery, assessed by the number of lymph nodes excised from the axilla, was also highly significantly associated with increased arm oedema ($p = 0.01$ and $p < 0.001$ in

the 12 and 22 fraction groups, respectively).

All of the above examples show how procedures that are not in themselves associated with significant morbidity may 'top up' the radiation-induced damage and make it clinically overt. This phenomenon may seriously confound the radiation dose-response relationship.

The Effect of Treatment Volume

The effect of treatment volume on the severity of normal-tissue damage has been demonstrated by a number of clinical studies. Figure 12.6 shows the incidence of late complications as a function of field size after radiotherapy for laryngeal carcinoma. The total dose was 60 Gy delivered in 30 fractions. Persistent oedema and pharyngo-cutaneous fistulae were documented; no prophylactic metronidazole was used (compare with Figure 12.8). A significant increase in the incidence of late complications was seen with increasing field size. Data on the volume effect in animal systems is dealt with in Section 13.4.

Other Co-factors Involved in Expression of Radiation Damage

The age of the patient significantly influences the incidence of normal-tissue damage in a number of clinical situations. Figure 12.7 shows

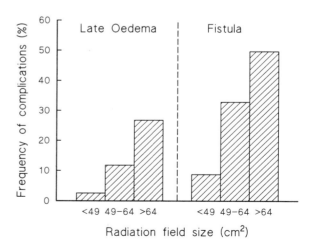

Figure 12.6 The incidence of late oedema and fistula as a function of the field size in the radiotherapy of laryngeal carcinoma (Overgaard, unpublished results).

an example of this. Dose-response relationships for the proportion of patients with moderate and severe impairment of shoulder movement after postmastectomy radiotherapy were documented according to patient age. In the clinical examination of these patients a relative measure of impaired shoulder movement was used and the ability to move the treated and the untreated shoulders was compared in individual patients. There was a significant tendency for the older patients to experience greater impairment.

The effect of metronidazole on the incidence of late radiation damage following radiotherapy for laryngeal cancer is shown in Figure 12.8 (Johansen *et al*, 1988). The incidence of pharyngo-cutaneous fistulae after laryngectomy in patients receiving primary radiotherapy increased substantially with increasing total dose. In this situation, fistulae may therefore be taken as an expression of normal-tissue injury after radiotherapy. The introduction of prophylactic metronidazole during the time of the study significantly reduced the incidence of this complication (p < 0.01).

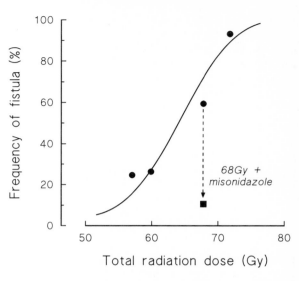

Figure 12.8 The risk of developing pharyngo-cutaneous fistulae after laryngectomy in patients receiving primary radiotherapy was drastically reduced by the prophylactic administration of metronidazole. From Johansen *et al* (1988), with permission.

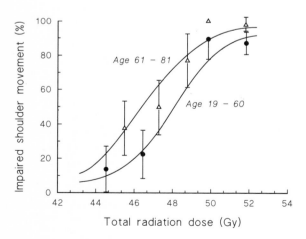

Figure 12.7 Dose-response relationships for moderate and severe impairment of shoulder movement after postmastectomy radiotherapy in relation to the age of the patient. (△) patients 61 to 81 years of age; (●) patients 19 to 60 years of age. All patients received 12 dose fractions. The effect of age is significant (p = 0.005). From Bentzen *et al* (1989a), with permission.

12.6 Quantative radiobiology

An increasing number of publications are concerned with the quantitative analysis of clinical radiobiological data. In addition to the evaluation, grading, and reporting of normal-tissue injury, a number of methodological problems must be addressed in such a study. These may roughly be grouped as clinical, dosimetric, and statistical:

Clinical aspects include the evaluation of endpoints using a well-defined system, identification of confounding factors as exemplified above and, especially in non-randomized studies, a careful consideration of the reasons for variability in treatment characteristics. Subsets of patients treated with low/high doses or in protracted overall time are likely not to be randomly selected.

Dosimetric aspects involve a detailed account of treatment technique and quality assurance procedures employed. Furthermore, the identification of biologically relevant dosimetric reference points and a proper evaluation of the doses to these points are required.

Statistical aspects include the choice of valid statistical methods that are appropriate for the data type in question and utilize the available information in an optimal way. Statistical tests for significance or, preferably, confidence limits on estimated parameters, should be specified. When negative findings are reported an assessment of the *statistical power* of the study should be given. Finally, the censoring (incomplete follow-up) and latency should be allowed for.

For an overview of the quantitative analysis of clinical data, see Bentzen *et al* (1988, 1993).

Key points

1. In any study of cancer treatment, the reporting of treatment-related morbidity using a well-defined scoring system is *essential*.
2. Previously published and generally used systems should be preferred to *ad hoc* systems.
3. Avoid throwing away valuable information. Graded responses should be reported using a clinically relevant grading system. The statistical methods should be chosen to exploit all of the available information.
4. Late radiation reactions occur over time-spans of several years. Actuarial statistical methods are needed for the statistically valid analysis of such data.
5. Patient characteristics, surgical and drug treatment, and other interventions, may influence the incidence and severity of radiotherapy sequelae.

Bibliography

Bentzen SM (1993). Quantitative clinical radiobiology. *Acta Oncol* 32:259-275.

Bentzen SM, Christensen JJ, Overgaard J and Overgaard M (1988). Some methodological problems in estimating radiobiological parameters from clinical data. Alpha/beta ratios and electron RBE for cutaneous reactions in patients treated with postmastectomy radiotherapy. *Acta Oncol* 27:105-116.

Bentzen SM, Overgaard M and Thames HD (1989 a). Fractionation sensitivity of a clinical endpoint: Impaired shoulder movement after post-mastectomy radiotherapy. *Int J Radiat Oncol Biol Phys* 17:531-537.

Bentzen SM, Overgaard M, Thames HD *et al* (1989 b). Early and late normal-tissue injury after postmastectomy radiotherapy alone or combined with chemotherapy. *Int J Radiat Biol* 56:711-715.

Bentzen SM, Thames HD, Travis EL *et al* (1989 c). Direct estimation of latent time for radiation injury in late-responding normal tissues: gut, lung and spinal cord. *Int J Radiat Biol* 55:27-43.

Bentzen SM, Turesson I and Thames HD (1990). Fractionation sensitivity and latency of telangiectasia after postmastectomy radiotherapy. A graded response analysis. *Radiother Oncol* 18:95-106.

Chasssagne D, Sismondi P, Horiot JC *et al* (1993). A glossary for reporting complications of treatment in gynecological cancers. *Radiother Oncol* 26:195-202.

Cosset JM, Henry-Amar M, Burgers JM *et al* (1988). Late radiation injuries of the gastrointestinal tract in the H2 and H5 EORTC Hodgkin's disease trials: Emphasis on the role of exploratory laparotomy and fractionation. *Radiother Oncol* 13:61-68.

Dische S, Warburton MF, Jones D and Lartigau E (1989). The recording of morbidity related to radiotherapy. *Radiother Oncol* 16:103-108.

Field SB and Upton AC (1985). Non-stochastic effects: compatibility with present ICRP recommendations. *Int J Radiat Biol* 48:81-94.

Holthusen H (1936). Erfahrungen über die Verträglichkeitsgrenze für Röntgenstrahlen und deren Nutzanwendung zur Verhütung von Schäden. *Strahlentherapie* 57:254-269.

Johansen LV, Overgaard J and Elbrønd O

(1988). Pharyngo-cutaneous fistulae after laryngectomy. Influence of previous radiotherapy and prophylactic metronidazole. *Cancer* 61:673-678.

Machin D and Gardner MJ (1989). Calculating confidence intervals for survival time analyses. In: *Statistics with Confidence* pp. 64-70. (Eds) Gardner MJ and Altman DG. British Medical Journal; London.

Miller AB, Hoogstraten B, Staquet M and Winkler A (1981). Reporting results of cancer treatment. *Cancer* 47:207-214.

Overgaard M, Bentzen SM, Christensen JJ and Hjøllund Madsen E (1987). The value of the NSD formula in equation of acute and late radiation complications in normal tissue following 2 and 5 fractions per week in breast cancer patients treated with postmastectomy radiotherapy. *Radiother Oncol* 9:1-12.

Perez CA and Brady LW (1992). Overview. In: *Principles and Practice of Radiation Oncology*, pp.1-63. (Eds) Perez CA and Brady LW. Lippincott; Philadelphia.

Sismondi P, Sinistrero G, Zola P *et al* (1989). Complications of uterine cervix carcinoma treatments: the problem of a uniform classification. *Radiother Oncol* 14:9-17.

Taylor JMG, Withers HR, Vegesna V and Mason K (1987). Fitting the linear-quadratic model using time of occurrence as the endpoint for quantal response multifraction experiments. *Int J Radiat Biol* 52:459-468.

Till JE (1988). Quality of survival. In: *Innovations in Radiation Oncology*. (Eds) Withers HR and Peters LJ. Springer-Verlag; Berlin.

Withers HR, Taylor JMG and Maciejewski B (1988). Treatment volume and tissue tolerance. *Int J Radiat Oncol Biol Phys* 14:751-759.

13

Radiobiology of normal tissues

Albert J. van der Kogel

13.1 Introduction

The timing and dose-dependence of the radiation response of normal tissues are largely determined by the proliferative organization of stem cells, proliferating cells and mature functional cells (Chapter 4). Time-dose-fractionation relationships for normal tissue tolerance are discussed in Chapters 7-9, including the clinical significance of the α/β ratio for acute- and late-responding tissues. In this chapter additional aspects of normal-tissue radiobiology will be discussed, such as the development of different types of injury, clonogenic assays for target-cell radiosensitivity, and two clinically important topics: volume effects and retreatment tolerance.

A general outline of the relation between tissue organization, time-to-response, and various factors determining the radiosensitivity of normal tissues is given in Figure 13.1. This diagram shows that many of the characteristics of normal tissues are predominantly determined by the stem cells and to a variable degree the proliferating precursor cells. The response of the bulk of the cells in a tissue, the mature functional cells, is important in determining the appearance and timing of a reaction. The response of stem cells is involved in other important factors such as:

- tissue sensitivity: tolerance dose, α/β ratio
- time-related recovery factors: repair half-time, repopulation, long-term recovery
- volume effects: cell migration, tissue compartments, injury probability

13.2 Pathogenesis of acute and late effects

The development of acute effects in rapidly renewing systems such as skin and the haemopoietic system is influenced by the existence of a hierarchical cell lineage. For these acute effects of radiation the identity of

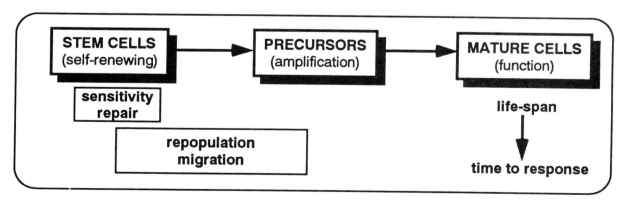

Figure 13.1 Relation between the proliferative organization of a tissue, the latent period to functional response, and tissue tolerance factors. Most of the factors determining tolerance are related to characteristics of the stem cells.

the *target cells* is usually clear, in contrast to some of the effects that have a long latent period. This is not necessarily restricted to slowly renewing cell systems, since for instance in the skin, in addition to the acute epidermal reactions, several late waves of injury occur such as fibrosis, atrophy and telangiectasia. Thus, different types of injury may develop sequentially in one organ, with different underlying mechanisms and different target cells. This obviously also complicates the issue of normal-tissue tolerance, as the various endpoints are associated with different tolerance doses.

In many tissues an 'early' wave of damage (which can vary in latency from a few weeks to many months depending on the turnover of functional cells) may be followed by a later wave of injury that often has a vascular basis (Figure 13.2). This will be illustrated for three tissues/organs: skin, lung, and central nervous system (CNS).

In the *skin*, two or three types of injury are recognized, each with a characteristic latent period: acute epidermal reactions (in particular desquamation), dermal necrosis, and late vascular reactions. The separate origin of the epidermal and dermal reactions in pig skin has been demonstrated by Hopewell and colleagues.

The development of late vascular reactions, such as telangiectasia, may take many years, as shown in Figure 13.3 by the investigations of Turesson and Notter (1986).

In the *lung*, at least two waves of injury are recognized: early pneumonitis and late fibrosis. On the basis of histological criteria, Travis (1980) described these two manifestations of radiation lung damage. The differential recovery characteristics of target cells involved in the two waves were clearly demonstrated by a comparison of single- and split-dose irradiations with different time intervals, using a functional assay (Figure 13.4; Travis and Down, 1981). With longer time intervals between two fractions, the incidence of pneumonitis subsided, while the late fibrosis still occurred. This also indicated the separate origin of late fibrosis, rather than being the late consequence of early pneumonitis.

In the *central nervous system*, several types of damage may develop, for which different recovery characteristics have also been described. A schematic representation of the pathogenesis of delayed injury in the CNS is shown in Figure 13.5. In this hypothetical scheme, the potential target cells involved in the two main pathways

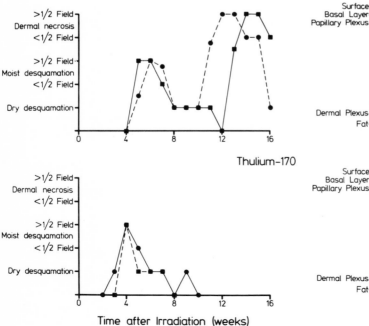

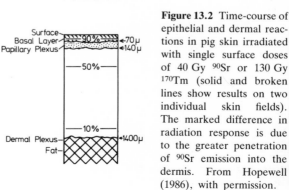

Figure 13.2 Time-course of epithelial and dermal reactions in pig skin irradiated with single surface doses of 40 Gy ^{90}Sr or 130 Gy ^{170}Tm (solid and broken lines show results on two individual skin fields). The marked difference in radiation response is due to the greater penetration of ^{90}Sr emission into the dermis. From Hopewell (1986), with permission.

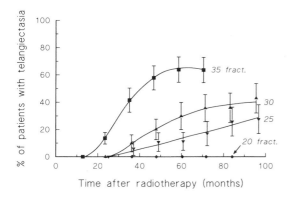

Figure 13.3 Time-course of the development of telangiectasia (grade $\geqq 2$) in human skin irradiated with daily 2 Gy fractions, 5 fractions per week. The curves show the effect of increasing dose. From Turesson and Notter (1986), with permission.

of the development of delayed damage, vascular and glial elements, are indicated (van der Kogel, 1991). As in the lung, different recovery patterns are observed for the two types of injury (early white-matter necrosis and late vascular damage) after split-dose irradiation of the rat spinal cord with different time intervals (Figure 13.6).

13.3 Assays of normal-tissue injury

Functional Assays and Lethality

For the examples in the previous section, functional and histological criteria were used to construct dose-response relationships for skin, lung and CNS injury. Besides these *functional* assays, two other categories of assay are those that employ *lethality* as an endpoint, and the *clonogenic* assays. Lethality endpoints have been used extensively in the past, and are based on death due to (more or less) specific tissue injury after whole- or partial-body irradiation. Examples of dose-lethality curves are shown in Figure 13.7, clearly demonstrating the large difference in radiation sensitivity of different tissues and organs. An example of dose-response curves obtained from functional assays is shown in Figure 13.8 for the irradiation of the mouse lung at different dose rates. The functional assay used was the measurement of respiratory frequency

with a whole-body plethysmograph. The results clearly demonstrate the large dose-rate effect for radiation pneumonitis in the mouse (Section 15.3).

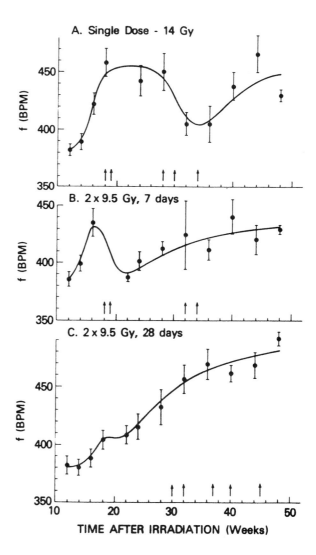

Figure 13.4 Evidence for two phases of radiation response in the mouse lung. Using breathing rate as a measure of damage, two waves of response are seen after single doses (panel A). Split-dose irradiation, especially with a gap of 28 days, reduces the severity of the first phase (acute pneumonitis), but has little effect on the second phase (fibrosis). Arrows indicate the death of individual mice. From Travis and Down (1981), with permission.

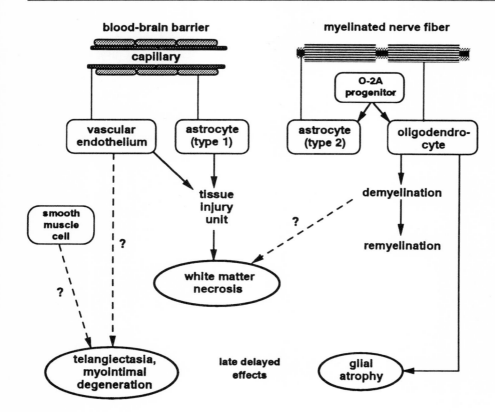

Figure 13.5 Schematic outline of the pathogenesis of early and late delayed types of injury in the central nervous system. Adapted from van der Kogel (1991), with permission.

Clonogenic Assays

The most direct way to assess the radiosensitivity and other characteristics of stem cells in tissues is by *in vivo* or *in vitro* clonogenic assays. There are three main types of clonogenic assay:

In situ assays, in which surviving stem cells are studied for their colony-forming ability in their original location. The tissue is irradiated with a carefully chosen radiation dose so that during regeneration individual colonies derived from surviving stem cells can be distinguished. A number of *in situ* assays have been developed by Withers and his colleagues, including assays for the skin, intestine, testis, and kidney. One of the most widely used of these *in situ* assays is the intestinal crypt-colony assay, usually performed in the mouse. For this assay the abdomen (or the whole mouse) is irradiated with a range of doses (single dose: approximately 10 – 16 Gy), which reduces the number of intestinal crypts containing at least one surviving stem cell to less than 100 per gut circumference. After 3.5 days the mouse is killed and the number of regenerating

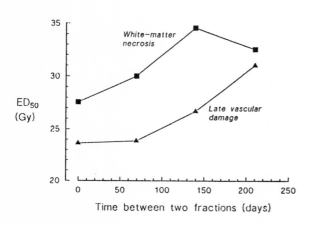

Figure 13.6 Recovery characteristics of two types of injury in the rat spinal cord (early white-matter necrosis and late vascular damage) after split-dose irradiation with different time intervals. Adapted from van der Kogel *et al* (1982), with permission.

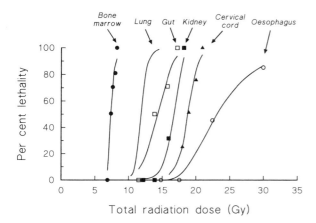

Figure 13.7 Dose-response curves following local irradiation of different normal tissues, illustrating the use of lethality assays. For the cervical cord the endpoint was paralysis. From Travis (1987), with permission.

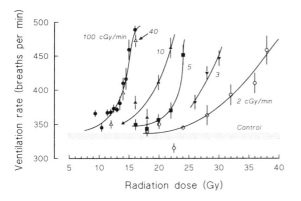

Figure 13.8 Dose-response curves for radiation damage to the mouse lung, demonstrating the dose-rate effect. In the mouse, breathing rate at 14 weeks is a good indicator of radiation pneumonitis. From Down *et al* (1986), with permission.

crypt colonies is counted in transverse sections of the intestine.

Transplantation assays, in which single-cell suspensions are made from the irradiated tissue and transplanted to suitable sites in immunologically identical animals. The classical example is the spleen-colony assay. In this assay the number of surviving bone-marrow stem cells is related to the number of colonies formed in the spleen of a previously irradiated host animal, 9 - 11 days

after injection of the cell suspension. Stem cells detected in this manner were termed by Till and McCulloch Colony-Forming Units (CFU) since their cellular identity was not known. Another example of a transplantation assay is the injection of a cell suspension made from an irradiated tissue (for instance, mammary gland, liver or thyroid) into a scapular or inguinal fat pad of recipient animals. After a few weeks, nodules resembling the original tissue develop in the fat pad and can be counted. The fat-pad assay has been developed by the group of Gould and Clifton (1977).

In vivo-in vitro assays

In which single-cell suspensions are made from the irradiated tissue and colony formation is assessed *in vitro*. These assays require the ability to identify the relevant cell types in tissue culture, also the necessary growth conditions allowing proliferation and differentiation of the tested stem cells or progenitor cells. This assay was first developed for the bone-marrow, but another recent example of such an assay is the glial-progenitor assay for CNS tissues (van der Maazen *et al*, 1990). In this assay, glial stem cells are isolated from perinatal or adult CNS tissues and cultured on monolayers of astrocytes. Using specific monoclonal antibodies, colonies derived from glial progenitor cells can be identified. In Figure 13.9, survival curves for perinatal or adult glial progenitors from different locations in the CNS show a different sensitivity for the various cells, indicating their different developmental stage and position in the differentiation lineage. This assay can also be applied to the study of long-term regeneration of glial-progenitors in the CNS. The lower panel in Figure 13.9 shows an example in the optic nerve after whole brain irradiation of the adult rat.

13.4 Normal-tissue tolerance: volume effects

Volume effects differ among the various organs of the body, depending on their structural organization (compartmentalization) as well as on the migration characteristics (rate and distance) of the target cells. The volume of tissue irradiated is an important factor determining the *clinical tolerance* of an organ (Figure 12.6), which can be quite different from the tissue sensitivity *per se*. Examples of this are the kidney or lung, both of which are among the most sensitive organs when totally irradiated ($TD_5 \approx 20$ Gy in 2 Gy fractions), but quite large partial volumes can be treated to far higher radiation doses. This is because there is considerable reserve capacity in these organs and only one quarter to one third of the functional organ volume is required.

The radiosensitivity of a tissue depends largely on its organization into separate functional units, as well as on the possibility of surviving clonogenic target cells migrating into and repopulating the irradiated tissue. Tissues with a high migratory capacity include skin, mucosae, and the intestinal tract, and in these tissues relatively small volumes can be treated to high doses, as repopulation takes place rapidly from the surrounding unirradiated tissue. However, once a critical migration distance is passed, central necrosis develops in the absence of adequate repopulation. Also, above a certain dose level, structural damage to connective tissue

and the vasculature may prevent regeneration. The high sensitivity of kidney and lung tissue may largely be related to their high degree of compartmentalization into functional subunits, the nephrons and the alveoli. Once all stem cells in such a subunit are sterilized it is unlikely that repopulation from neighbouring subunits will occur.

Compartmentalization is less pronounced in the skin and CNS, although the spinal cord has been suggested to be an example of a *series* organ, responding according to a 'sliced salami' model (Yaes and Kalend, 1988). In this model, an organ is assumed to be organized as a series of functional subunits. Inactivation of any one subunit causes loss of function of the whole organ. With the same radiation dose to a larger volume, the probability of inactivation of a single unit increases. In such a statistical model, the probability of inactivation is only related to the total irradiated volume, regardless of the spatial distribution of functional subunits. This is clearly not the case for small volumes for which cell migration plays a dominant role, as in skin and intestine, and perhaps also in spinal cord.

In organs with a *parallel* organization of their functional units (kidney, lung), a large number can be inactivated without any consequence for the overall organ function. This leads to a paradoxical situation in normal-tissue tolerance: a whole organ with a high tolerance may be lost by inactivation of a small part (e.g. spinal cord), while an organ with a very low tolerance (e.g. kidney, lung) may sustain the loss of more than half of its functional mass without serious repercussions.

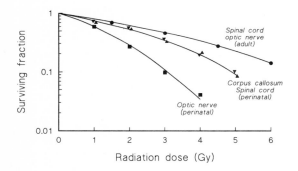

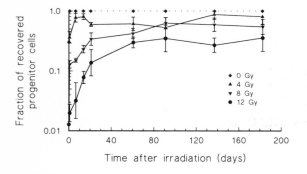

Examples of Volume Effects: Skin and Spinal Cord

In skin, the migration of surviving basal cells from the periphery of the irradiated field is thought to be an important factor in the volume effect for small irradiated fields. The field-size effect in pig skin has been demonstrated after irradiation with circular ^{90}Sr sources, showing a steep increase in isoeffective dose for the induction of moist desquamation with decreasing diameter of the plaques (Figure 13.10). Field sizes larger than 22.5 mm did not show a further change in the dose-response curve.

A similar volume dependence is seen in the rat spinal cord (Figure 13.11). The rate of cell renewal

Figure 13.9 Radiation damage and recovery in the CNS system. Upper panel: dose-survival curves for glial progenitor cells in perinatal or adult rats. Lower panel: long-term regeneration of glial progenitor cells (types 0–2A) in the adult rat optic nerve after whole-brain irradiation. From van der Maazen *et al* (1991; 1992), with permission.

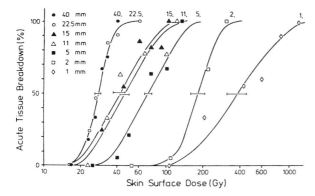

Figure 13.10 The volume effect in pig skin. The skin was irradiated with circular ^{90}Sr sources ranging in diameter from 1.0 to 40 mm. The percentage of skin fields showing moist desquamation is shown as a function of the skin surface dose. From Hopewell *et al* (1986), with permission.

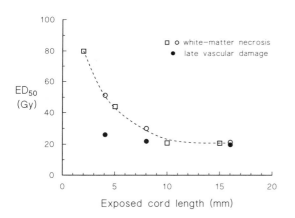

Figure 13.11 The volume effect in rat spinal cord. Data are shown on the ED_{50} for induction of white-matter necrosis from two studies. Full symbols indicate values for late vascular damage, suggesting less volume dependence. From Hopewell (1987) and van der Kogel (1991), with permission.

is much slower than in skin and also the development of injury occurs much later (5–7 months). The steep volume effect for the induction of white-matter necrosis suggests that cell migration is an important factor, analogous to the situation in skin and other rapidly renewing cell systems. The target cells may be the glial progenitor cells (*see* Figure 13.5), vascular endothelial cells, or even cooperative units of glial and endothelial cells.

13.5 Normal tissue tolerance: retreatment

In rapidly proliferating tissues, repopulation already starts during a conventionally fractionated treatment, contributing to a higher tolerance of the tissue. After the end of a fractionated course, proliferation continues and in tissues such as skin and intestine this may result in almost complete recovery. After that time re-irradiation can be performed to a full tolerance dose, as shown in the skin and the intestinal tract by various investigators. However, this is the situation in the rapidly renewing epithelial component of these tissues. Some dose-fractionation schedules preferentially spare the acute effects but not the late effects that arise from damage to the connective-tissue component. In such situations the overall tolerance may be determined by late effects (e.g. fibrosis or telangiectasia).

In late responding tissues the situation is more complex. In mouse *lung*, a dose-dependent recovery has been observed (Figure 13.12). This was complete for retreatment at 2 months after an initial treatment that did not exceed 70% of the tolerance dose. After a higher initial dose (10 Gy), recovery was much reduced and seemed only to be temporary.

In the *spinal cord* a modest but significant long-term recovery seems to occur, and the retreatment tolerance again depends upon the magnitude of

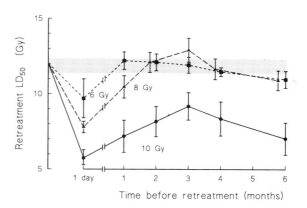

Figure 13.12 Retreatment tolerance of the mouse lung. The vertical scale gives the LD_{50} for retreatment at the indicated times after priming treatment with 6, 8, or 10 Gy. The shaded area shows the range of LD_{50} values for untreated animals. Adapted from Terry *et al* (1988), with permission.

the initial dose. In rat spinal cord, the total tolerated dose in two treatments separated by a minimum of 6 months is about 130–140% BED (relative to 100% as a single treatment). This finding is supported by a study in the monkey spinal cord (Figure 13.13). The ED_{50} for myelopathy in a single course (2.2 Gy per fraction) was 76 Gy. In a retreatment study, animals were first irradiated with a dose of 44 Gy, followed by retreatment at two years, resulting in a total cumulated ED_{50} in excess of 110 Gy.

In retreatment situations, tissue structure and proliferative organization are also likely to be important factors, as indicated by the lack of long-term regeneration in the kidney. In this organ a steady progression of injury seems to occur even after doses well below clinical tolerance. In a study of the mouse kidney, tolerance to re-irradiation *decreased* compared to the expected tolerance immediately after an initial treatment (Stewart and Oussoren, 1990).

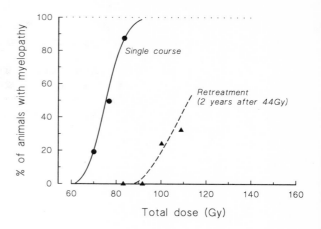

Figure 13.13 Retreatment tolerance of the monkey spinal cord. After an interval of 2 years a further 35–40 Gy can be delivered for the same level of damage. All treatments were given with 2.2 Gy per fraction. From Ang *et al* (1993), with permission.

Key points

1. *Time to response* in normal-tissue injury is mainly determined by the lifespan of the mature cells. *Tolerance* is determined by the characteristics of the stem cells (their sensitivity, recovery, and proliferation), also by the proliferative structure of the tissue.
2. The *volume paradox* of normal-tissue tolerance: a tissue with an intrinsically high tolerance may fail as a result of the inactivation of a small segment (as in the spinal cord), while a tissue with an intrinsically low tolerance (kidney, lung) may lose a substantial number of its functional units without impact on clinical tolerance.
3. *Retreatment tolerance*: rapidly renewing tissues such as skin or intestine show almost complete recovery within 2–3 months of an initial treatment, and can be retreated almost to full tolerance. Slowly renewing tissues generally show more limited recovery, which depends on the size of the initial dose (e.g. lung, CNS). There may be no recovery at all or even a gradual loss of tolerance in kidney.

Bibliography

Ang KK, Price RE, Stephens LC *et al* (1993). The tolerance of primate spinal cord to re-irradiation. *Int J Radiat Oncol Biol Phys* 25:459-464.

Down JD, Easton DF and Steel GG (1986). Repair in the mouse lung during low dose-rate irradiation. *Radiother Oncol* 6:29-42.

Gould MN and Clifton KH (1977). The survival of mammary cells following irradiation *in vivo*: a directly generated single dose survival curve. *Radiation Res* 72:343-352.

Hopewell JW (1986). Mechanisms of the action of radiation on skin and underlying tissues. *Br J Radiol*, Suppl. 19:39-51.

Hopewell JW, Morris AD and Dixon-Brown A (1987). The influence of field size on the late tolerance of the rat spinal cord to single doses of x-rays. *Br J Radiol* 60:1099-1108.

Stewart FA and Oussoren Y (1990). Re-irradiation of mouse kidneys: a comparison of re-treatment tolerance after single and frac-tionated partial tolerance doses. *Int J Radiat Biol* 531-544.

Terry NHA, Tucker SL and Travis EL (1988). Residual damage in mouse lung assessed by pneumonitis. *Int J Radiat Oncol Biol Phys* 14:928-939.

Till JE and McCulloch EA (1961). A direct meas-urement of the radiation sensitivity of normal mouse bone marrow. *Radiat Res* 14:213-222.

Travis EL (1980). The sequence of histological changes in mouse lung after single doses of x-rays. *Int J Rad Oncol Biol Phys* 6:345-347.

Travis EL (1987). Relative radiosensitivity of the human being. *Adv Radiat Biol* 12:205-238.

Travis EL and Down JD (1981). Repair in mouse lung after split doses of X rays. *Radiat Res* 87:166-174.

Travis EL and Terry NHA (1989). Cell depletion and initial and chronic responses in normal tissues. In: *Radiation Tolerance of Normal Tissues. Front Radiat Ther Oncol*, pp. 41-59. (Eds) Vaeth JM and Meyer JL. Karger, Basel.

Turesson I and Notter G (1986). Dose-response and dose-latency relationships for human skin after various fractionation schedules. *Br J Cancer* 53 (Suppl VII):67-72.

van der Kogel AJ (1991). Central nervous system radiation injury in small animal models. In: *Radiation Injury to the Nervous System*, pp. 91-112. (Eds) Gutin PH, Leibel SA, Sheline GE. Raven Press: New York.

van der Kogel AJ, Sissingh HA and Zoetelief J (1982). Effect of x-rays and neutrons on repair and regeneration in the rat spinal cord. *Int J Rad Oncol Biol Phys* 8:2095-2097.

van der Maazen RWM, Verhagen I and van der Kogel AJ (1990). An *in vitro* clonogenic assay to assess radiation damage in rat CNS glial progenitor cells. *Int J Radiat Biol* 58:835-844.

van der Maazen RWM, Kleiboer BJ, Verhagen I and van der Kogel AJ (1991). Irradiation in vitro discriminates between different O-2A progenitor cell subpopulations in the perinatal CNS. *Radiat Res* 128:64-72.

van der Maazen RWM, Verhagen I, Kleiboer BJ, and van der Kogel AJ (1991). Repopulation of O-2A progenitor cells after irradiation of the adult rat optic nerve analysed by an in vitro clonogenic assay. *Radiat Res* 132:82-86.

Yaes RJ and Kalend A (1988). Local stem cell depletion model for radiation myelitis. *Int J Radiat Oncol Biol Phys* 14:1247-1259.

14

The radiobiology of tumours

G. Gordon Steel

14.1 The clinical picture: tumour control probability

The level of success with radiotherapy for cancer varies considerably from one disease and tumour stage to another. It is common clinical experience that some tumours are highly curable, others not. A quantitative description of this picture is provided by a comparison of tumour control probability curves. The collection shown in Figure 14.1 was made by Dr. J.M. Deacon. The curves are taken from the clinical literature; they are of variable reliability because the data do not come from randomized clinical trials, which would generally be unethical over such a wide range of dose levels. A variety of fractionation schedules were used (also a range of field sizes) and the results have been brought together on a single dose scale by calculating the NSD dose.

Overall, it can be seen that doses required for

50% tumour control range widely, varying from NSD values of around 6–8 Gy for some lymphomas to over 20 Gy for some epithelial tumours. Gliomas are well-known to be refractory and it is not possible to give a high enough radiation dose to approach 50% tumour control, nor even to see a clear dose-response relationship. The picture would be similar with osteosarcomas. The steepness of each dose-response curve reflects a number of variables, which include:

(i) an underlying Poisson relationship. If the average number of clonogenic tumour cells that survive treatment is m, then the probability that no cells survive and that the tumour is cured is e^{-m}. Tumour control probability therefore has a sigmoid dependence on m, with a finite maximum slope;
(ii) variability in curability among tumours of the same type, arising from differences in cellular radiosensitivity, repopulation, hypoxia, etc;
(iii) inter-patient variation in the quality of radiation dose delivery.

The steepness of tumour control curves has been quantified in a variety of ways which have been reviewed by Mijnheer *et al* (1987) and Brahme (1988). Widely used is the γ_{50} value; this is the percentage change in tumour control probability for a 1% change in dose. As a result of point (i) above, γ_{50} cannot exceed a value of about 6.5; for uniform types of mouse tumour it can be ≈ 4.5; and for human tumours values range from roughly 1 to 5 with a mean of ≈ 2.6 (Suit *et al*, 1992; Brahme, 1988).

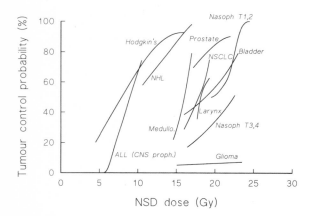

Figure 14.1 Dose-response curves for tumour control taken from a variety of clinical studies. From J.M. Deacon, unpublished.

14.2 Experimental tumour systems

Research into the radiation response of tumours has been performed on a wide variety of tumour cell systems. *In vivo* studies have mainly been carried out on tumours in experimental animals, usually in mice and rats. In addition to studies carried out on permanent *in vitro* tumour cell lines, *in vitro* techniques have often been used to investigate the radiosensitivity of cells from experimental tumours (so-called *in vivo–in vitro* experiments) or on cells taken directly from human tumours. The range of cell systems that have been used may be described under the following headings, arranged roughly in order of increasing closeness to cancer in man:

In Vitro Cell Lines

Although it is possible to grow cells from normal tissues in cell culture systems the cultures usually fail after perhaps 20-30 passages. This is known as the *Hayflick limit*. It is clearly a disadvantage for most laboratory research that cultures should die out and it has been overcome in three main ways. Firstly, some normal-cell cultures have been grown through the Hayflick limit and have become immortal. They retain some characteristic features of normal-tissue cells (contact-inhibition of growth in crowded cultures or failure to grow in immune-deficient mice, etc.) and they are usually not known to be virally transformed. Widely used examples are CHO (Chinese hamster ovary) cells and V79 fibroblasts (also from hamster). Secondly, there are normal-tissue cells that have been virally transformed (for instance by simian virus, SV40). These usually lose contact-inhibition and retain viral sequences in their genome. The third approach is to use human or animal tumour cells. Tumour cells appear not to be subject to the Hayflick limit and can often be grown continuously without deterioration. A wide variety of cell lines have been used, including HeLa (derived from a human cervix carcinoma), L5178Y mouse lymphoma cells, and the human tumour cell lines referred to in Section 14.5 below. All types of 'permanent' cell lines are subject to genetic drift and the various sublines in different laboratories may not be identical. *See* Freshney (1987) for a general text on tissue culture.

Multicellular Spheroids

Some cell lines readily form aggregates in tissue culture that can grow up to a diameter of a fraction of a millimetre. They have been widely studied as *in vitro* models of tumours; they of course have no vascular system but depend on diffusion of oxygen and other nutrients through the surface of the 'spheroid'. Small spheroids are fully oxygenated but as they grow they develop a hypoxic core. In larger spheroids 3 or more concentric zones can sometimes be distinguished among which cell proliferation, oxygenation, and drug and radiation sensitivity may vary (Durand and Sutherland, 1973).

Transplanted Tumours in Experimental Animals

A wide variety of tumours have been conditioned to repeated transplantation in laboratory animals. Some of these arose spontaneously; some were induced by chemicals, radiation or viruses. During repeated passage, usually subcutaneously, they grow faster and more uniformly and often lose differentiated characteristics. They are attractive as reproducible and convenient *in vivo* tumour systems but may in some respects have deviated away from the original primary tumour. Well-known examples are L1210 leukaemia, Lewis lung tumour, B16 melanoma, R1 rhabdomyosarcoma (*see* Kallman, 1987).

A matter of some importance is the immune status of the grafts. Tumours grown in non-inbred strains of animals or in an inbred colony that differs from that in which they arose will inevitably be subject to variable host rejection. If the tumours grow fast they may beat the developing rejection processes and the investigator may imagine that rejection is unimportant. But if the tumour is treated with radiation or cytotoxic drugs the influence of the immune response on residual tumour may become significant; more importantly, if the antitumour effects of two agents are compared and one is more immune-suppressive than the other, misleading results can be obtained. This is especially the case if tumour cure is used as the endpoint, for immune responses are particularly effective against a small amount of tumour remaining after therapy.

Primary Animal Tumours

The word *autochthonous* is sometimes used for tumours that are studied in the host within which they arose. They may be *spontaneous*, or *induced* by radiation, carcinogenic chemicals, viruses, or other means. A primary tumour would be expected to bear greater resemblance to human tumours than one that has been transplanted many times: its immune status should be more realistic and it will not have undergone the growth acceleration and other changes that occur on repeated transplantation. The main drawbacks are that spontaneous tumours require large numbers of animals to be kept for a long period of time and are therefore expensive; secondly, if potent carcinogens are used to increase the induction frequency the resulting tumours tend to be immunogenic. Mammary tumours arising spontaneously in C3H mice and their isotransplants have been used for some important radiobiological studies (Suit *et al*, 1965, 1992; Suit and Maeda, 1967).

Human Tumour Xenografts

A xenograft is a transplant from one species to another. In the cancer field this usually refers to a human tumour grown in a laboratory animal. If the recipient animal has a normal immune system then a xenograft should not grow, but there are two main ways in which growth has been achieved. First, animal strains have been developed that are congenitally immune-deficient. Best known are *nude mice*, which in addition to being hairless also lack a thymus. Many human tumours will grow under the skin of nude mice (Sparrow, 1980). Secondly, it is possible to severely immune-suppress mice to the point where they will accept human tumour grafts. It is important to recognize that neither type of host completely fails to reject the human tumour cells: rejection processes are still present and these complicate the interpretation of *in situ* therapeutic tumour studies. Nevertheless, xenografts do maintain many of the biological and therapeutic properties of their source tumours, and they constitute a valuable type of experimental system (Steel *et al*, 1983).

Clinical Radiobiology

The ultimate experimental system is the cancer patient. Testing of new treatments and randomized clinical trials have an essential role in the development of new therapies. In addition, although the scope for experiment on patients is limited, there are some radiobiological experiments which, while not of direct benefit to the individual patient, can ethically be carried out

with appropriate informed consent. Examples are measurements of the distribution of oxygen concentration in tumours, and the testing of chemical radiosensitizers by measuring the response of metastases within the same patient that are irradiated before or after drug administration (Ash, 1980).

14.3 Endpoints for measuring radiation effects on tumours

Three principal methods have been used to document and compare the effects of radiation and cytotoxic drugs on experimental tumours:

Tumour Growth Delay

This is especially useful for tumours growing subcutaneously, the size of which can be measured accurately with callipers. A group of tumours are selected to have closely similar size. They are divided into groups and given different treatments, one group being left untreated. Tumour volume is then followed at regular intervals. The usual pattern is that shown in Figure 14.2A: a period of regression followed by regrowth. In order to measure growth delay, we select an endpoint (such as twice or four times the treatment size), determine the average time that treated and control tumours take to reach this size, and by subtraction find the delay.

Results obtained with different radiation doses can then be plotted as a *dose-response curve* (Figure 14.2B). If we wish to evaluate the effect on the tumour of some modification of treatment (adding a radiosensitizer, changing inspired oxygen level, etc.) we would perform a larger experiment in which both modified and unmodified tumours are studied together. Thus we would obtain two dose-response curves and a good way of indicating the extent of modification is to calculate a *Dose Modifying Factor (DMF)*. This can be read off as the ratio of radiation doses that give the same effect: (without modification)/(with modification). If the modification is truly *dose modifying*, then the DMF value should be the same at all levels of effect. It is then better to calculate the DMF (by computer) by asking what value would allow the two curves to be most nearly superimposed. A variety of terms similar to dose modifying factor have also been used and calculated in the same way: Oxygen Enhancement Ratio (OER), Sensitizer Enhancement Ratio (SER), Thermal Enhancement Ratio (TER), etc.

Comparison of growth delay among tumours of different growth rate leads to uncertainties in interpretation. One approach (Kopper and Steel, 1975) is to calculate a *specific growth delay*:

$$\text{Specific growth delay} = \frac{\text{TD}_{treated} - \text{TD}_{control}}{\text{TD}_{control}}$$

where TD indicates the time within which treated or control tumours double in volume. Specific growth delay corresponds to number of volume doubling times saved by treatment. Since the doubling time for repopulation by clonogenic cells may not bear a constant relation to volume doubling time, this approach should be regarded as only roughly satisfactory. There is no ideal solution to the problem of comparing therapeutic response among tumours of different growth rate.

Tumour Control

As radiation dose is increased there will come a point where some tumours fail to regrow. We can therefore evaluate a modifying agent by determining its effect on this 'curative' radiation dose. The radiation dose that controls 50% of tumours is usually called the TCD_{50} and a DMF can be calculated by determining the ratio of TCD_{50} values (without/with) the modifier. It is important when using this assay to observe the tumour-bearing mice for a long enough time to detect almost all possible recurrences. Death of animals from metastases may frustrate this and the assay is therefore not appropriate for tumours that frequently metastasise. A further drawback is that the assay is greatly affected by any host immune reaction against the tumours (Section 5.6). The TCD_{50} assay has been widely and successfully used by Suit and his colleagues (Suit *et al*, 1965).

The use of this assay in evaluating the radiosensitization by misonidazole of first generation transplants of C3H mouse mammary tumours is illustrated in Figure 14.3 (Fowler *et al*, 1976). The objective was to ask: "What

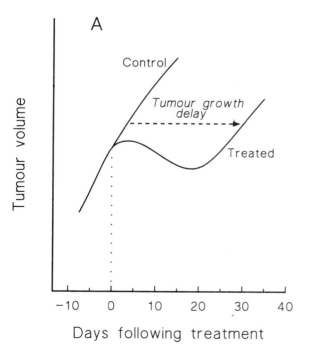
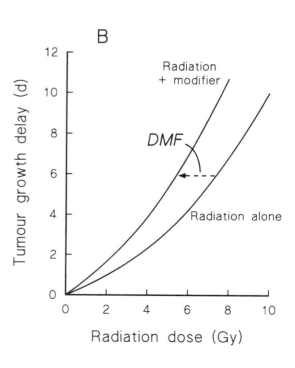

Figure 14.2 (A) illustrating the measurement of tumour growth delay, and **(B)** the calculation of a dose modifying factor (DMF).

duration of fractionated radiotherapy gives the best therapeutic response, in the presence or absence of the sensitizer?" Figure 14.3A shows examples of the dose-response curves for tumour control with and without the administration of the sensitizer 30 minutes before irradiation. Dose-response curves for the early skin reaction in the feet of mice were documented in parallel experiments. These allowed the radiation dose (with or without sensitizer and for any duration of treatment) that gave a fixed level of skin damage to be identified. For fractionated treatment there was no sensitization of skin; the level of tumour control that corresponded to each of these doses (for instance, D) could then be read off from the corresponding tumour control curve. Figure 14.3B shows (in outline) the results: tumour control probability *for a fixed level of skin damage* as a function of the duration of fractionated treatment. Without misonidazole short treatments were bad; there was an optimum duration of around 8 days. Adding misonidazole greatly improved the results of short schedules but had little effect on the longer ones. The explanation may be one that is important for clinical radiotherapy: reoxygenation is incomplete for short treatment times and a radiosensitizer may counteract this deficiency; long treatment times may allow reoxygenation to occur but they may be sub-optimal because of tumour cell repopulation.

Cell Survival

Cell survival studies have for many years underpinned the cellular basis of tumour response to treatment. In comparison with the other two endpoints described above, clonogenic assays have the advantage of removing the cells into a growth environment that is uniform and unaffected by treatment; there is therefore less opportunity for artefacts due to the effects of treatment on the host animal. Clonogenic cell survival is dealt with in Chapters 5 and 6.

14.4 Some conclusions from the *in vivo* radiobiology of experimental tumours

The large number of radiobiological studies done on animal tumours during the 1970s and 1980s provided the basis for many important concepts, including the following:

The Tumour-Size Effect

Large tumours are more difficult to cure than small tumours but this is mainly due to the number of clonogenic cells that have to be killed. A course of radiotherapy that can achieve a surviving frac-

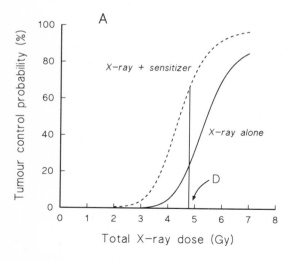

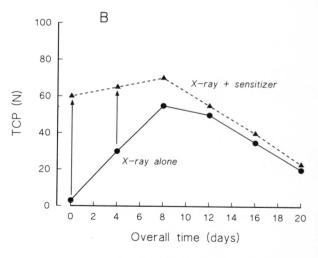

Figure 14.3 Tumour control in the evaluation of optimum fractionation with a radiosensitizer. **(A)** examples of tumour control curves for a selected duration of treatment; **(B)** tumour control probability, TCP(N), for a fixed level of early skin damage. The effect of the sensitizer (arrows) was greatest for short overall treatment times. A diagrammatic representation of the results of Fowler *et al* (1976), with permission.

tion of say 10^{-9} could be curative in a tumour that has less than 10^9 clonogenic cells, but probably not in one that has 10^{12} (Figure 2.1; Section 5.6). The more intricate question is whether, in addition to this obvious effect, the clonogenic cells in large tumours are also *less sensitive* to therapy.

There is good evidence that this is the case. Stanley *et al* (1977) treated Lewis lung tumours with γ-radiation, BCNU or cyclophosphamide at a wide range of tumour sizes and produced the results shown in Figure 14.4. As tumour size increased, there was in each case a steep decline in cellular sensitivity (a rise in cell survival) over the size range from 1–100 mm³. This could have been due to the internal vascular supply becoming progressively poorer in the growing tumours, decreasing the access of chemotherapeutic agents and increasing the proportion of cells that were hypoxic and therefore resistant to radiation treatment.

Accelerated Repopulation

The notion that clonogenic cells which survive radiation treatment may repopulate the tumour quickly was suggested by the classic study of Hermens and Barendsen (1969). They irradiated the rat R1 rhabdomyosarcoma with a single 20 Gy dose of x-rays and measured both tumour volume and the fraction of surviving clonogenic cells over the following few weeks (Figure 14.5). Tumour volume showed a slight regression, followed by regrowth. Surviving fraction immediately after irradiation was around 10^{-2} and it remained at that level for 4 days. It then increased rapidly to reach unity at post-irradiation days 10 – 12. Although this appears to demonstrate rapid tumour repopulation, it should be noted that surviving fraction does not take into account the loss of viable cells from the tumour which presumably was increasing during this 12-day period.

More reliable, therefore, are the results of Stephens *et al* (1978) who in the Lewis lung tumour carefully measured not only the surviving fraction but also the number of viable cells per tumour and were thus able to make an estimate of the *total clonogenic cells per tumour* (Figure 14.6). Following single radiation doses in the range 15–35 Gy there was clear evidence for accelerated repopulation: the speed of repopulation was greater following the larger doses.

An important notion that is well illustrated by

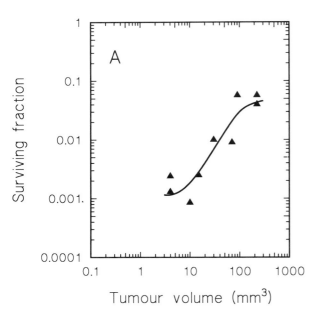
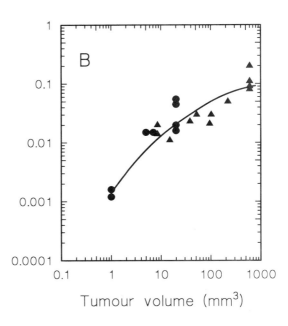

Figure 14.4 Variation with tumour size of cell survival in the Lewis lung tumour treated with (**A**) 75 mg/kg cyclophosphamide or (**B**) 10 Gy γ-rays. (▲) subcutaneous tumours; (●) lung tumours. From Stanley *et al* (1977), with permission.

the data in Figure 14.5 is that a treatment that pro-duces only slight and temporary regression may depress surviving fraction by as much as 2 decades (99% clonogenic cell kill). It is the slow rate of tumour regression that prevents this from being revealed in the volume change (Section 2.5).

The Tumour-Bed Effect

Careful measurement of the growth rate of experi-mental tumours that recur following radiation treatment has often shown that it is slower than the growth rate of untreated tumours of the same size. This is called the *tumour-bed effect*. A similar phenomenon is the reduced growth rate of tumours transplanted into previously irradiated subcutaneous sites. It is thought that both of these effects are due to radiation damage to stromal (including vascular) tissues. The reason why *accelerated repopulation* and *retarded regrowth* can occur together is because the former is seen in surviving clonogenic cells at a time when the tumour may be shrinking, while the latter is a property of the volume growth rate of irradiated tumours. *See* Begg and Terry (1985) and Chapter 7 of the book edited by Kallman (1987).

Hypoxic Fraction

The term 'hypoxic fraction' refers to the fraction of *clonogenic tumour cells* that have a radiosen-sitivity that is characteristic of hypoxic cells. The standard way in which it has been measured is as follows. A group of animals bearing transplanted tumours are divided into say 6 groups that are irradiated while breathing air and a further 6 groups that are killed 15 min *before* irradiation, thus making the tissues hypoxic. The radiation doses will be chosen to range up to the upper limit at which cell survival can still be detected. After irradiation *in vivo*, cell survival is studied using an *in vitro* or *in vivo* assay. The result will be as shown in Figure 14.7. In air-breathing animals the survival curve will be biphasic, reflecting the radiosensitivity of a mixture of oxic and hypoxic cells. In the killed animals, only the hypoxic component will be seen. The fact that the two survival curves are parallel confirms that they are both characteristic of hypoxic cells. If we draw a

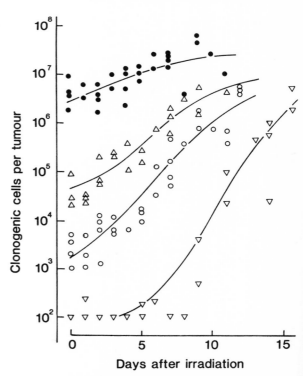

Figure 14.6 Estimated number of clonogenic cells per tumour in the Lewis lung tumour following various doses of γ-radiation: △15 Gy. ○25 Gy; ▽35 Gy. From Stephens *et al* (1978), with permission.

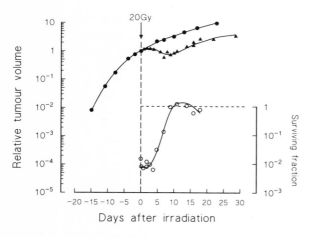

Figure 14.5 Response of the R1 tumour to 20 Gy x-rays showing: **(A)** the volume response and **(B)** the surviving fraction of clonogenic cells. From Hermens and Barendsen (1969), with permission.

vertical line at any point where the lines are parallel, then the ratio (survival in air-breathing mice)/(survival in dead mice) gives the *hypoxic fraction* of the tumours in air-breathing mice (Section 11.2).

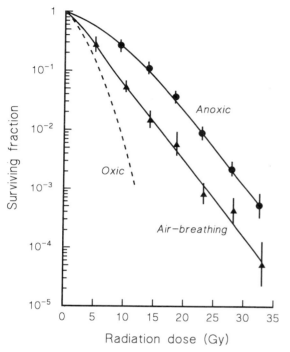

Figure 14.7 Measurement of hypoxic fraction in the KHT mouse sarcoma. From Hill and Bush (1977), with permission.

Reoxygenation

The time-course of changes in the hypoxic fraction of a tumour before and after irradiation is illustrated in Figure 14.8. Tumour nodules whose diameter is less than about 1 mm have been found to be fully oxygenated (Stanley *et al*, 1977). Above this size the hypoxic fraction often increases until it may range up to perhaps 50% of clonogenic cells (Sutherland and Franco, 1980). Irradiation of a tumour will inevitably kill more oxic than hypoxic cells and if the radiation dose is large enough the hypoxic fraction will then approach 100%. The *number* of surviving hypoxic cells will be low but their *fraction* of all surviving clonogenic cells will be high. The term reoxygenation refers to the process by which these hypoxic cells become better supplied with oxygen. Reoxygenation has been studied by measuring the hypoxic fraction (as described above) at various times after a priming dose of radiation. The experiments are difficult, since they involve assaying the increase in cell kill from adding one dose to another. The results of these studies have indicated that some tumours reoxygenate quickly (hypoxic fraction falling from 100% to 10% within approximately one day); other tumours reoxygenate slowly (taking a week or more). Biological mechanisms of reoxygenation are discussed in Section 11.4.

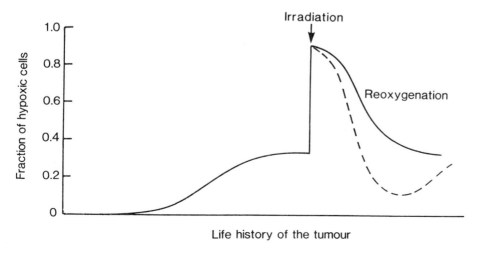

Figure 14.8 The time-course of changes in the hypoxic fraction during the life history and response to irradiation of a tumour.

14.5 The radiobiology of human tumour cells

The Initial Slope of the Cell Survival Curve

A key question in radiation biology applied to radiotherapy is: How radiosensitive are human tumour cells, and how does this relate to clinical radiocurability? Prior to 1980 there was little information on this but interest was aroused by Fertil and Malaise (1981) who surveyed the published literature on *in vitro* human tumour cell survival curves and found evidence for a correlation with clinical response. This survey was repeated by Deacon *et al* (1984) who summarized data on 51 non-HeLa human tumour cell lines. These covered 17 different histopathological tumour types which (on the basis of data of the sort shown in Figure 14.1) were placed into 5 categories of local tumour radiocurability: **A**: lymphoma, myeloma, neuroblastoma; **B**: medulloblastoma, small-cell lung cancer; **C**: breast, bladder, cervix carcinoma; **D**: pancreas, colo-rectal, squamous lung cancer; **E**: melanoma, osteosarcoma, glioblastoma, renal carcinoma. The placing of tumour types in this list is somewhat uncertain and the underlying clinical data do not allow this to be done unequivocally. However, the ranking **A → E** broadly reflects clinical experience. The *in vitro* data for each cell line were analyzed to determine the surviving fraction at 2 Gy (which was termed SF_2), chosen as a measure of the *initial slope* of the cell survival curves. The result is shown in Figure 14.9. Within each category of clinical radioresponsiveness there was a considerable scatter (not surprising in view of the many different sources, cell lines, and techniques used) but in confirmation of Fertil and Malaise's conclusions there was a significant trend in the data towards Group **A** having lower and Group **E** having higher SF_2 values. This important conclusion underlies the belief that the steepness of the initial slope is a significant factor in the clinical response of tumours to radiotherapy.

Initial Slope and Tumour Cure

Cell lines in Group **A** of Figure 14.9 have SF_2 values that average around 0.2 or less, while those in Group **E** cluster around 0.5. Is this difference large enough to be of clinical significance? It may be, for the reasons shown in Figure 14.10. Imagine treating a tumour whose SF_2 is 0.5 with

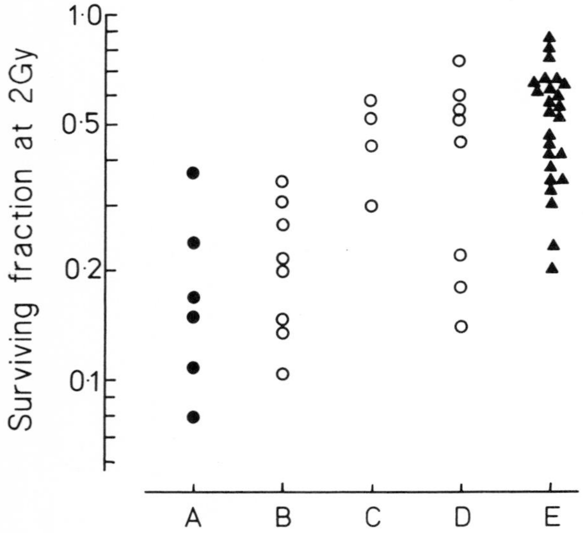

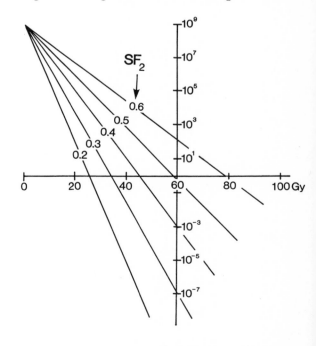

Figure 14.9 Surviving fraction at 2 Gy for 51 human tumour cell lines, arranged in 5 categories of clinical radioresponsiveness. From Deacon *et al* (1984), with permission.

Figure 14.10 Effect of multiple fractions of 2 Gy given to tumours whose SF_2 values range from 0.2 to 0.6.

a succession of 2 Gy radiation doses. If the surviving fraction per dose remains constant, then the survival from 30 doses will be $(0.5)^{30} \approx 10^{-9}$. For an SF_2 of 0.2 the overall survival would be below 10^{-20}. Looking horizontally in the figure, the first tumour requires a total dose of roughly 60 Gy to reduce an initial 10^9 clonogenic cells down to one cell, whereas the second tumour requires roughly 25 Gy. This is a very simplistic argument which assumes constant effect per fraction and ignores the effects of tumour hypoxia; what it indicates is that the steepness of the initial slope could be an important determinant of the success of multifraction irradiation.

Cell Survival Curves for Human Tumour Cells

The survival curves shown in Figure 14.11 illus-

trate the range of radiosensitivity commonly found among human tumour cell lines. The doses that correspond to a survival of 10^{-2} differ by approximately a factor of three. As will be shown below (Section 15.2) the range of steepness of the *initial slopes* of these curves is even wider. The full lines in Figure 14.11 are linear-quadratic curves fitted to the data. With these and other data sets the fit is good: there is a clear initial slope (in contrast to the prediction of the multi-target equation, Figure 6.1) and the data are consistent with a continuously bending curve.

Since there may be a subcellular basis for regarding the separate terms of the linear-quadratic equation as mechanistically different (Section 24.1), it is interesting to examine their relative contributions to cell killing. We may separate them thus:

Linear or *alpha* component $= \exp(-\alpha d)$
Quadratic or *beta* component $= exp(-\beta d^2)$

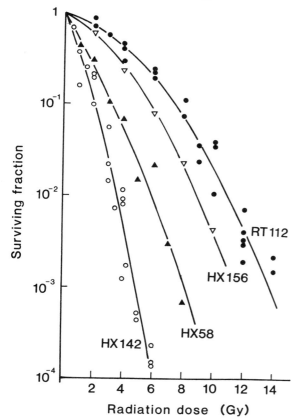

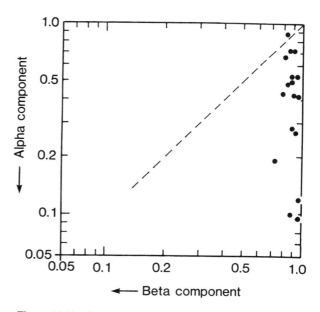

Figure 14.11 Cell survival curve for 4 representative human tumour cell lines irradiated at high dose rate. HX142, neuroblastoma; HX58, pancreas; HX156, cervix; RT112, bladder carcinoma. From Steel (1991), with permission.

Figure 14.12 Contributions to the surviving fraction at 2 Gy from the linear and quadratic components of radiation cell killing, for 17 human tumour cell lines. From Steel and Peacock (1989), with permission.

Having fitted the data with the linear-quadratic equation, as shown in Figure 14.11, we know the values for α and β, and for any chosen dose we can calculate these components. This has been done in Figure 14.12 for 17 human tumour cell lines (Steel and Peacock, 1989). The chosen dose is 2 Gy, a typical dose per fraction in clinical radiotherapy. It can be seen that the calculated points lie down the right-hand border of this diagram: the dispersion in radiosensitivity among these cell lines at 2 Gy is entirely due to differences in the steepness of the *linear* component of cell killing. The

small amounts of cell kill due to the beta component (distance of the points from the right-hand boundary) do not seem to correlate with sensitivity.

The conclusion is one that derives from most of the models of radiation cell killing: cell killing at clinically realistic doses is dominated by the steepness of the linear component. The nature of this linear component is therefore a matter of considerable interest, and this is dealt with in Chapter 24.

Key points

1. Human tumours differ in radiocurability, and the initial slope of the cell survival curve for oxic tumour cells is one of the underlying factors.
2. Radiobiological studies on tumours in experimental animals have identified some of the important processes in tumour radiobiology: for instance hypoxia, reoxygenation, repopulation, the effect of tumour size, and the tumour-bed effect.
3. Cell survival curves for human tumour cells are well fitted by the linear-quadratic equation. Survival at radiation doses of $\leq$ 2Gy is dominated by the linear term in this equation.

Bibliography

Ash DV (1980). Growth delay studies in patients with multiple metastases. *Brit J Cancer* 41(suppl IV):17-20.

Begg AC and Terry NHA (1985). Stromal radiosensitivity: influence of tumour type on the tumour bed effect assay. *Brit J Radiol* 58:93-96.

Brahme A (1988). Accuracy Requirements and Quality Assurance of Electron Beam Therapy with Photons and Electrons. *Acta Oncologica Supplement* 1.

Durand RE and Sutherland RM (1973). Dependence of the radiation response of an *in vitro* tumor model on cell cycle effects. *Cancer Res* 33:213-219.

Fowler JF, Sheldon PW, Denekamp J and Field SB (1976). Optimum fractionation of the C3H mouse mammary carcinoma using X-rays, misonidazole or neutrons. *Int J Radiat Oncol Biol Phys* 1:579-592.

Freshney RI (1987). *Culture of Animal Cells*. Alan Liss Inc., New York.

Hermens AF and Barendsen GW (1969). Changes of cell proliferation characteristics in a rat rhabdomyosarcoma before and after X-irradiation. *Eur J Cancer* 5:173-189.

Hill RP and Bush RS (1977). A new method of determining the fraction of hypoxic cells in a transplantable murine sarcoma. *Radiat Res* 70:141-153.

Kopper L and Steel GG (1975). The therapeutic response of three human tumour lines maintained in immune-suppressed mice. *Cancer Res* 35:2704-2713.

Mijnheer BJ, Battermann JJ and Wambersie A (1987). What degree of accuracy is required and can be achieved in photon and neutron therapy? *Radiother Oncol* 8:237-252.

Sparrow S (1980). *Immunodeficient Animals for Cancer Research*. Macmillan; London.

Stanley JA, Shipley WU and Steel GG (1977). Influence of tumour size on hypoxic fraction and therapeutic sensitivity of Lewis lung tumour. *Brit J Cancer* 36:105-113.

Steel GG, Courtenay VD and Peckham MJ (1983). The response to chemotherapy of a variety of human tumour xenografts. *Brit J Cancer* 47:1-13.

Steel GG and Peacock JH (1989). Why are some human tumours more radiosensitive than others? *Radiother Oncol* 15:63-72.

Stephens TC, Currie GA and Peacock JH (1978). Repopulation of gamma-irradiated Lewis lung carcinoma by malignant cells and host macrophage precursors. *Brit J Cancer* 38:573-582.

Suit HD, Shalek RJ and Wette R (1965). Radiation response of C3H mouse mammary carcinoma evaluated in terms of radiation sensitivity. In: *Cellular Radiation Biology*. Williams & Wilkins; Baltimore.

Suit HD and Maeda M (1967). Hyperbaric oxygen and radiobiology of a C3H mouse mammary carcinoma. *J Nat Cancer Inst* 39:639-52.

Suit HD, Skates S, Taghian A *et al* (1992). Clinical implications of heterogeneity of tumor response to radiotherapy. *Radiother Oncol* 25:251-260.

Sutherland RM and Franco AJ (1980). On the nature of the radiobiologically hypoxic fraction in tumours. *Int J Radiat Oncol Biol Phys* 6:117-120.

Further reading

Deacon J, Peckham MJ and Steel GG (1984). The radioresponsiveness of human tumours and the initial slope of the cell survival curve. *Radiother Oncol* 2:317-323.

Fertil B and Malaise EP (1981). Inherent radiosensitivity as a basic concept for human tumor radiotherapy. *Int J Radiat Oncol Biol Phys* 7:621-629.

Hall EJ (1988). *Radiobiology for the Radiologist*. Lippincott; Philadelphia.

Kallman RF (1987). *Rodent Tumor Models* Pergamon; New York.

Steel GG (1991). Cellular sensitivity to low dose-rate irradiation focuses the problem of tumour radioresistance. *Radiother Oncol* 20:71-83.

15

The dose-rate effect: brachytherapy

G. Gordon Steel

15.1 Mechanisms underlying the dose-rate effect

The dose rates used for most radiobiological studies on cells and tissues tend to be in the range 1–5 Gy/min, as are dose rates used clinically for external-beam radiotherapy. As dose rate is lowered, the time taken to deliver a particular radiation dose increases; it then becomes possible for a number of biological processes to take place *during* irradiation and to modify the observed radiation response. These processes are best described by the *4 Rs of Radiobiology*: recovery (or repair), reassortment, repopulation, and reoxygenation (Section 5.9).

Figure 15.1 illustrates the operation of three of these processes in producing the dose-rate effect. The range of dose rates over which each has an effect depends upon its speed. Repair is the fastest

of these processes (half-time ≈ 1 h) and when the exposure duration is of the order of 1 hour considerable repair will take place. Repair thus will modify radiation effects over the dose-rate range from around 1 Gy/min down to ≈ 1 cGy/min. Even in the range of clinical external-beam dose rates, small effects on tolerance may arise from changes in dose rate. In contrast, repopulation is a much slower process. Doubling times for repopulation in human tumours or normal tissues cannot be less than one day; the range is probably very wide, from a few days to weeks or months (Section 9.4). Only when the exposure duration becomes a considerable fraction of a day will significant repopulation occur during irradiation. Repopulation, either in tumours or normal tissues, will therefore influence cellular response over a much lower range of dose rates, below say 2 cGy/min, depending upon the cell proliferation

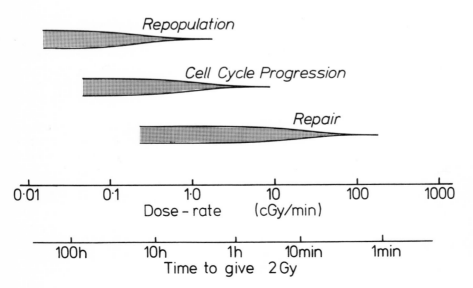

Figure 15.1 The range of dose rates over which repair, reassortment, and repopulation modify radiosensitivity depends upon the speed of these processes. From Steel *et al* (1986), with permission.

rate. Reassortment (i.e. cell-cycle progression) will modify response over an intermediate range of dose rates, as will reoxygenation in tumours.

15.2 Dose-rate effect on cell survival

As radiation dose rate is lowered in the range 1 Gy/min down to 1 cGy/min, the radiosensitivity of cells decreases and the shouldered cell survival curves observed at high dose rate gradually become straighter. This is illustrated in Figure 15.2. At 150 cGy/min the survival curve has a marked curvature; at 1.6 cGy/min it is almost straight (on the semi-log plot) and seems to extrapolate the initial slope of the high dose-rate curve. The amount of sparing associated with the dose-rate reduction can be expressed by reading off the radiation doses that give a surviving fraction of say 0.01: these values are 7.7 Gy at 150 cGy/min and 12.8 Gy at 1.6 cGy/min. The ratio of these doses 12.8/7.7 = 1.6 has been called the *dose-recovery factor (DRF)*.

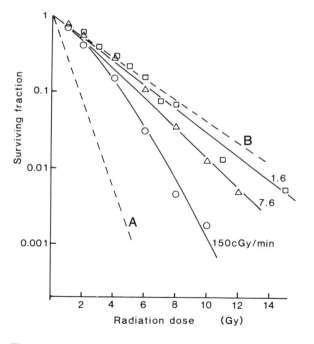

Figure 15.2 Cell survival curves for a human melanoma cell line irradiated at dose rates of 150, 7.6 or 1.6 cGy/min. The data are fitted by the LPL model, from which the lines A and B are derived (*see text*). From Steel *et al* (1987), with permission.

For four selected human tumour cell lines, Figure 15.3 shows the survival curves at these two dose rates. These four sets of data have been chosen to illustrate the dose-rate effect within the range of radiosensitivities seen among human tumour cells (Steel *et al*, 1987). At high dose rate there is a range of approximately 3 in the radiation dose that gives a survival of 0.01. At low dose rate the curves fan out and become straight or nearly so: the range of $D_{0.01}$ values is now roughly seven. Low dose-rate irradiation discriminates better than high dose rate between cell lines of differing radiosensitivity.

15.3 Dose-rate effect in normal tissues

Most normal tissues show considerable sparing as dose rate is reduced. An example is shown in Figure 15.4. The thorax of conscious mice was irradiated with ^{60}Co γ-rays and damage to the lung was measured using a breathing-rate assay (Down *et al*, 1986). The radiation dose that produced acute pneumonitis in 50% of the mice (i.e. the ED_{50}) was 13.3 Gy at 100 cGy/min but it increased to 34.2 Gy at the lower dose rate of 2 cGy/min (DRF = 2.6). Note that a similar degree of sparing could be achieved by fractionated high dose-rate irradiation using 2 Gy per fraction (and even more sparing at 1 Gy per fraction). Note also that at 2 cGy/min the curve is still rising rapidly. It was not possible in these experiments to go down to dose rates below 2 Gy/min because of the difficulty of immobilizing the mice for long periods of time.

The data in Figure 15.4 have been fitted by the incomplete repair model (Thames, 1985; Sections 8.6, 15.4). This model simulates the effect of recovery on tissue sensitivity; it does not take account of cell proliferation during irradiation. The model fits the data well and it also allows extrapolation down to low dose rates. It predicts that dose-sparing due to recovery will continue to increase down to about 0.01 cGy/min at which the ED_{50} is 59 Gy and the recovery factor (DRF value) is 4.4. Proliferation of stem-cells in the lung will lead to even greater sparing at very low dose rates.

The comparison between a single low dose-rate exposure (2 cGy/min) and fractionated high dose-rate irradiation (2 Gy/fraction) allows an important conclusion to be drawn. If the fractions are delivered once per day then the overall time to deliver an ED$_{50}$ dose of 34 Gy is 34 days. The same effect is produced by a single low dose-rate treatment in 28 hours. Continuous low dose-rate exposure is the *most efficient* way of achieving tissue recovery in the shortest overall time. It minimises the effects of proliferation, which is an advantage in terms of damage to tumour cells but a disadvantage for normal-tissue tolerance.

Figure 15.5 shows similar data from a number of other studies of the dose-rate effect on normal tissues in mice. Considerable sparing of the intestine is observed, especially below 1 cGy/min where proliferation has a marked effect. In contrast, there is little or no sparing of haemopoietic tissues. The dose-rate effect on mouse lethality (LD$_{50}$, indicated by the full line without points) is comparatively slight, probably because this is predominantly due to damage to bone marrow, also with a component of damage to the intestine.

15.4 Isoeffect relationships between fractionated and continuous low dose-rate irradiation

A variety of theoretical descriptions of the dose-rate effect have been made but for clinical application the most widely used is the incomplete repair model of Thames (1985). The calculations of Dale (1985) make the same basic assumptions, although the formulation is slightly different. The basic equation of the incomplete repair model is:

$$E = \alpha D + \beta D^2.f(t) \qquad \text{(Eqn 15.1)}$$

where E is the level of effect, α and β are parameters of the linear-quadratic equation, D is the total dose, and $f(t)$ is a function of time (both the time between fractions and the duration of continuous exposure). Note that the time-dependent

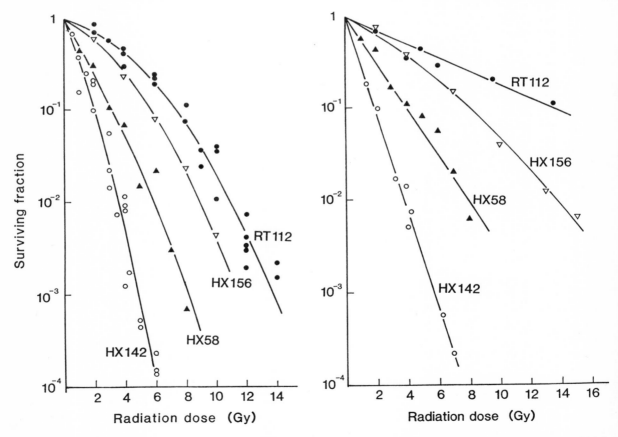

Figure 15.3 Cell survival curves for 4 human tumour cell lines irradiated at 150 cGy/min (left) or 1.6 cGy/min (right). HX142–neuroblastoma, HX58 – pancreas ca., HX156–cervix ca., RT112–bladder ca. From Steel (1991), with permission.

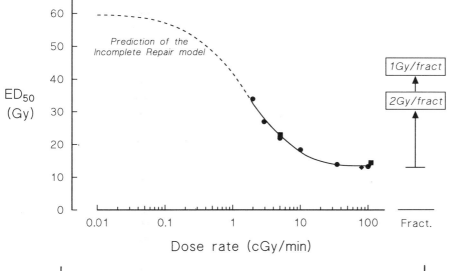

Figure 15.4 The dose-rate effect for pneumonitis in mice. The full line fitted to the data was calculated on the basis of the incomplete repair model; the broken line shows its extrapolation to very low dose rates. The boxes on the right show the ED_{50} values for fractionated irradiation. From Down *et al* (1986), with permission.

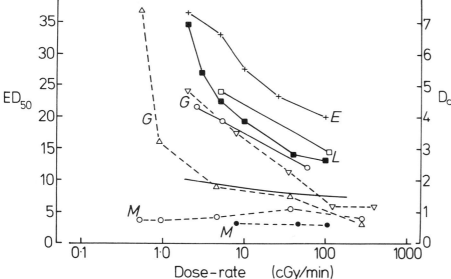

Figure 15.5 The dose-rate effect in normal tissues of the mouse: L = lung, G = gut, E = epilation, M = bone marrow. Full lines refer to left-hand scale, dashed lines to right-hand scale. See Steel *et al* (1986) for sources.

recovery factor modifies only the quadratic term in the LQ equation, a feature that is supported by experimental data (Wells and Bedford, 1983; Steel *et al*, 1987; Figure 15.2).

For the case of *continuous* exposure, the value of f(*t*) depends upon the half-time for recovery (τ) and the duration of exposure (T) according to the relation:

$$f(t) = 2[1-(1-e^{-\mu T})/\mu T]/\mu T \qquad \text{(Eqn 15.2)}$$

where $\mu = 0.693/\tau$

(Thames, 1985).

This model allows isoeffect relationships to be calculated, of which examples are shown in Figure 15.6. On the left is the fractionated case. The line in this chart corresponds to Equation 8.4; the interfraction intervals have here been assumed to be long enough to allow complete recovery although the model can handle shorter intervals. The right-hand panel in Figure 15.6 shows isoeffect curves for continuous exposure at any dose rate, on the assumption that the half-time for recovery is 1.0, 1.5 or 2.0 hours. This illustrates the dependence of the isoeffect curve for continuous exposure on the speed of recovery: the curve shifts

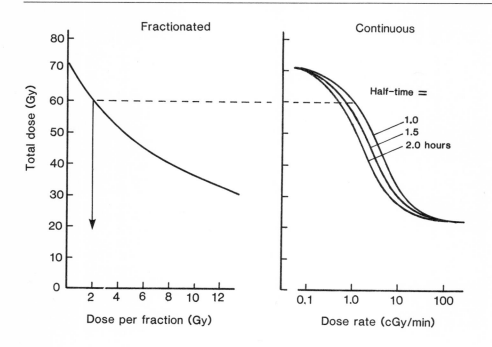

Figure 15.6 Isoeffect curves calculated on the incomplete repair model (Thames, 1985) either for fractionated or continuous radiation exposure (the two panels are mutually isoeffective). α/β ratio is 10 Gy, half-time for recovery 1.0, 1.5 or 2.0 hours, extrapolated response dose (BED) is 72 Gy. Adapted from Steel (1991), with permission.

laterally to lower dose rates as the half-time is prolonged. Unfortunately the recovery half-time is seldom known in clinical situations, which limits the precision of calculations of this sort.

The curves in the two panels of Figure 15.6 are mutually isoeffective. They are both calculated for the same effect level and for the same values of α and β (the α/β ratio is 10 Gy), chosen to give an extrapolated dose of 72 Gy at infinitely small dose per fraction or infinitely low dose rate. This example illustrates the equivalence that is predicted by the mathematical models between a particular continuous dose rate and a corresponding dose per fraction. For the parameters assumed here, a dose rate of around 1-2 cGy/min (roughly 1 Gy/h) is equivalent to fractionated treatment with approximately 2 Gy per fraction, for both of which the isoeffective dose is 60 Gy.

An alternative approach to the description of the dose-rate effect is the Lethal-Potentially Lethal (LPL) model of Curtis (1986). This is a mechanistic model which is described in Section 6.6. It has theoretical advantages for studies that seek to describe the cellular mechanisms of radiation cell killing but is less appropriate for clinical calculations than the empirical equations of Thames and Dale referred to above.

Effect of Cell Proliferation

The isoeffect relationships shown in Figure 15.6 assume no cell proliferation during treatment. They probably apply reasonably well to late-responding normal tissues and, as indicated above, there should be no effect of proliferation during continuous exposure to dose rates above about 1 cGy/min. But in the proliferating cell system of a tumour or an early-responding normal tissue the isoeffect dose for any treatment that extends over longer than a day or two will be higher than predicted. The effect of proliferation during fractionated irradiation is dealt with in Sections 8.7 and 9.3. At the present time there is no consensus on how this should be accounted for in tolerance calculations. Calculations will be performed here in terms of the Biologically Effective Dose (BED, as described in Section 10.1). If we assume constant proliferation rate, then for fractionated irradiation with full recovery between fractions:

$$\text{BED} = D[1 + d/(\alpha/\beta)] - K_r.T \qquad \text{(Eqn 15.3)}$$

where d is the dose per fraction and $D = n.d$ is the

total dose. For a single continuous exposure:

$$\text{BED} = D[1 + f(t).D/(\alpha/\beta)] - K_r.T \quad \text{(Eqn 15.4)}$$

where D is the total dose, and $f(t)$ is the time-dependent function given above. The effect of proliferation is described in both these equations by the term $K_r.T$, where T is the period of continuous irradiation. K_r has units of Gy.day^{-1} and can be regarded as the loss of biological effectiveness (BED) per day as a result of proliferation. Although repopulation may not begin at its full rate from the very start of treatment (Section 8.7), the assumption here is that it occurs at a constant rate during irradiation.

Unfortunately, as described in Sections 8.7 and

10.1, the magnitude of K_r depends not only on the rate of repopulation in the tissue (doubling time T_r) but also on its radiosensitivity:

$$K_r = 0.693/(\alpha T_r)$$

where α is the coefficient of the linear term in the LQ equation. K_r will be greater for short doubling times, but it will also be greater for radioresistant tumours where α is small. Since the absolute values of α and T_r are not well known, these calculations may only be used as a guide to the relationships involved.

Figure 15.7 shows the results of illustrative calculations of the therapeutic advantage of altered fractionation schedules, using the above equations. Following Dale (1989), we have assumed that 30 fractions of 2 Gy (total dose 60 Gy) is at the limit of *late* normal-tissue tolerance. The α/β ratios are taken to be 3 Gy for late normal-tissue damage and 10 Gy for tumour response (Fowler, 1989). The BED values for tumour and normal tissues are:

$$\text{BED}_{\text{late}} = 60 (1 + 2/3) = 100 \text{ Gy}$$
$$\text{BED}_{\text{tumour}} = 60 (1 + 2/10)-(0.6 \times 39) = 48.6 \text{ Gy}$$

We are assuming no proliferation in the late-reacting normal tissues but that repopulation in the tumour is associated with a K_r-value of 0.6 Gy/day (overall time 39 days including weekends).

For modified fractionation, we vary the fraction number (for simplicity assumed to include weekends) and first calculate by Equation 15.1 the corresponding tolerance doses per fraction ($\alpha/\beta = 3$ Gy). Assuming that these are also the daily doses to the tumour, we then calculate $\text{BED}_{\text{tumour}}$ values. This gives the tumour BED values that correspond to a fixed level of normal-tissue damage ($\text{BED}_{\text{late}} = 100$ Gy). In Figure 15.7A it can be seen that for no repopulation ($K_r = 0$) the curve rises continuously. This is the well-known gain from using large fraction numbers and small fraction sizes. For 30 fractions, $\text{BED}_{\text{tumour}}$ is 72 Gy. As K_r is increased, repopulation counteracts this therapeutic gain and for $K_r = 0.6$ Gy/d the curve is almost flat: repopulation is just balancing the gain due to recovery between fractions. For larger K_r values, there is a *disadvantage* in using large numbers of daily fractions. K_r values in excess of 2.0 Gy/day are unlikely in human tumours, though they may occur for tumours in experimen-

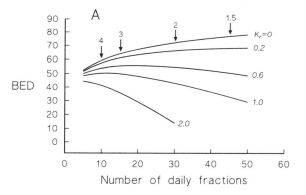

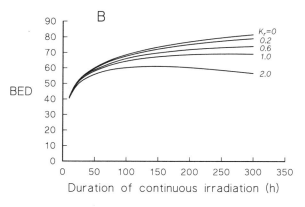

Figure 15.7 Tumour response for a fixed level of late normal-tissue damage as a function of (**A**) fraction number, or (**B**) exposure time in a single continuous dose. These curves are recalculated and redrawn after Dale (1989), as described in the text. The arrows in panel **A** indicate the dose per fraction at various points along the curve for no tumour cell proliferation ($K_r = 0$).

tal animals. Dale (1989) has also performed similar calculations for multiple fractions per day.

The effects of continuous irradiation can be calculated in a similar way. For any dose rate we calculate using Equation 15.2 the treatment time that is equivalent to a BED_{late} of 100Gy without repopulation ($\alpha/\beta = 3$ Gy). The half-time for recovery has been taken as 1.5 hours. Then once again with $\alpha/\beta = 10$ Gy we obtain BED_{tumour} values (Figure 15.7B). Within the range of parameters used, lowering the dose rate almost always gives a therapeutic advantage, especially where the effect of proliferation is small. Proliferation has less effect in panel B than panel A of Figure 15.7, reflecting the distinctive advantage of continuous treatment: overall time is minimised, and so also is the detrimental effect of tumour-cell repopulation.

15.5 Radiobiological aspects of brachytherapy

The principal reasons for choosing interstitial or intracavitary radiotherapy in preference to external-beam treatment relate to dose delivery and dose distribution rather than to radiobiology. Irradiation from an implanted source *within* a tumour carries a distinct geometrical advantage for sparing the surrounding normal tissues that will inevitably tend to receive a lower radiation dose.

Variation in Cell Killing around an Implanted Radioactive Source

The non-uniformity of radiation field around an implanted source has important radiobiological consequences. Close to the source the dose-rate is high and the amount of cell killing will be close to that indicated by the acute-radiation survival curve. As we move away from the source, two changes take place: cells will be less sensitive at the lower dose rates, and within a given period of implantation the accumulated dose will also be less. These two factors lead to a very rapid change of cell killing with distance from the source. Within tissues (tumour or normal) that are close to the source the level of cell killing will be so high that cells of any radiosensitivity will be killed. Further out, the effects will be so low that even the most radiosensitive cells will survive. Between

these extremes there is a critical zone in which differential cell killing will occur. As shown by Steel *et al* (1989), for cells of any given level of radiosensitivity there will be cliff-like change from high to low local cure probability, taking place over a radial distance of a few millimetres (Figure 15.8). The distance of the cliff from the source is determined by the radiosensitivity of the cells at low dose rate, nearer for radioresistant cells and further away for radiosensitive cells (Steel, 1991).

Figure 15.9 contrasts this situation with external-beam radiotherapy where the aim is

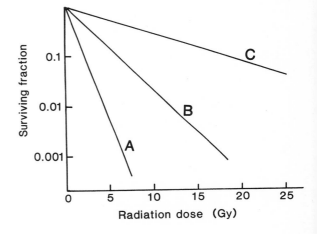

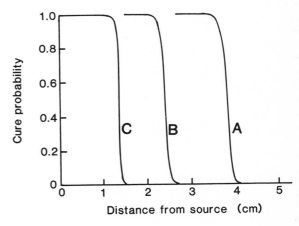

Figure 15.8 The likelihood of cure varies steeply with distance from a point radiation source. The radius at which failure occurs depends upon the steepness of the survival curve at low dose rate (upper panel). From Steel *et al* (1989), with permission.

to deliver uniform radiation dose across the tumour. Only in a narrow zone around an implanted source (where the surviving fraction changes from say 10^{-20} to 10^{-6}) will radiobiological considerations be of interest or importance in relation to tumour control. The same principle will apply to normal-tissue damage: serious damage to normal structures depends on making sure that they are outside the corresponding 'cliff'.

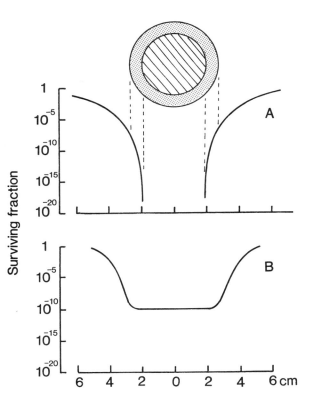

Figure 15.9 Variation of cell kill around a point source of radiation. The source gives 0.87 Gy/min at 2 cm (i.e. 75 Gy in 6 d); there are 10^9 cells per cm³, for which $\alpha = 0.35$ Gy^{-1}, $\beta = 0.035$ Gy^{-2}, half-time for recovery is 1 hour (Steel *et al*, 1989). The hatched area indicates the volume within which the surviving fraction is below 10^{-20}. The stippled area indicates the volume where survival is between 10^{-20} and 10^{-6}, which is the critical region for tumour control. For comparison, panel B shows the type of profile that would be aimed for with external-beam radiotherapy.

Is there a Radiobiological Advantage in Low Dose-rate Radiotherapy?

The question of whether low dose-rate irradiation itself carries a therapeutic advantage is an interesting one; there is a considerable volume of literature on the dose-rate effect both in tumours and in normal tissues on the basis of which it would be difficult to claim an overall benefit or disadvantage. As shown in Figure 15.3, cells that are the least sensitive to radiation and have the largest shoulder on the cell survival curve will show the greatest degree of dose-sparing (these are not necessarily cell lines of low α/β ratio, for Peacock *et al* (1992) have shown that human tumour cell lines, including those shown in Figure 15.3, have similar α/β ratios). This does not, however, answer the therapeutic question. There is no doubt that low dose-rate irradiation is radiobiologically better than a single large fraction at high dose rate; the question is whether it is better than conventional fractionation.

As is illustrated in Figure 15.6, there is, on the basis of the incomplete repair model, an equivalence between dose per fraction in fractionated radiotherapy and dose rate for a single continuous exposure. Roughly speaking, a dose rate of 1 Gy/h produces the same amount of cell killing as 2 Gy/fraction. This equivalence depends upon the half-time for recovery but it is relatively independent of the α/β ratio (Fowler, 1989). In radiobiological terms, these two treatments should be equally effective. Lowering the (fractionated) dose per fraction will spare late-responding normal tissues whose α/β ratio is low, as also will lowering the dose rate (continuous) below 1 Gy/h.

By the same argument, the use of high continuous dose rates is in radiobiological terms sub-optimal. That high dose-rate intracavitary therapy is widely thought to be acceptable may result from two factors:

(1) the lower *volume* of normal tissue irradiated to a dose that discriminates between tissue sensitivities (i.e. the annular region referred to in relation to Figure 15.9).

(2) the practical benefits to patient management of short treatment times.

The clearest *advantage* for low dose-rate irradiation is that for a given level of cell killing, and without hazarding late-responding normal tissues, this treatment will be complete within the *shortest overall time* (Section 15.4). Tumour-cell repopulation will therefore be minimized. This could confer a therapeutic advantage for the treatment of rapidly-repopulating tumours.

A potential *disadvantage* of low dose-rate irradiation is that because of the short overall treatment time there may be inadequate time available for the reoxygenation of hypoxic tumour cells and therefore greater radioresistance due to hypoxia.

Pulsed Brachytherapy

The availability of computer-controlled high dose-rate afterloading systems provides the opportunity to deliver interstitial or intracavitary radiotherapy in a series of pulses. The gaps between pulses allow greater freedom for the patient and increased safety for nursing staff. In principle, any move away from continuous exposure towards closely spaced dose fractions carries a radiobiological *disadvantage*. This is equivalent to fractionation with a larger dose per fraction and the theoretical and experimental evidence that this will lead to a relative increase in late normal-tissue reactions is strong (Section 9.2). The magnitude of this effect has been considered by Brenner and Hall (1991) who conclude that for gaps between pulses of up to 60 minutes the radiobiological deficit may be acceptable.

A further warning about the use of high dose-rate afterloading systems relates to overall time. High dose-rate afterloading systems create the temptation to shorten the overall time and, as indicated above, this could lead to greater radioresistance due to hypoxia.

Key points

1. A larger radiation dose is usually required to produce a particular biological effect at low dose rate (≈ 1 Gy/h) compared with high dose rate (≈ 1 Gy/min).
2. Low dose-rate irradiation discriminates better than high dose-rate irradiation between effects on cells of differing radiosensitivity.
3. The dose-rate effect observed between 1 Gy/min and 1 cGy/min is predominantly due to *repair* during irradiation; the effect seen below 1 cGy/min is mainly due to *cell proliferation* during irradiation.
4. Continuous low dose-rate exposure is the most efficient way of achieving full recovery from radiation damage in the shortest overall time. It minimizes the effects of proliferation, which is an advantage in terms of damage to tumour cells but a disadvantage for the tolerance of acutely responding normal tissues.
5. High continuous dose rates (i.e. above say 2 Gy/h) are biologically equivalent to the use of a large dose per fraction in fractionated radiotherapy; greater late damage to normal tissues for a given level of tumour response is therefore to be expected. This disadvantage may be offset in brachytherapy by the lower *volume* of normal tissue irradiated to high dose.
6. Cell killing varies steeply around an implanted radiation source. Close to the source, all cells will be killed. The *radius* at which tumour control will fail depends critically on the radiosensitivity of tumour cells at low dose rate.

Bibliography

Brenner DJ and Hall EJ (1991). Fractionated high dose rate *versus* low dose rate regimens for intracavitary brachytherapy of the cervix. *Brit J Radiol* 64:133-141.

Curtis SB (1986). Lethal and potentially lethal lesions induced by radiation – a unified repair model. *Radiat Res* 106:252-270.

Dale RG (1985). The application of the linear-quadratic dose-effect equation to fractionated and protracted radiotherapy. *Brit J Radiol* 58:515-528.

Dale RG (1989). Time-dependent tumour

repopulation factors in linear-quadratic equations–implications for treatment. *Radiother Oncol* 15:371-382.

Down JD, Easton, DF and Steel GG (1986). Repair in the mouse lung during low dose-rate irradiation. *Radiother Oncol* 6:29-42.

Peacock JH, Eady JJ, Edwards SM *et al* (1992). The intrinsic α/β ratio for human tumour cells: is it a constant? *Int J Radiat Biol* 61:479-487.

Steel GG, Down JD, Peacock JH and Stephens TC (1986). Dose-rate effects and the repair of radiation damage. *Radiother Oncol* 5:321-331.

Steel GG, Kelland LR and Peacock JH (1989). The radiobiological basis for low dose-rate radiotherapy. In: *Brachytherapy 2*, pp.15-25. Proceedings of the 5th International Selectron Users' Meeting 1988 (Ed) Mould RF, Nucletron International BV, Leersum, The Netherlands.

Thames, HD (1985). An 'incomplete-repair' model for survival after fractionated and continuous irradiation. *Int J Radiat Biol* 47:319-339.

Wells RL and Bedford JS (1983). Dose-rate effects in mammalian cells. IV: Repairable and nonrepairable damage in noncycling C3H 10T$_{1/2}$ cells. *Radiat Res* 94:105-134.

Further reading

Fowler JF (1989). Dose-rate effects in normal tissues. In: *Brachytherapy 2*, pp.26-40. Proceedings of the 5th International Selectron Users' Meeting 1988 (Ed) Mould RF, Nucletron International BV, Leersum, The Netherlands.

Steel GG (1991). Cellular sensitivity to low dose-rate irradiation focuses the problem of tumour radioresistance. (The ESTRO Breur Lecture). *Radiother Oncol* 20:71-83.

Steel GG, Deacon JM, Duchesne GM *et al* (1987). The dose-rate effect in human tumour cells. *Radiother Oncol* 9:299-310.

16

Particle Beams in Radiotherapy

Michael C. Joiner

16.1 Introduction

Radiotherapy is usually given with ^{60}Co γ-rays, or high-energy x-rays produced by linear accelerators at energies of 10 or more megavolts. These are uncharged electromagnetic radiations, physically similar in nature to radio waves or visible light except that the photons ('packets' of energy) are energetic enough to ionize molecules in tissues that they penetrate. It is this ionization that results in the biological effects seen in radiotherapy. Although there is *some* energy-dependence, the biological effect per unit dose of these radiations is similar. Electron beams are quantum-mechanically similar to and produce similar biological effects to x-rays. Two other classes of radiations for use in radiotherapy are often referred to as:

Light particles – e.g. protons, neutrons and alpha-particles.

Heavy particles – e.g. fully-stripped carbon, neon, silicon or argon ions.

These light and heavy particles may have a greater effect per unit dose compared with the conventional radiations. The *charged* particles have, in addition, very different depth-dose absorption profiles compared with the uncharged particles (neutrons) or conventional electromagnetic radiations, and this enables more precise dose distributions to be achieved in radiotherapy. This chapter focuses on these newer types of radiation for use in cancer therapy.

16.2 Microdosimetry

It is possible to build up a picture of the submicroscopic pattern of ionizations within a cell nucleus using special techniques for measuring ionization in very small volumes, together with computer simulations: the field of *microdosimetry*. Figure 16.1 shows examples of microdosimetric calculations of ionization tracks from γ-rays or α-particles passing through a cell nucleus (Goodhead, 1988;

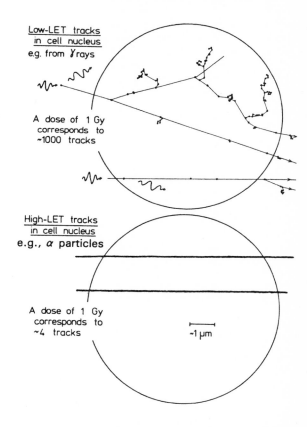

Figure 16.1 The structure of particle tracks for low-LET radiation (above) and α-particles (below). The circles indicate the typical size of mammalian cell nuclei. Note that the tortuous tracks of low-energy secondary electrons are greatly magnified. From Goodhead (1988), with permission.

1989). At the scale of the cell nucleus, the γ-rays deposit much of their energy as single isolated ionizations or excitations and much of the resulting DNA damage can be efficiently repaired by enzymes within the nucleus (Section 24.1). About 1000 of these sparse tracks are produced per gray of absorbed radiation dose. The α-particles produce fewer tracks but the intense ionization within each track leads to more severe damage where the track intersects vital structures such as DNA. The resulting DNA damage may involve several adjacent base pairs and will be much more difficult or even impossible to repair; this may be the reason why these radiations produce steeper cell survival curves and allow less cellular recovery than x-rays.

Linear Energy Transfer (LET) is the term used to describe the density of ionization in particle tracks. LET is the average energy (in keV) given up by a charged particle traversing a distance of 1 μm. In Figure 16.1 the γ-rays have an LET of about 0.3 keV μm^{-1} and may be described as low-LET radiation. The α-particles have an LET of about 100 keV μm^{-1} and are an example of high-LET radiation.

16.3 Biological effects depend upon LET

As LET increases, radiations produce more cell killing per gray. Figure 16.2 shows the survival of human T1g cells plotted against dose for eight different radiations, with LET varying from 2 keV μm^{-1} (250 kVp x-rays) to 165 keV μm^{-1} (2.5 MeV α-particles). The radiations become more efficient per gray at killing cells as the LET increases. As LET increases, the survival curves also become straighter with less shoulder, which indicates either a higher ratio of lethal to potentially lethal lesions (in lesion-interaction models) or that high-LET radiation damage is less likely to be repaired correctly (in repair saturation models; *see* Chapter 6). For particles of identical atomic composition, LET generally increases with decreasing particle energy. However, notice that 2.5 MeV α-particles are *less* efficient compared with 4.0 MeV α-particles even though they have a higher LET; this is due to the phenomenon of overkill indicated in Figure 16.3.

The *Relative Biological Effectiveness (RBE)* of a high-LET radiation is defined as:

$$ RBE = \frac{\text{dose of reference radiation}}{\text{dose of high-LET radiation}} $$

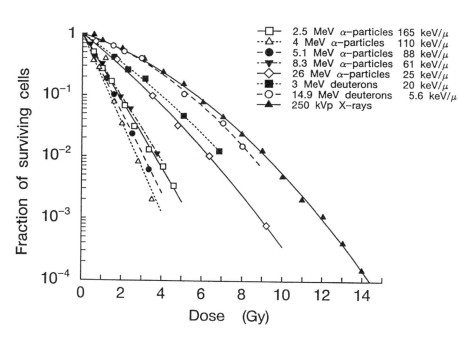

Figure 16.2 Survival of human kidney cells exposed *in vitro* to radiations of different LET. From Barendsen (1968), with permission.

to give the same biological effect. The *reference low-LET* radiation is usually 250 kVp x-rays. Figure 16.3 shows RBE values for the T1g cells featured in Figure 16.2. Curves have been calculated at cell survival levels of 0.8, 0.1 and 0.01, illustrating the fact that RBE is not constant but *depends on the level of biological damage* and hence on the dose level. RBE rises to a maximum at an LET of about 100 keV μm^{-1}, then falls for higher values of LET due to *overkill*. For cells to be killed, energy must be deposited in a number of critical sites in the cell (Section 6.3). Sparsely-ionizing, low-LET radiation is inefficient because more than one particle may have to pass through the cell to kill it. Densely ionizing, very high-LET radiation is also inefficient because it deposits more energy than necessary in critical sites. These cells are *overkilled* and per gray there is then less likelihood that *other* cells will be killed, leading to a reduced biological effect. Radiation of optimal LET deposits just enough energy to inactivate the critical targets. This optimum LET is usually around 100 keV μm^{-1} but it does vary between different cell types and depends on the *spectrum* of LET values in the radiation beam as well as the mean LET.

As LET increases, the Oxygen Enhancement Ratio (OER, Section 11.1) decreases. The measurements shown as an example in Figure 16.4 were again made with cultured T1g cells of human origin (Barendsen, 1968). The sharp reduction in OER occurs over the same range of LET as the sharp increase in RBE (Figure 16.3).

16.4 Relative biological effectiveness (RBE) depends on dose

As indicated in Figure 16.3, the RBE is higher if measured at lower radiation doses, corresponding to higher levels of cell survival. Figure 16.5 shows in more detail the RBE for 4.0 MeV α-particles plotted against dose of 250 kVp x-rays, for the T1g human cells irradiated *in vitro*. The data points were derived from Figure 16.2 by reading off from the α-particle survival curve the dose required to achieve the same cell survival as obtained for each x-ray dose tested. The RBE for the 4.0 MeV α-particles increases with decreasing dose because the low-LET x-ray survival response is more curved and has a bigger shoulder compared with the high-LET survival response. If linear-quadratic equations are used to model both the

low and the high-LET responses, RBE can also be predicted mathematically from the α/β ratios and the ratio $\alpha_{\text{high-let}}/\alpha_{\text{low-let}}$. This prediction is shown by the solid line.

RBE can also be measured *in vivo*. In normal tissues this may be done by comparing the relationships between *functional damage* and dose for high- and low-LET radiations. Figure 16.6A

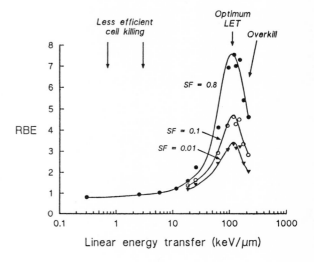

Figure 16.3 Dependence of RBE on LET and the phenomenon of overkill by very high LET radiations. From Barendsen (1968), with permission.

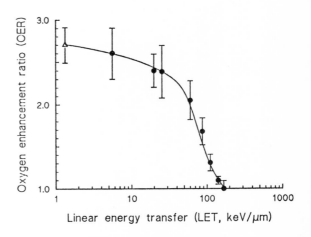

Figure 16.4 The oxygen enhancement ratio (OER) decreases with increasing LET. Closed circles refer to monoenergetic α-particles and deuterons and the open triangle to 250 kVp x-rays. From Barendsen (1968), with permission.

shows the results of an experiment to study the loss of renal function in mice after external-beam radiotherapy. This was done by measuring the increased retention of ^{51}Cr-radiolabeled EDTA in the plasma 1 hour after injection; normally-functioning kidneys completely clear this substance from the body within this time. For neutrons (produced by bombarding beryllium with 4MeV deuterons, designated d(4)-Be), fractionation makes almost no difference to the

tolerance doses but for x-rays a much higher total dose is required to produce renal damage when the treatment is split into 2, 5 or 10 fractions. This difference in the fractionation response for high- and low-LET radiations *in vivo* reflects the shape of the survival curves for the target cells in the tissue: almost straight for neutrons, and downwards-bending for x-rays (Figure 16.2). In this situation RBE is calculated from the ratio of x-ray and neutron total doses required to produce the same biological effect *in the same number of fractions*. This is plotted against x-ray dose per fraction in Figure 16.6B. It can be seen that the *in vivo* RBE increases with decreasing dose per fraction in exactly the same way as for cells *in vitro* shown in Figure 16.5.

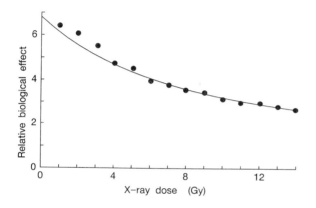

Figure 16.5 RBE of 4 MeV α-particles increases with decreasing dose for cell lines irradiated *in vitro*. RBE values were calculated from the cell survival data shown in Figure 16.2. The full line is calculated as described in the text.

16.5 Response of different tissues to high-LET radiation

The response to neutrons shown in Figure 16.6A suggests that for a fixed level of biological effect there should be much less change in total dose with fractionation for high-LET radiation compared with low-LET radiation. Figure 16.7 summarizes isoeffect curves relating total dose to dose per fraction for early-responding (dashed lines) and late-responding (full lines) tissues exposed

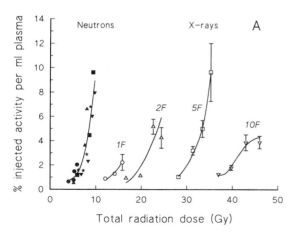

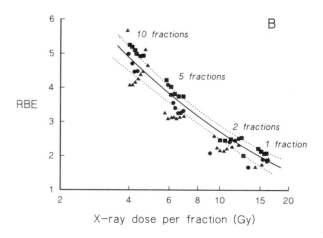

Figure 16.6 The RBE for kidney damage increases with decreasing dose per fraction. RBE values are derived from graphs similar to panel **A**, which shows dose-effect curves for ^{51}Cr-EDTA clearance following irradiation with 1, 2, 3, 5 and 10 fractions of neutrons or 1, 2, 5 and 10 fractions of x-rays. The RBE values in panel **B** were obtained with various renal-damage endpoints: isotope clearance (circles); reduction in haematocrit (squares); increase in urine output (triangles). From Joiner and Johns (1987), with permission.

to fractionated neutron irradiation (Withers *et al*, 1982). This figure should be compared with Figure 9.1 which shows these relationships for a similar range of tissues exposed to fractionated X- or γ-rays. The following conclusions can be drawn from this comparison:

1) There is little change in isoeffective total dose with fractionation for neutrons, either in early- or late-responding tissues. This reflects the almost straight survival curves for the target cells for high-LET radiation;

2) For photons, the total dose increases more steeply with decreasing dose per fraction for late-responding than early-responding tissues, reflecting the smaller α/β ratios for late tissues (Section 8.5). RBE therefore rises rapidly with decreasing dose per fraction for late-responding tissues and more gradually for early-responding tissues;

3) Comparing the same tissues exposed to both photons and neutrons, RBE values for late tissue responses are *not* intrinsically higher than for early responses, but because of their faster increase as the dose is reduced the RBE values for late tissue response *tend* to be higher than for early tissue response at low doses per fraction, especially at or below 2 Gy per (x-ray) fraction.

To emphasize this last point, Figure 16.8 demonstrates the rise in neutron RBE (compared with x-rays) with decreasing dose per fraction in skin (an early-responding tissue) and kidney (a late-responding tissue). In this example the RBE for d(16)-Be neutrons in kidney was greater than in skin at an x-ray dose per fraction of 2 Gy, but *lower* for a more modern, more highly penetrating, p(62)-Be neutron therapy beam. Therefore compared with conventional photon therapy, late renal damage would be increased relative to acute reactions (and perhaps relative to tumour response) by treating with a low-energy neutron beam, but late renal injury would actually be spared on the high energy machine. It is very important to understand that these relationships are specific to these tissues and these neutron beams. Similar relationships between other early-responding and late-responding tissues may not follow the same pattern and so must be evaluated individually in each case and for each treatment site to determine whether neutrons would deliver a therapeutic gain. It is not true that late reactions are *always* worse after neutron therapy for the same level of acute injury, but they may be in some cases.

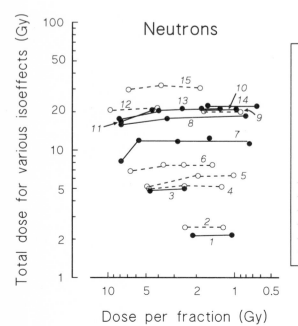

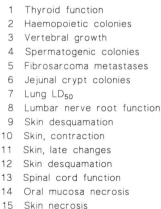

Figure 16.7 Summary of published data on isoeffect curves for neutrons as a function of dose per fraction in various tissues of mice and rats. Broken lines indicate data on early-responding tissues; full lines are for late-responding tissues. Compare with Figure 9.1. From Withers *et al* (1982), with permission.

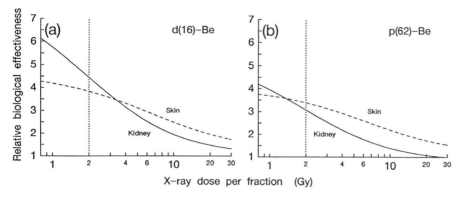

Figure 16.8 Comparison of RBE values for mouse skin and kidney exposed to two different neutron beams. From Joiner (1988), with permission.

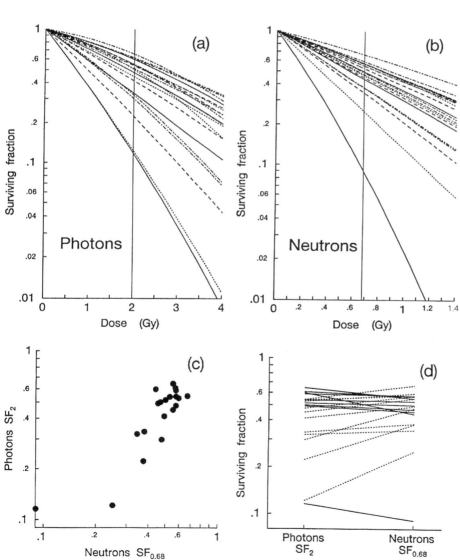

Figure 16.9 Response of 20 human tumour cell lines to (a): 4 MVp photons, or (b): p(62.5)–Be neutrons. The vertical lines show the photon (2 Gy) and neutron (0.68 Gy) doses that give the same *median* cell survival; the average RBE is therefore 2/0.68 = 2.94. Panel (c) shows that the range of cell survival at the reference neutron dose of 0.68 Gy is less than the range of photon SF_2 values. In 9/20 of the cell lines (panel d) neutrons gave lower cell survival than photons at these doses.

16.6 The biological basis for high-LET radiotherapy

We have seen (Figure 16.4) that the differential radiosensitivity between poorly oxygenated and well oxygenated cells is reduced by using high-LET radiations. Therefore, tumour sites in which hypoxia is a problem in radiotherapy (some head and neck tumours, for example) might benefit from high-LET radiotherapy in the same way as from chemical hypoxic-cell sensitizers (Section 19.3).

The effect of low-LET radiation on cells is strongly influenced by their position in the cell cycle, with cells in S-phase being more radioresistant than cells in G2 or mitosis (Section 5.8). Cells in stationary (i.e. plateau-phase) also tend to be more radioresistant than cells in active proliferation. Both of these factors act to increase the effect of fractionated radiotherapy on more rapidly cycling cells compared with those cycling slowly or not at all, because the rapidly cycling cells which survive the first few fractions are statistically more likely to be caught later in a sensitive phase and so be killed by a subsequent dose. This differential radiosensitivity due to cell-cycle position is considerably reduced with high-LET radiation (Chapman, 1980) and is a reason why we might expect high-LET radiotherapy to be beneficial in some slowly growing, x-ray resistant tumours.

A third biological rationale for high-LET therapy is based on the observation that the *range* of radiation response of different cell types is reduced with high-LET radiation compared with x-rays. This is shown in Figure 16.9, panel (c), which summarizes the *in vitro* response of 20 human cell lines to photon and neutron irradiation (Britten *et al*, 1992). This reduced range of response affects the benefit expected, which is the balance between tumour and normal-tissue responses. Thus, if tumour cells are already more radiosensitive to x-rays than the critical normal-cell population, high-LET radiation should not be used since this would reduce an already favourable differential. Possible examples are seminomas, lymphomas and Hodgkin's disease. However, if critical normal cells are more sensitive than the tumour cells, high-LET radiation might reduce this difference in radiosensitivity and thus would selectively 'protect' the normal cell population to x-rays; high-LET radiation would be an advantage

in this case. Figure 16.9, panel (d), shows that tumour response would be improved, relative to the average response of all tumours, in perhaps 40% of cases by using high-LET treatment. However, only if normal-tissue response is increased *less* than the tumour response would this give a therapeutic benefit.

These radiobiological arguments lead us to expect that high-LET radiotherapy might be of benefit to some cancer patients but not to others. Clinical trials of neutrons that have so far been performed have generally failed to detect such an advantage in the whole cancer patient populations that have been studied. If high-LET therapy is going to be of clinical use, it should therefore only be given to patients who are likely to respond poorly to conventional x-ray therapy, based on the results of assays for tumour oxygenation, cell kinetics and radiosensitivity. The principles of these predictive assays are described in Chapter 23. Table 16.1 demonstrates hypothetically the importance of patient selection for neutron therapy. Suppose that 200 patients enter a trial of high-LET *versus* photon therapy with 100 patients in each arm. 80% of the patients respond equally well to the two treatments (and we suppose a 50% cure rate) but the other 20% do better with the high-LET therapy, and this small subgroup responds with a 70% cure rate after high-LET and 30% cure after photons. The results for the total group fail to achieve significance; if the subgroup of 40 patients had been selected out they would have demonstrated a margin in favour of neutrons. It would be even more confusing if the majority (160) of the patients actually did *worse* with high-LET therapy: suppose 45% were cured with high-LET but 55% were cured with photons. Now the whole trial (Table 16.1B) reveals nothing at all but would still conceal an important subgroup. Rational patient selection is thus an important principle in relation to any modality that may improve treatment in only a minority of cases.

In spite of the potential difficulties demonstrated by Table 16.1, some clinical indications for fast neutron therapy have emerged. These have been summarized by Wambersie and Barendsen (1989) as listed in Table 16.2. Neutrons may be of some benefit in treating x-ray resistant tumours, slowly-growing tumours and some advanced cancers that perhaps contain a high proportion of hypoxic cells. Wambersie estimated that up to 10% of patients currently receiving radiotherapy

Table 16.1 Hypothetical clinical trials which show the importance of patient selection in determining the value of high-LET radiotherapy

A	Total number	Successful response to		
		Neutrons	Photons	*p* value
Subgroup	40	14	6	0.03
Remainder	160	40	40	-
Total	200	54	46	0.3

B	Total number	Successful response to		
		Neutrons	Photons	*p* value
Subgroup	40	14	6	0.03
Remainder	160	36	44	0.3
Total	200	50	50	-

From Bewley (1989).

Table 16.2 Summary of clinical indications for fast neutron therapy

1. Salivary gland tumours (locally extended)
2. Prostatic adenocarcinoma (locally extended)
3. Soft-tissue sarcoma (slowly-growing, inoperable)
4. Paranasal sinuses (adenocarcinoma, adenoid cystic ca.)
5. Some tumours of the head and neck (locally extended etc.)
6. Melanoma (inoperable, recurrent)

From Wambersie and Barendsen (1989).

would benefit from neutron therapy using modern isocentric machines, *if those patients could be identified reliably*.

16.7 The physical basis for charged-particle therapy

With conventional x-ray therapy, absorbed dose increases very rapidly within the short distance in which electronic equilibrium ('build-up') occurs, and then decreases exponentially with increasing penetration. Figure 16.10A shows central-axis depth doses from ^{60}Co γ-rays and from x-rays generated by a 6 MV linear accelerator (Fowler, 1981). Neutrons are also uncharged and their depth dose characteristics are similar. Modern high-energy neutron therapy beams have a penetration that is comparable to 6 MV x-rays. The only rationale for neutron therapy is therefore radiobiological, as discussed earlier.

In contrast, ion beams (i.e. incident beams of *charged* particles) *increase* their rate of energy deposition as they slow down with increasing penetration, finally stopping and releasing an intense burst of ionization called the Bragg peak. As an example, curve *1* in Figure 16.10B shows the depth-dose distribution of a primary beam of 160 MeV protons. The broad peak is obtained by superimposing on curve *1* four other beams of different intensities and ranges (curves *2, 3, 4, 5*), achieved by passing the primary beam through a rotating wheel with sectors of different thickness of plastic sheet. This spread-out peak (*Sum*) can be adjusted to cover the tumour volume and therefore increase the ratio of tumour-to-normal tissue dose compared with conventional photon therapy (Raju, 1980).

Figure 16.11 shows some possible treatment plans with heavier ion beams of helium and carbon nuclei, using carcinoma of the pancreas as an example. The improvement given by the He ions over 18 MV x-rays is as dramatic as the comparison between 18 MV and 250 kVp x-rays. The mean doses to the spinal cord and kidney are almost zero for He ions, 50% for 18 MV x-rays and 70% for 250 kVp x-rays. Uniformity over the

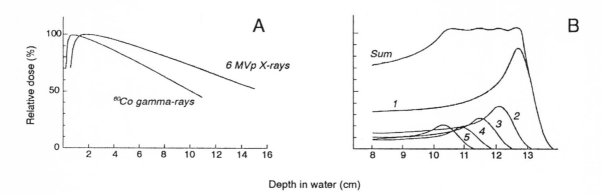

Depth in water (cm)

Figure 16.10 The different depth-dose characteristics of (**A**) photons and (**B**) proton beams of different intensities and ranges, achieved by passing a primary beam (*1*) through plastic absorbers.

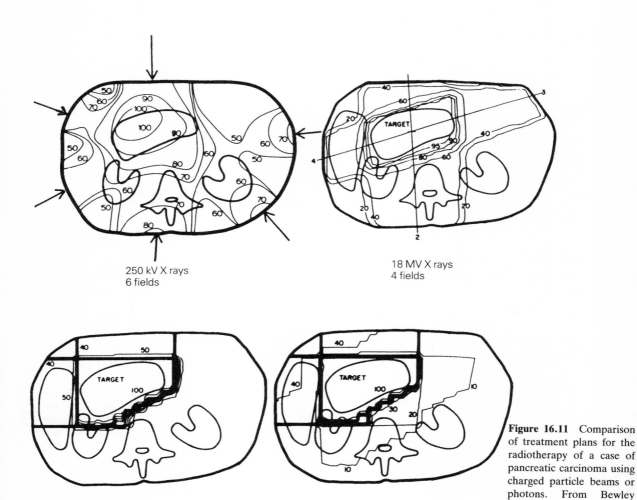

250 kV X rays
6 fields

18 MV X rays
4 fields

He ions

C ions

Figure 16.11 Comparison of treatment plans for the radiotherapy of a case of pancreatic carcinoma using charged particle beams or photons. From Bewley (1989), with permission.

tumour is 2 to 3%, 5% and 15% respectively.

Carbon ions give a similar dose distribution to He ions but in addition they have a higher LET and RBE in the Bragg peak which in suitable tumours (see above) might confer a therapeutic advantage (Figure 16.12). The LET of a charged particle is proportional to the square of its charge divided by the square of its velocity. Therefore in the Bragg peak, where the particles are slowing down rapidly, heavy ions such as carbon, neon and silicon have very high LET, with the potential for a greatly increased biological effect. To illustrate this, Figure 16.12 shows depth-dose curves for beams of heavy ions accelerated to two different energies giving maximum penetrations in tissue of about 14 or 24 cm. In each case the solid line represents the pattern of dose produced by

a ridge filter designed to spread out the Bragg peak to cover imaginary tumours of 4 or 10 cm respectively. This is a similar 'peak spreading' technique as described in Figure 16.10B. However, the dotted line shows the distribution of *equivalent photon dose*, which is physical dose × RBE. The RBE values are those for Chinese hamster cells corresponding to an x-ray dose of about 2 Gy (Blakely, 1982). This demonstrates that for heavy ions (*not* high-energy protons or helium ions) the physical advantage of better dose distribution in the spread-out Bragg peak can be further enhanced by the biological advantage from the higher LET.

Figure 16.13 conveniently summarizes the relative physical and radiobiological properties of different radiations and charged particles (Fowler, 1981). Protons have superb depth-dose distributions and have radiobiological properties similar to x-rays: it is highly probable that light-ion beams of protons and perhaps helium will play a key role in better radiotherapy during the next 20 years. Neutrons have no dose-distribution advantage over megavoltage x-rays but may be useful because of their high LET. The heavy ions give better dose distributions than x-rays, also a higher LET, depending on the particle. Argon ions have a high LET but in practice they break up so readily that only limited penetration is useful. Carbon, neon and silicon ions seem to be the most promising of the heavy ions at the present time and if heavy ion therapy has a future it will probably be with these particles.

16.8 Summary of therapeutic conclusions

Neutrons are the commonest type of particle beam so far used for radiotherapy but the clinical results obtained are controversial. Some benefits have been claimed, as indicated in Table 16.2. Much of the clinical work with heavy ions has taken place at the Lawrence Berkeley Laboratory in California. Some benefit in some tumours has been claimed although the high cost of this treatment means that it will be restricted to a few large centres each serving a large population (Wambersie and Barendsen, 1989). Proton beams are probably the most attractive radiation at the present time. They are not excessively expensive and have greatly improved dose distributions compared with photons.

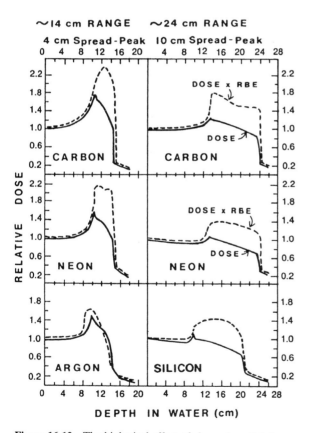

Figure 16.12 The biological effect of charged particle beams is increased further in the Bragg peak. Depth-dose curves are shown for three types of ion beam, each with a 4 cm or 10 cm spread peak. Full lines show the dose distribution; broken lines show the *equivalent photon dose* (i.e. dose × RBE). From Blakely (1982), with permission.

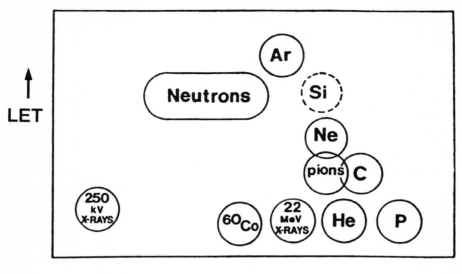

Quality of dose distribution ⟶

Figure 16.13 The radiations available for radiation therapy differ in the quality of beam that they produce, also in RBE. From Fowler (1981), with permission.

Key points

1. X- and γ-rays are sparsely ionizing radiations with a low Linear Energy Transfer (LET). Some particle radiations (e.g. neutrons, α-particles or heavy ions) have a high LET.
2. High-LET radiations are *biologically* more effective per gray than low-LET radiations. This is measured by the Relative Biological Effectiveness (RBE). For most high-LET radiations at therapeutic dose levels, RBE is in the range of 2 to 10.
3. RBE increases as the LET increases up to about 100 keV μm^{-1} above which RBE decreases because of cellular overkill. The Oxygen Enhancement Ratio (OER) also decreases rapidly over the same range of LET.
4. RBE increases as the dose is reduced *in vitro*, or the dose *per fraction* is reduced *in vivo*. In late-responding tissues, this increase occurs more rapidly than in early-responding tissues.
5. High-LET radiations may be clinically useful in selected cases.
6. Heavy particles such as He, C and Ne ions, have a high LET and in addition they have improved physical depth-dose distributions.
7. Proton beams provide the best improvement in dose distribution for the lowest cost; their RBE is similar to photons.

Bibliography

Barendsen GW (1968). Responses of cultured cells, tumours and normal tissues to radiations of different linear energy transfer. *Current Topics Rad Res Quart* 4:293-356.

Blakely EA (1982). Biology of Bevelac beams: cellular studies. In: *Pion and Heavy Ion Radiotherapy: Pre-clinical and Clinical Studies.* pp.229-250. (Ed) Skarsgard LD. Elsevier, New York.

Britten RA, Warenius HM, Parkins C and Peacock JH (1992). The inherent cellular sensitivity to 62.5MeV neutrons of human cells differing in photon sensitivity. *Int J Radiat Biol* 61:805-812.

Chapman JD (1980). Biophysical models of

mammalian cell inactivation by radiation. In: *Radiation Biology in Cancer Research*, pp.21-32. (Eds) Meyn RE and Withers HR. Raven Press; New York.

Goodhead DT (1989). The initial physical damage produced by ionizing radiation. *Int J Radiat Biol* 56:623-634.

Joiner MC (1988). A comparison of the effects of p(62)-Be and d(16)-Be neutrons in the mouse kidney. *Radiother Oncol* 13:211-224.

Joiner MC and Johns H (1987). Renal damage in the mouse: the effect of d(4)-Be neutrons. *Radiat Res* 109:456-468.

Raju MR (1980). *Heavy Particle Radiotherapy*. Academic Press; New York.

Wambersie A and Barendsen GW (1989). Is there a future for high-LET radiotherapy: the radiobiological arguments. In: *Proc. EULIMA Workshop on the Potential Value of Light Ion Beam Therapy*, pp.3-31. (Eds) Chauvel P and Wambersie A. EUR 12165 EN, Commission of European Communities; Luxembourg.

Withers HR, Thames HD and Peters LJ (1982). Biological bases for high RBE values for late effects of neutron irradiation. *Int J Radiat Oncol Biol Phys* 8:2071-2076.

Further reading

Alpen EL (1990). *Radiation Biophysics*. Prentice-Hall, London.

Bewley DK (1989). *The Physics and Radiobiology of Fast Neutron Beams*. Adam Hilger; Bristol.

Fowler JF (1981). *Nuclear Particles in Cancer Treatment*. Adam Hilger; Bristol.

Goodhead DT (1988). Spatial and temporal distribution of energy. *Health Physics* 55:231-240.

Hall EJ (1982). The particles compared. *Int J Radiat Oncol Biol Phys* 8:2137-2140.

Hall EJ (1988). *Radiobiology for the Radiologist*. Chapter 13, Lippincott; Philadelphia.

17

Chemotherapy from the standpoint of radiotherapy

Adrian C. Begg

17.1 Introduction

In considering the biological basis of chemotherapy we have to deal with a variety of cytotoxic agents, not just one agent (ionizing radiation) as with radiotherapy. There are many different drugs and drug analogues, often with different mechanisms of action. Despite this complexity, the basic principles of chemotherapy are in many respects similar to those of radiotherapy. Important factors such as the achievement of multi-log tumour cell kill (Section 5.6), the concept of therapeutic gain (Section 1.6), the often limited effectiveness due to cellular resistance (Section 5.7), and the limited value of tumour regression compared with disease-free survival as an indicator of tumour response (Section 2.5), are common to both therapies. In addition, quantitative experimental methods for measuring cell kill, tumour response, and normal-tissue response, can usually be applied to both forms of therapy.

There are also marked differences between chemotherapy and radiotherapy. Firstly, radiotherapy is primarily a local treatment, in which accurate dose delivery can achieve a high level of specificity for damage to the tumour, with sparing of normal tissues. Chemotherapy is usually employed to treat systemic disease. As a sole treatment modality, chemotherapy at the present time is markedly less effective than radiotherapy (Section 1.1). Chemotherapy at the present time is curative when used as a single modality only in a small minority of diseases (e.g. some lymphomas and leukaemias, teratomas). Surgery and radiotherapy are considerably more successful as single-treatment modalities. Chemotherapy is therefore most often used in combination with surgery or radiotherapy. Severe organ toxicity (often to the bone marrow or intestinal epithelium) limits the dosage that can be delivered, resulting in a small therapeutic margin.

Natural or acquired drug resistance is also cited as a common cause of treatment failure. For radiotherapy, acquired resistance is rare, although inherent resistance often limits tumour control. Several ways of overcoming drug resistance have been tried, including alternating or switching drug types, and administration of agents that potentiate uptake or reduce efflux. Several ways of increasing the administered drug dose have been investigated, including the use of rescue agents (including growth factors for bone marrow) and drug targeting by regional infusion or by using a carrier (e.g. antibodies or liposomes) with greater specificity for the tumour than the free drug. A continuing search is under way for new drugs, including analogues of existing drugs, with greater effectiveness, less toxicity and without cross-resistance; also agents against particular biological targets such as hypoxic cells or cells at low pH, oncogenes, or specific enzyme systems. This chapter will cover a few of these aspects.

17.2 Drug classification

Drug Type

Drugs can be classified in several ways. The first is by drug type (Table 17.1). This classification divides drugs according to both their mode of action and their source: it is thus a mixed classification that is convenient rather than instructive. *Alkylation* and *antimetabolite* describe in general terms how the drugs act, whereas *natural products* describes where the drugs came from. There are also drugs that do not fit any of these categories.

Drug Action

Cytotoxic drugs can also be classified on the basis of dose-response curves for cell killing. This approach originated in the work of Bruce *et al* (1966), and is sometimes called the *Bruce*

Table 17.1 Four general categories of cytotoxic agent used in cancer chemotherapy

Alkylating agents	Nitrogen mustard, chlorambucil, melphalan, cyclophosphamide, busulphan, nitrosoureas
Antimetabolites	Methotrexate, 5-fluorouracil, cytosine arabinoside, 6-thioguanine, 6-mercaptopurine
Natural products	Adriamycin, daunorubicin, actinomycin D, bleomycin, mitomycin C, taxol, vinblastine, VP16
Miscellaneous:	Cisplatin, DTIC, procarbazine (*prob. alkylating activity*)

Classification. Cell survival curves for the treatment of slowly and rapidly proliferating cells are compared. This classification arose from the concept (not universally true) that tumour cells proliferate faster than the stem cells in normal tissues. The classification shown in Figure 17.1 is based on the killing of rapidly proliferating lymphoma cells compared with relatively slowly proliferating normal haematopoietic cells, both treated *in vivo* in mice. Three classes of cytotoxic agent were distinguished:

Proliferation non-specific agents (class I).

The rapidly and slowly proliferating cells are similarly sensitive. In the work of Bruce *et al* nitrogen mustard and gamma-radiation fell into this category.

Cell-cycle phase-specific agents (class II).

The cell survival curves fall to a plateau. Following a brief drug exposure, an agent that kills cells only in a particular phase of the cycle will show such a plateau in the dose response curve, the height of which corresponds to the fraction of resistant cells that are present. Examples are methotrexate, hydroxyurea, vinblastine.

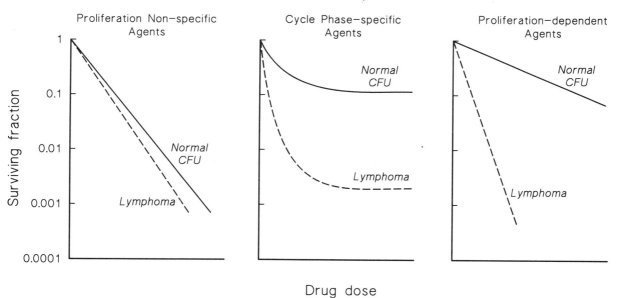

Figure 17.1 Dose-response curves for slowly proliferating normal bone marrow stem cells (full lines) and rapidly proliferating lymphoma cells (dashed lines) in mice, illustrating three categories of cytotoxic agent. From Bruce *et al* (1966), with permission.

Proliferation-dependent agents (class III).

Rapidly proliferating cells are much more sensitive to these agents, but both have roughly exponential survival curves. Examples are cyclophosphamide, 5-fluorouracil.

This classification is more useful than drug type, since it leads to concepts of drug scheduling. For instance, phase-specific agents must be infused or given repeatedly, since single doses will be ineffective; the level of cell kill with these agents depends critically on the *treatment duration*. The classification also throws light on drug resistance in kinetically heterogeneous tumour cell populations where slowly proliferating or resting cells may fail to be killed. The tendency for proliferating cells to be more sensitive to drug treatment than resting cells is illustrated in Figure 17.2 (van Putten, 1974). This shows the effects on

resting and regenerating mouse bone marrow of 8 cytotoxic agents. Note the large differences in sensitivity shown by these data and that in most cases proliferating cells are more sensitive than non-proliferating cells.

Cycle-phase specificity

Many agents, even though not completely cycle-phase specific, vary in their killing efficiency through the cell cycle (Table 17.2). This includes x-radiation which, in contrast to drugs, is usually *less* efficient in killing late S-phase cells (Section 5.8). Most agents also delay the progress of cells through the cell cycle. Note that the phase at which cells are blocked is not necessarily the phase of maximum killing; an example is vincristine which blocks cells in mitosis but which has maximal cell killing in the S-phase. The most common delay points are at entry into the S-phase (i.e.

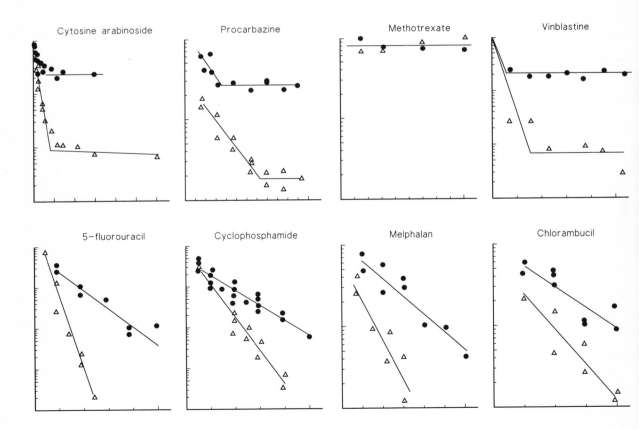

Figure 17.2   Survival curves for resting (●) and rapidly regenerating (△) mouse bone marrow cells treated with eight different cytotoxic agents. From van Putten (1974), with permission.

the G_1/S boundary) and entry into M (the G_2/M boundary). Phase specificity for cell killing is usually determined by assessing cloning efficiency for cultured cells synchronized in different phases. Flow cytometry also provides a useful means for detecting drug-induced progression delay.

Table 17.2 Predominant phase of the cell cycle for blocking or cell kill

Drug	Cell killing	Progression delay
Actinomycin D	G_1/S, M	G_1, G_1/S, G_2
Adriamycin	Late S, M	S, G_2
BCNU	G_1/S	Late S, G_2
Bleomycin	G_2, M	S/G_2, G_2
Cisplatin	G_1, G_2	S G_2, G_1/S
5-Fluorouracil	All phases	G_1/S
Hydroxyurea	S	G_1/S
Methotrexate	Early G_1, G_1/S, S	G_1/S
Mitomycin C	G_1, G_2, M	S/G_2
Mitozantrone	G_1, G_2	G_2
Etoposide	S, G_2	S, G_2
Vincristine	S	M
Radiation	G_1/S, G_2, M	G_1, S, G_2

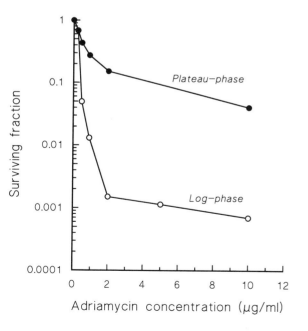

Figure 17.3 Survival curves for log-phase and plateau-phase CHO cells treated with adriamycin. Adapted from Humphrey and Barranco (1975), with permission.

Survival curve plateaus cannot always be explained by phase specificity. Figure 17.3 shows survival curves for CHO cells treated *in vitro* with adriamycin either when the cells were in exponential growth (*log-phase*) or when crowding of the cultures had led to growth arrest (*plateau-phase*). The curves level out at a lower survival in log-phase cells than plateau-phase. But the resistant component at a survival of around 10^{-3} in the log-phase cells is too low to represent one phase of the cell cycle, though large enough to cause treatment failure. Another possibility is the existence of a small fraction of mutant drug-resistant cells.

17.3 Drug toxicity

Drugs often show specific toxicity to one particular organ, which limits the dose that can be administered. Table 17.3 lists the major toxicities of some of the most commonly used chemotherapeutic agents. Bone marrow depression is a common dose-limiting toxicity; nausea and vomiting are also common, although less likely to limit the treatment dose. Note that several of the limiting toxicities occur in nonproliferating or slowly proliferating organs (e.g. kidney for cisplatin, lung for bleomycin) illustrating the fact that proliferation rate is not the only determinant of the cytotoxic effects of chemotherapy. The same is true for tumours, where there are many examples of cell lines with similar proliferation rates but markedly different sensitivities to a particular drug.

Table 17.3 Specific toxicities of chemotherapy agents

Adriamycin	–	heart
Bleomycin	–	lung
Carboplatin	–	bone marrow
Cisplatin	–	kidney
Cyclophosphamide	–	bladder
Cycle–specific agents	–	bone marrow

17.4 Combination chemotherapy

Rationales for Combining Drugs

Most cancer chemotherapy involves the administration of several different types of drug. Some of the reasons for choosing which drugs to use in combination are listed in Table 17.4. Rationale #1 aims at avoiding excessive normal-tissue toxicity, whereas the other 4 rationales are aimed specifically at increasing tumour response.

When combining drugs with non-overlapping toxicities, drugs are chosen with some evidence of effectiveness as single agents in that disease site. It is clearly important to choose the most effective agents that can be so combined, in order to maximize additive cell killing in the tumour. This approach may thus lead to an increased tumour 'dose' where it is not possible to increase the dose of any single agent without unacceptable toxicity. If there is interaction between the drugs in producing normal-tissue toxicity, such that the dose of each must be lowered compared with that given as a single agent, the combination therapy is likely to be less effective.

Combination of two drugs with different mechanisms of action (rationale #2) is an empirical approach based on the hope that cells not sensitive to one drug type will be sensitive to the other. In contrast, choosing drugs that complement each other biochemically (rationale #3) is a scientifically sound approach which attempts to maximize tumour cell kill and minimize the chance of developing drug resistance. Potentiation of drug uptake (rationale #4) has been shown to work in cell culture and in some animal tumours, although there have been few clinical studies of this. Rationale #5 is based on attacking pharmacologically resistant subpopulations (e.g. non- or slowly cycling cells; hypoxic cells). This approach is analogous to giving hypoxic radiosensitizers or hypoxic cytotoxic agents with radiotherapy (Section 19.8).

For rationales #2–5, it is important that any increased tumour response is not matched by an equal increase in toxicity, which would leave the therapeutic ratio unchanged. For rationales #2–4

in particular, there is no *a priori* reason why an increased effect would not also occur in normal tissues.

Hypoxic-specific Cytotoxins

Hypoxic cells are often far from blood vessels, and thus may be difficult to kill for two separate reasons: they may be non-cycling and therefore resistant to many drugs, and they may be exposed to lower drug levels than are achieved close to blood vessels. Compounds have therefore been developed which are specifically toxic to hypoxic cells. Three examples are shown in Figure 17.4; in each case the oxic cells are *less* sensitive than the hypoxic cells. These compounds are usually nitro-compounds which undergo reduction to a toxic product only under hypoxic conditions. Clinical trials with some of these compounds are under way. They could be combined with radiation and with drugs which specifically kill the well-oxygenated, cycling cells, from which a therapeutic benefit may be expected.

17.5 Drug resistance

Biochemical Mechanisms

Drug resistance is a major cause of chemotherapy failure. Two types of drug resistance can be distinguished: *inherent* and *induced*. Induced drug resistance is most apparent when patients who originally showed a good response to a first course of chemotherapy have a much reduced or no response to the same therapy when given for recurrent disease. Drug resistance in cultured tumour cells can be induced by repeated treatments for most drug types. In some cases this leads to 100-fold larger drug dose being required for the

Table 17.4   Rationales for cytotoxic drug combinations

Rationale:		Example:
1.	Non–overlapping toxicities	–	cisplatin (kidney) + 5–FU (bone marrow)
2.	Different mechanisms	–	antimetabolite + alkylating agent
3.	Biochemical complementation	–	inhibition of 2 enzymes on same or converging pathway
4.	Potentiation of uptake	–	amphotericin B + alkylating agents
5.	Separate subpopulations	–	cycling + non–cycling; oxic + hypoxic

same level of cell killing. In contrast, it is usually impossible to induce radiation resistance in the laboratory by repeated radiation exposures.

Many causes of induced drug resistance have been elucidated, including reduced drug uptake, decreased activation, and increased inactivation (Figure 17.5). Examples of the types of resistance found with some drugs are listed in Table 17.5. Some drugs elicit *multidrug resistance (MDR)*, in which resistance induced to one drug results in cross-resistance to a group of others. The mechanism usually involves production by the resistant cells of higher levels of a membrane p-glycoprotein which is involved in the active efflux of drugs from the cell. Adriamycin and VP16 belong to the class of agents that elicit MDR. It is now recognized that there are other forms of multidrug resistance not involving p-glycoprotein.

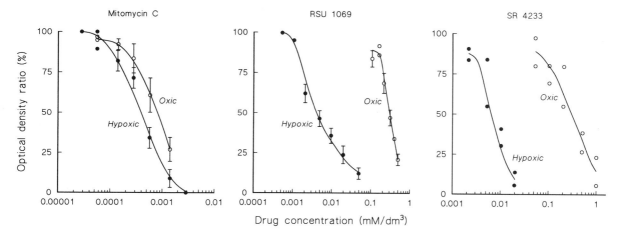

Figure 17.4 Dose-effect curves for V79 cells treated under oxic or hypoxic conditions with three different cytotoxic agents. The vertical axis is optical density of cell cultures, a measure of surviving fraction. Redrawn from Stratford and Stephens (1989), with permission.

Table 17.5 Probable mechanisms associated with resistance to commonly used anticancer drugs

Mechanism	Drugs
Increased proficiency of repair of DNA	cisplatin, cyclophosphamide, melphalan, mitomycin C, nitrogen mustard, nitrosoureas
Decrease cellular uptake, or increase in drug efflux	Act D, ADM, daunomycin, melphalan, 6–mercaptopurine, methotrexate, nitrogen mustard, vincristine, vinblastine
Increased level of 'target' enzyme	methotrexate
Alterations in 'target' enzyme	5–FU, 6–mercaptopurine, methotrexate, 6–thioguanine
Decreased drug activation	cytosine arabinoside, ADM, 5–FU, 6–mercaptopurine, 6–thioguanine
Increased drug degradation	bleomycin, cytosine arabinoside, 6–mercaptopurine
Alternative biochemical pathways	cytosine arabinoside

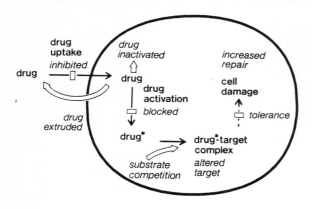

Figure 17.5 Mechanisms of drug resistance. From Borst (1991), with permission.

Pharmacological Resistance

One cause of inherent resistance is inadequate penetration of drug within tumours, leaving pharmacological sanctuaries or 'cold spots', where drug concentrations are low and insufficient to cause cell killing. Figure 17.6 shows a multicellular tumour spheroid grown in culture and treated with adriamycin. Fluorescence from the drug is limited to the outer cell layers, leaving a large fraction of clonogenic inner spheroid cells relatively untouched. Similar patterns of heterogeneity in drug distribution can be expected in solid tumours *in vivo*.

17.6 Drug targeting

Failure to achieve adequate tumour drug concentrations is a major reason for failure with chemotherapy. To simultaneously increase tumour drug concentrations and reduce normal-tissue drug levels is therefore an important objective. Drug targeting to the tumour is one way of achieving this and Table 17.6 lists several methods which

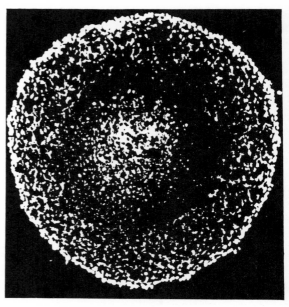

Figure 17.6 A multicellular spheroid that has been exposed to adriamycin and then examined under UV light. The outer layer of cells shows intense fluorescence, which declines with distance into the spheroid. Non-specific fluorescence is also visible in the necrotic central region. From Sutherland *et al* (1979), with permission.

attempt to do this. So far, most of these methods can be applied in limited situations only. The development of toxic monoclonal antibodies is often limited by poor access into solid tumours, breakdown of the antibody, and by the difficulty of finding an antibody that binds to *all* clonogenic tumour cells but not to critical normal tissues. Liposomes or microspheres must be trapped to a high level in the specific tumour under treatment; they must not bind the drug too tightly or too loosely which would result in no release or premature release of drug. Intratumoural injection is a crude approach to drug delivery that can only be applied to accessible tumour foci. Approaches such as these are being tackled by many labora-

Table 17.6 Drug targeting methods

1.	Regional chemotherapy	–	arterial perfusion, i.p. chemotherapy
2.	Liposomes	–	containing drugs such as adriamycin
3.	Microspheres	–	albumin or polymers + cisplatin
4.	Monoclonal antibodies	–	bound to a toxin such as ricin
5.	Intratumoural injection	–	of cisplatin, radiosensitizers, etc.

tories although they have yet to lead to major treatment successes and widespread use.

17.7 The therapeutic significance of tumour regression

Responses to chemotherapy in the clinic are often measured and reported as partial and complete regressions. As indicated in Section 5.6, it is important to appreciate the amount of killing necessary to achieve marked regression compared with the total killing necessary to achieve cure. Killing 3 logs of tumour cells may result in a *complete response (CR)*, despite the presence of 8–9 logs of cells which remain to be killed and which will in all probability lead to tumour recurrence (Figure 17.7). This figure is the chemotherapy counterpart of Figure 2.8. It illustrates the concept of complete remission and the later development of induced drug resistance. Success and failure in cancer chemotherapy often depend on the killing of a small residual minority of clonogenic tumour cells (say 10^6 per tumour), cells whose biological characteristics and drug-sensitivity may differ from the rest of the cells that are successfully killed.

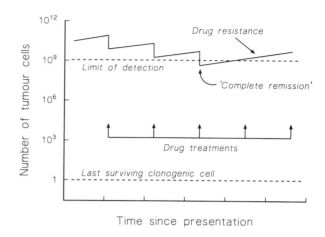

Figure 17.7 The response of a tumour to repeated courses of chemotherapy, followed by the development of drug resistance.

Key points

1. The primary role of chemotherapy at present is as an adjuvant therapy. It is successful as a single modality only in a few disease sites.
2. Inherent and induced drug resistance are common causes of treatment failure and they arise from a variety of causes. Induced resistance to radiation is rare, although inherent resistance can often limit tumour response.
3. Complete and partial regressions are frequently observed following chemotherapy, but are often followed by relapse. These responses are consistent with 2–3 decades of tumour cell killing but usually less than the 9 or more decades required for long-term tumour control.
4. For chemotherapy to become a more powerful modality, tumour specificity must be significantly increased and effective ways to combat drug resistance must be found.

Bibliography

Bruce WR, Meeker BE and Valeriote FA (1966). Comparison of the sensitivity of normal haemopoietic and transplanted lymphoma colony-forming cells to chemotherapeutic agents administered *in vivo*. *J Nat Cancer Inst* 37:233-245.

Stratford IJ and Stephens MA (1989). The differential hypoxic toxicity of bioreductive drugs determined *in vitro* by the MTT assay. *Int J Radiat Oncol Biol Phys* 16:973-976.

Sutherland RM, Eddy HA, Bareham B *et al* (1979). Resistance to adriamycin in multicellular spheroids. *Int J Radiat Oncol Biol Phys* 5:1225-1230.

van Putten LM (1974). Are cell kinetic data relevant for the design of tumour chemotherapy schedules? *Cell Tissue Kinet* 7:493-504.

Further reading

Borst P (1991). Genetic mechanisms of drug resistance. *Acta Oncol* 30:87-105.
Fox BW and Fox M (Eds) (1984). *Antitumor Drug Resistance*. Springer Verlag; Berlin.

Goldie JH and Coldman AJ (1984). The genetic origin of drug resistance: implications for systemic therapy. *Cancer Res* 44:3643-3653.
Humphrey RM and Barranco SC (1975). *Pharmacological Basis of Cancer Chemotherapy*. p95. Williams & Wilkins; Baltimore.
Kartner N and Ling V (1989). Multidrug resistance in cancer. *Scientific American* 260:26-33.
Tannock IF and Hill RP (Eds) (1987). *The Basic Science of Oncology*. Pergamon Press; New York, chapters 17-19.

18

Combination of radiotherapy and chemotherapy

G. Gordon Steel

18.1 The objectives of combined modality therapy

The biological problems presented by combined modality therapy are considerable. Radiotherapy by itself induces complex changes both in tumours and in the adjacent normal tissues and in spite of decades of intensive research into radiation biology it is still not possible to explain precisely why radiotherapy succeeds in some cases and not in others. The response to chemotherapy is similarly complex: in addition to many of the factors that determine response to radiation treatment we also have problems of drug delivery, drug resistance, and metabolism (Chapter 17). The combination of radiotherapy and chemotherapy involves the combined complexity of *both* modalities, plus the interactions between them. This chapter seeks to provide a framework within which these processes can be examined. In general, what we seek is an improved therapeutic strategy, which may be defined as follows.

An Improved Therapeutic Strategy:

A combination of drugs and radiation that gives a greater tumour response than either of the component single agents, the combination and single-agent treatments being evaluated at a comparable level of overall toxicity.

This definition is illustrated by Figure 1.4. In experimental animals it is practicable to obtain dose-response curves for effects on tumours and on dose-limiting normal tissues. Using these dose-response curves it is possible to identify an improved therapy quite reliably. In clinical studies it is usually impracticable to examine dose-response curves over the range of responses used in experimental animals, although Figure 12.3 is an example. Restrictions on the size of clinical trials also limit the number of dose and treatment groups that can be compared simultaneously.

The strategy outlined in Figure 18.1 is the minimum scale of study necessary to show a therapeutic gain and to answer the question: Could an observed gain in tumour control by combined modality therapy also have been obtained merely by increasing the radiation dose? A three-arm trial is envisaged, with two radiation doses (D_1 and D_2), the third arm consisting of the lower radiation dose plus chemotherapy. By 'dose' we here mean some measure of intensity of fractionated radiation treatment, for instance the total radiation dose. We also assume that 'toxicity' can be ascribed a numerical value, plotted on the vertical scale; this is a gross over-simplification, for as will be indicated below the addition of chemotherapy may not only enhance radiation-induced damage but will almost certainly introduce new toxicities as well. The toxicity of the combined arm is equivalent to a radiation dose X (lower panel). The tumour response that could have been *expected* from this dose (alone) can be found by interpolation as shown by the broken lines. If the *actual* tumour response is greater than this, then a therapeutic gain has been identified. Whether this gain is significantly different from zero will depend on the precision of all six experimental points in this analysis (three tumour, three toxicity). Clearly, to achieve sufficient precision will require a very large clinical trial. But if this cannot be done, or if this minimum three-arm study cannot be performed, then the *existence* of a therapeutic gain will be in doubt.

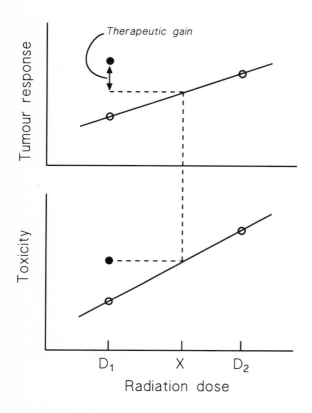

Figure 18.1　Scheme for the identification of an improved therapeutic strategy, in clinical research (see text).

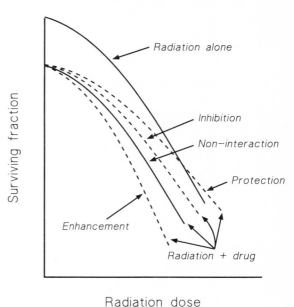

Figure 18.2　A terminology for the description of interactive processes between a cytotoxic drug and radiation. From Steel (1979), with permission.

steepened, then this may be called *enhancement* of response; if it is made shallower, this is *inhibition*, and in the extreme case where the combination gives less effect than radiation alone, this is *protection*. For the reasons outlined below we avoid the use of the ambiguous terms *synergism* or *additive*.

The Concept of Interactive and Non-interactive Combinations

This distinction is central to the discussion of biological mechanisms in combined modality treatment. *Non-interactive* describes a situation where each modality appears to exert its own individual effect; *interactive* refers to a situation where there is evidence that one modality modifies the effect of the other.

A suggested terminology of interactive processes is described in Figure 18.2. If the result of adding a cytotoxic drug is to move the dose-response curve for radiation alone without changing its shape, then the combination is *non-interactive*. If the radiation dose-response curve is

18.2　Exploitable mechanisms in the combination of radiotherapy and chemotherapy

The processes that may lead to a therapeutic gain can be described under four headings (Steel and Peckham, 1979).

Spatial Cooperation

This term describes the use of radiotherapy and chemotherapy to hit disease in different anatomical sites. The commonest situation is where radiation is used to treat the primary tumour and chemotherapy is added as an adjuvant to deal with systemic spread (Figure 18.3). There is an analogous situation in the leukaemias where chemotherapy is the main-line treatment and radiotherapy is brought in to deal with disease in a 'seclusion site' such as the brain.

This is an important aspect of combined modality treatment and there is some evidence for its practical efficacy (Rosen *et al*, 1974; Bleyer and Poplack, 1985). But it should be stressed that this combined use of drugs and radiation envisages no *interaction* between them: the two modalities are used separately to treat disease in spatially different anatomical locations. The optimum clinical approach will be to give the best radiotherapy and the best chemotherapy, seeking to *avoid* interactions between them.

The successful exploitation of spatial cooperation depends critically on the effectiveness of the available chemotherapy. As an illustration of this, consider a situation in which a small amount of disease has spread outside the radiation field. Radiotherapy alone will fail. If only 0.1g of tumour is missed by radiation this could contain 10^8 cells of which upwards of 10^6 might be clonogenic. Current evidence (Tannock, 1989) suggests that in the common solid tumours chemotherapy seldom achieves a surviving fraction of 10^{-6} and in those cases this adjuvant use of chemotherapy will fail even to control this very small amount of disseminated disease. For spatial cooperation to succeed more widely we need better drugs.

Independent Cell Kill

This term describes the simple concept that if two therapeutic modalities can both be given at full dose, then *even in the absence of interactive processes* the tumour response should be greater than that achieved with either alone.

For the hypothetical example of treatment of a lung tumour, Table 18.1 illustrates the idea behind this approach. Radiation produces a $(+++)$ tumour response and is limited (for example) by radiation pneumonitis. Chemotherapy also produces a tumour response $(++)$ but is limited by intestinal or bone marrow damage. Even if the antitumour effects of these two treatments are *subadditive* $(++++$ instead of the expected $+++++)$ the overall antitumour effect may well be greater than either drug or radiation alone. Clearly, *any* extra tumour response produced by the chemotherapy will improve on radiation alone. The cost of this advantage is that the patient has to tolerate a wider range of toxic reactions and a critical factor in the reasoning is the assumption that radiation lung damage is not enhanced by the addition of chemotherapy (still $+++$ for lung toxicity). If this is not the case and lung damage is increased, then to maintain an iso-toxic treatment the radiation dose would have to be reduced and this might well lead to the loss of the extra small gain in tumour response. In order to exploit *independent cell kill* successfully it is thus vital to select effective antitumour drugs that do not exacerbate radiation damage to critical normal tissues within the radiation field.

Table 18.1 Concept of independent toxicity leading to simple addition of antitumour effects as a mechanism in combined modality therapy

	Associated toxicity			Response of bronchial tumour
	Intestinal	Bone marrow	Lung	
Drug	+++	+	−	++
Combination	+++	+	+++	++++

To what extent is it possible to find effective chemotherapy that does not make radiation-induced normal-tissue damage worse? There is a large experimental literature on this, including some important reviews (Phillips and Fu, 1976; von der Maase, 1986; Steel, 1988). The extent to which chemotherapy enhances radiation damage varies widely among drugs and among the normal tissues studied. In some cases there is little or no

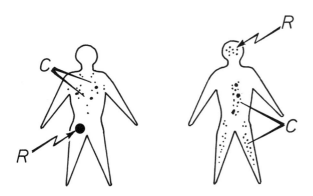

Figure 18.3 The concept of spatial cooperation. R = radiotherapy; C = chemotherapy.

enhancement; in others there is severe enhancement and radiation dose would have to be reduced by up to perhaps 50 per cent to keep the toxicity the same. The guidelines given by Phillips and Fu are probably still useful:

(i)   beware of the cytotoxic antibiotics (actinomycin, bleomycin, adriamycin) which enhance radiation damage in a variety of tissues;

(ii) beware of drugs that have a recognized toxicity to the tissues that are being irradiated (examples are cyclophosphamide in the lung, and various proliferation-dependent agents in the intestine);

(iii) avoid *concurrent* treatment with drugs and radiation (see below).

Most of the evidence for drug-induced enhancement of radiation toxicity has concentrated on early-responding normal tissues and there are few experimental studies on the enhancement of late reactions. If interactions are mediated by effects on cell proliferation, then they may be less prominent in late-responding tissues. But it would be a mistake to depend upon this, as evidenced by the enhancement of spinal cord damage in the rat when intravenous methotrexate was used with irradiation (van der Kogel and Sissingh, 1985).

Independent cell kill is an obvious and promising way in which chemotherapy may improve on the results of radiotherapy alone. Note that, as with *spatial cooperation*, this mechanism does not require interactive processes between drugs and radiation: in fact in critical normal tissues these are specifically to be avoided in order to retain tolerance to radiotherapy.

Protection of Normal Tissues

We now move to strategies in combined modality therapy that *do require* interaction, as defined above. First, can we identify chemotherapeutic drugs that, when used in conjunction with radiation, reduce the damage to dose-limiting normal tissues? This would seem unlikely, for two toxic agents usually tend to produce more damage than either alone. However, there are well-documented situations in experimental animals in which certain cytotoxic drugs increase the resistance of normal tissues to radiation or to a second cytotoxic treatment. W.W. Smith observed this with colchicine and the vinca alkaloids over 30 years ago, and Millar *et*

al (1978) studied this phenomenon in detail. Cyclophosphamide, cytosine arabinoside, chlorambucil and methotrexate were found to be effective radioprotective agents. An important characteristic of this phenomenon is its dependence upon timing. Maximal radioprotection of animal survival was achieved when cytosine arabinoside was given 2 days before irradiation but the optimum gap for cyclophosphamide was 3 days. A similar protection phenomenon has been found in which a priming treatment with one cytotoxic drug can protect against a large dose of another (Millar and McElwain, 1978).

Studies of the mechanism of this remarkable phenomenon have concentrated upon the bone marrow and intestinal epithelium. In the marrow it has been shown that the most effective of the 'protective' agents, cytosine arabinoside, did not modify stem-cell radiosensitivity; it stimulated enhanced repopulation by surviving stem cells. In the small intestine (Phelps and Blackett, 1979), microcolony survival experiments have shown that cytosine arabinoside given 12 hours before irradiation greatly increased the survival of intestinal stem cells, perhaps by enhancing the repair of radiation damage.

Although attempts have been made to exploit this phenomenon in high-dose combination chemotherapy (Hedley *et al*, 1978), its critical dependence on timing has precluded its exploitation in fractionated radiotherapy.

Enhancement of Tumour Response: the Concept of Supra-additivity

This is often perceived to be the principal aim of adding chemotherapy to radiotherapy. Is it possible to obtain a greater tumour response than would be expected on the basis of simple addition of antitumour effects? This is, both conceptually and experimentally, a very difficult problem. If dose-response curves are linear, the additivity of two agents has a simple and unique meaning. When, as is usually the case in cancer therapy, dose-response curves are far from linear, the nature of an additive response is controversial.

It has been argued (Steel and Peckham, 1979) that when dose-response curves are non-linear there is no unique description of an additive response. Take, for example, the dose-response curve shown in Figure 18.4. The dose D gives an effect E_1. On the assumption of *additivity* we would expect that if we give two such doses at the same time (dose *2D*) we would get twice the effect: *2E₁*. In fact, it can be seen from the dose-response curve that a dose *2D* actually gives an effect *E₂*. There is an apparent *supra-additive* effect equal to (E_2-2E_1). Such a result is therapeutically uninteresting: it derives purely from the shape of the survival curve. If one of the two doses were in fact a cytotoxic drug, what we wish to know is whether the response is *greater than E_2*, which would be an interesting case of synergism. This example illustrates the fact that when dose-response curves are non-linear great care is needed in the description of additivity; there is an area of uncertainty whose magnitude depends upon the non-linearity of the responses. The extent of the uncertainty is best judged by the use of an isobologram (Figure 18.5). This is an iso-effect plot which indicates the separate doses of two agents that in combination (using any chosen timing) give the iso-effect. The lines in

Figure 18.5 enclose the range of situations which *under some assumed analysis of the dose-response curves* might be regarded as additive (Steel and Peckham, 1979). Only a combination that gives an experimental point to the left of this boundary can confidently be described as *supra-additive*. The 'envelope of additivity' in this diagram should not be regarded as a new and more reliable definition of additivity: it is an expression of the *uncertainty* in this concept.

18.3 Possible mechanisms leading to interactions between the effects of drugs and radiation

A wide variety of biological mechanisms have been proposed to explain interactive processes between radiation and cytotoxic drugs. Some of these are as follows:

Inhibition of Repair of Radiation Damage

Many drugs have the property of inhibiting the repair of radiation damage (Kelland and Steel, 1988a). Some of these are antimetabolites that are of no interest as cytotoxic agents in their own right (3-aminobenzamide, cordycepin, caffeine, etc). Others have been used as anti-cancer agents (actinomycin-D, adriamycin, hydroxyurea, Ara-C, *cis*-platinum, etc). All of these agents are cytotoxic at sufficiently high drug concentrations. For experimental studies on repair inhibition it is usual to choose a non-toxic drug dose in order to simplify the analysis. In clinical treatment this is clearly unnecessary: provided the drug has some beneficial anticancer effect in its own right it will probably be best to employ it in high dose. Repair inhibition has been detected in a number of ways: removal of the shoulder on the cell survival curve, inhibition of split-dose recovery, inhibition of delayed-plating recovery, etc. Sensitization has been detected at low radiation doses and at low dose rate (Kelland and Steel, 1988b) which is of considerable therapeutic interest. However, there is little evidence so far that *selectivity* for effects on tumours rather than on normal tissues can be achieved. It must be borne in mind that as a result of local ischaemia, the tissue levels of a systemically administered drug are often

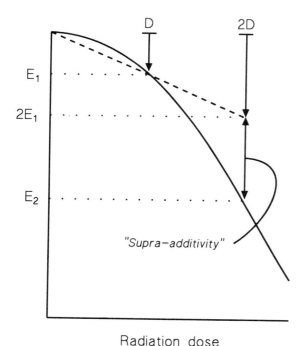

Figure 18.4 A non-linear dose-response curve can give a spurious impression of supra-additivity. In this example (two simultaneous doses of radiation given to mammalian cells in tissue-culture) the effect plotted on the ordinate is log(surviving fraction).

lower in tumours, or in parts of tumours, than in normal tissues, which *depend for their tolerance of radiation on their ability to repair*. Selectivity is therefore essential.

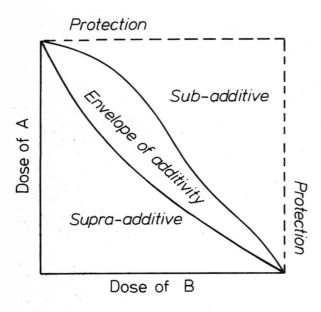

Figure 18.5 An isobologram is an isoeffect plot of the doses of two agents that together give a fixed biological effect. If dose-response curves are non-linear, there is a region of uncertainty about the existence of 'additivity'. From Steel and Peckham (1979), with permission.

Cell Synchronization

Many cytotoxic drugs show some degree of selectivity in killing cells at certain phases of the cell cycle (Mauro and Madoc-Jones, 1970; Table 17.2). Some agents show maximum effect on cells that are undergoing DNA synthesis. Radiation also has a cell-cycle dependence, often with peaks of *resistance* in the S-phase and in G_1 (Section 5.8). There is therefore an attractive possibility of complementary action between drugs and radiation. As has been found with kinetically optimized drug-drug combinations, it is unfortunately the case that this approach to synergism only works well with rapidly cycling cells. Positive effects have been found in cell cultures and fast-growing experimental tumours but the existence of slowly growing or resting cells in human tumours could

possibly explain why synchronization therapy has been disappointing (Tubiana *et al*, 1975; Tannock, 1989).

Recruitment

It follows from the above that response to therapy might be improved if non-proliferating cells could be stimulated to come into cycle. This has mainly been explored in combination chemotherapy. There is evidence (reviewed by Steel, 1977) that the growth fraction of some experimental tumours is increased by a suitable priming treatment. The resulting therapeutic benefit has not been large. There is also an academic point that tumours consist of dynamic cell populations and the non-dividing cells probably have a limited life-span; as a result, if the growth fraction rises after treatment this may not indicate that some non-proliferating cells have begun to cycle but rather that the rate of production of non-proliferating cells has been reduced (i.e. a lower rate of decycling). If so, this response is still therapeutically useful, but *recruitment* is a misleading term for it.

Enhanced Repopulation

Any effective cytotoxic treatment reduces the total number of viable tumour cells and, per-haps by improving the nutritional status of the remainder, may lead to accelerated repopulation (Section 9.3). In the combined modality situation it is logical to use radiation to debulk the tumour and then seek to use proliferation-specific drugs to exploit the kinetic response. There is some evidence that chemotherapy given a few days after radiotherapy does lead to greater effects on experimental tumours (Steel, 1988). Unfortunately, this strategy is also the most damaging to normal tissues that repopulate rapidly after irradiation.

It has also been suggested that enhanced repopulation may lead to a therapeutic *detriment* in combined modality therapy (Withers *et al*, 1988). If chemotherapy is given first it may switch on repopulation during a subsequent course of radiotherapy and thereby reduce its effectiveness.

Reduction of the Hypoxic Fraction

The debulking of a tumour by chemotherapy might lead to a reduction in the hypoxic fraction and improved response to radiotherapy. Although this has been postulated, there is little evidence for benefit being achieved in this way. It is also possible that the first few fractions of a course of radiation treatment will have a similar effect, which is the well-known phenomenon of reoxygenation (Section 14.4).

Debulking

This is probably the most promising basis for expecting a benefit from combined chemotherapy/radiotherapy. A tumour that has shrunk in response to one treatment may more easily be cured by a second, purely because there are fewer cells to be killed. In simple terms, this is what has been described above as *independent cell kill* and should not be confused with synergism. Debulking may also lead to improved oxygen supply or increased proliferation which, as indicated above, may lead to greater cell kill from subsequent radiotherapy. More promising, however, is the possibility that debulking by chemotherapy may allow the field size of subsequent radiotherapy to be reduced and the dose thus to be increased.

18.4 Time dependence of interactive effects between drugs and radiation

The mechanisms described in the previous section are widely varied, difficult to relate to actual therapeutic response, and in some cases hypothetical. The *time-line method* is an experimental approach that cuts through these difficulties. It is basically an empirical search for the optimum treatment with two agents. It can be applied to tumours or normal tissues in experimental animals, also to cells in tissue culture. The method was first described by Vietti *et al* (1971). Using mouse leukaemic cells growing *in vivo*, they selected fixed doses of 5-fluorouracil and radiation, then gave them both to groups of mice, changing only the time interval between them (Figure 18.6). In each group of mice they measured the survival of leukaemic cells, termed CFU in the figure. The data described an intricate response curve, with minimum CFU survival when 5-fluorouracil was given up to 8 hours *after* radiation. When the interval between the treatments (in either order) was over 40 hours, the level of cell kill was close to what would be

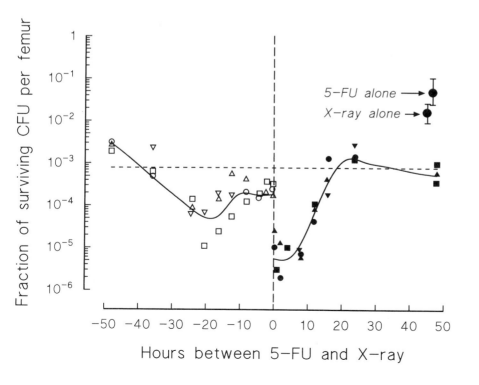

Figure 18.6 A time-line for the interaction of 5-fluorouracil (5-FU) and x-radiation in the treatment of mouse leukaemia. Radiation was given at time zero; points to the left of zero are for drug before radiation; points to the right are for drug after radiation. From Vietti *et al* (1971), with permission.

expected by adding the log cell kill from the separate treatments. The form of this time-line has not been fully explained but from a thera-peutic point of view its implications are obvious: it allows the optimum timing of the treatments to be identified.

Three further examples of time-line experi-ments are shown in Figure 18.7. Panel A shows a time-line for the interaction of cyclophosphamide and pelvic irradiation in mice. Radiation was given at time zero; each experimental point derives from a group of mice that were given cyclophosphamide (200 mg/kg) at some time up to 4 weeks before or 4 weeks after irradiation. Various radiation doses were used in order to derive the dose-enhancement factor (DEF: the ratio of radiation dose without drug to the radiation dose with drug, to give a fixed level of radiation damage). A DEF of 1.0 indicates no enhancement of radiation damage as a result of giving the drug. When DEF = 1.2, the radiation dose in the presence of the drug would have to be reduced by 17% (1/1.2 = 0.83) to produce the same amount of damage as with radiation alone. In this example there is massive enhancement of intestinal damage as a result of drug treatment. The peak DEF is 1.5 for cyclophosphamide given 3 days after irradiation. When the time interval between drug and radiation (or *vice versa*) was increased to 4 weeks, there was little enhancement of damage: the effect of the first treatment seems to have been forgotten. The minimum in DEF seen at -2 days is interesting. This may well reflect the protection phenomenon referred to in Section 18.2; in this case there is no protection (DEF > 1.0) but in the absence of this effect the DEF would have been around 1.3.

Figure 18.7B, from the same study, shows the results with three further chemotherapeutic agents. They gave similar responses: no enhance-ment of damage for drug given more than 5 days before radiation, a peak at +3 days, and a tendency to return towards no effect for drug given 14 days after irradiation.

Figure 18.7C is a rare example of a clinical time-line. This reports experience at the Royal Marsden Hospital (1976-1981) in treating testicu-lar teratomas with combination chemotherapy (VB, PVB, or BEP) together with radiation (Yarnold *et al*, 1983). Normal-tissue damage was scored as the percentage of patients with subcutaneous fibrosis or gastrointestinal damage. The group that were treated with chemotherapy

approximately 3 months after irradiation showed a high probability of damage and although the time-scale differs between man and mouse, the form of the time-line is roughly similar to those shown in the other two panels.

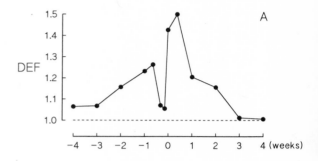

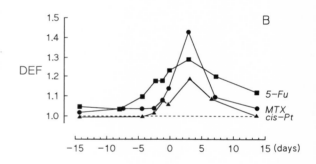

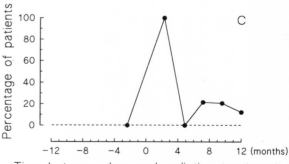

Time between drug and radiation treatment

Figure 18.7 A: time-line for the interaction of cyclophosphamide (200mg/kg) and pelvic irradiation in mice. B: time-lines for the interaction of 5-fluorouracil, methotrexate, or *cis*-platinum and pelvic irradiation in mice. C: time-line for normal-tissue damage in patients treated for testicular teratoma with radiation and combination chemo-therapy. A and B from Pearson and Steel (1984); C from Yarnold *et al* (1983), with permission.

The time-line approach has been used extensively in studies on normal-tissue damage in mice (von der Maase, 1986; reviewed by Steel, 1988). The broad picture is that there is great variation in the enhancement of normal-tissue damage, but most chemotherapeutic drugs enhance damage in some normal tissue for some particular timing. Short time intervals between drugs and radiation most frequently lead to maximum damage. Increasing the time interval tends to reduce the interaction. There are some drugs, of which *cis*-platinum is an example (Figure 18.7B), for which no enhancement of damage occurs provided the time intervals are chosen carefully.

Most of the experimental experience with the time-line approach applied to normal-tissue damage has been with early-reacting tissues. Although one might anticipate that time-dependent phenomena would be less marked in late-reacting normal tissues, this is not the case in the mouse lung (Collis and Steel, 1983) nor in the spinal cord (van der Kogel and Sissingh, 1985) where proliferation-dependent cytotoxic drugs significantly enhance radiation damage. Table 18.2 summarises the results of two research groups in studying the enhancement by chemotherapy of lung damage in mice. It illustrates the large differences in enhancement due to different drugs, with cyclophosphamide and the cytotoxic antibiotics at the top of the list. The interactions fall off with increasing time between treatments, in either sequence.

The time-line method has also been applied in the search for the optimum timing of combined modality treatment in transplanted mouse tumours. It has not been possible to examine long time intervals between drug and radiation because of the rapid growth of these tumours. Overall, the results do not encourage the attempt to exploit time-dependent phenomena in the combined modality treatment of cancer: a peak of tumour response has seldom been seen and when a peak is seen in one tumour system it has not been confirmed in others (Steel, 1988).

The overall conclusion of these studies is therefore disappointing: time-dependent interactions

Table 18.2 Lung damage in mice as a result of combined treatment with radiation and drugs

Drug	Drug administration[a]			Source[b]
	Before	**Concurrent**	**After**	
Cyclophosphamide	+ +	+ + +	+ +	C
	−	+ + +	−	M
Bleomycin	+ +	+ +	+ +	C
	−	+ + +	−	M
	+ +			S
Adriamycin	−	+ + +	+ +	C
	−	+ + +	−	M
	+			S
Actinomycin D	−	+		C
	+			S
Methotrexate	+	−	−	C
	−	−	−	M
	−			S
5–Fluorouracil	−	−	−	M
Vincristine	+	+	+	C
CCNU	−	−	+	C
cis–Platinum	−	−	−	C
	−	−	−	M
Mitomycin C	−	+	−	M

+ + +, severe enhancement of lung damage; + + moderate enhancement; + slight enhancement (doubtful significance);–no enhancement.

[a] Before = 7–28 days before radiation; after = 7–28 days after radiation.

[b] C = Collis (1981), Collis and Steel (1983); M = von der Maase (1986); S = Steel *et al* (1979).

are more commonly seen in the normal tissues of experimental animals than in experimental tumours. The take-home message for the 'mouse radiotherapist' is thus to avoid short time intervals between drugs and radiation; by doing so it will be possible to keep the drug and radiation doses high and thus to gain maximum benefit from *spatial cooperation* and *independent cell kill*.

18.5   The good news and the bad news

The four mechanisms in combined modality therapy that have been described here differ in their exploitability, both in laboratory and clinical studies. Table 18.3 is an attempt to summarize the general picture. *Spatial cooperation* and *independent cell kill* can easily be demonstrated in experimental animals. We have shown, for instance, that if Lewis lung tumours are implanted into the legs of mice and allowed to grow to a measurable size, the local tumour can be cured with high probability by irradiation (Steel *et al*, 1978); most of the mice, however, die of disseminated disease. Cyclophosphamide is very effective against this tumour, and when given in conjunction with local irradiation of the implant leads to cures in a high proportion of the

mice. Increased cure and increased growth delay in primary implants as a result of *independent cell kill* by cytotoxic drugs and radiation also have been observed widely. Evidence has been cited above for the observation in mice of the phenomenon of protection of normal-tissue damage. In spite of the described difficulties in identifying supra-additive tumour responses, some examples of this do exist.

In clinical studies, the gains from adding chemotherapy to radiotherapy have been small and the scope for identifying mechanisms of improvement is therefore limited (Tannock, 1989; Tubiana, 1989). Those gains that have been made can be attributed either to *spatial cooperation* or to *independent cell kill*. There appear to be no clinical results that require supra-additive effects on the tumours to be invoked for their explanation. We can therefore summarize the clinical picture by saying that where gains have so far been observed by adding drug therapy to radiotherapy they have come from direct cell killing (rather than interactive processes), either within the irradiated field or outside it.

This review of concepts that have come out of the extensive laboratory studies that have been made on combined modality therapy thus leads to 'good news' and 'bad news'. The good news is that clear therapeutic benefit can be obtained by adding chemotherapy to radiotherapy. The benefits are probably obtained by simple addition of the antitumour effects of drugs and radiation, either in the tissues that are irradiated or in *spatial cooperation* between effects on irradiated and non-irradiated disease. The benefits are probably proportional to the effectiveness of the chemotherapeutic drugs themselves. Only when these can achieve multi-decade tumour cell kill is there likely to be a detectable clinical benefit. The bad news is that the large amount of time and effort that has been put into identifying sophisticated mechanisms of synergism between drugs and radiation has so far failed to give useful clinical benefits.

Table 18.3 Summary of evidence for exploitation of four mechanisms in the combination of radiotherapy and chemotherapy

	Evidence in mice	Evidence in men
Spatial cooperation	+++	++
Independent cell kill	+++	+
Protection of normal tissues	++	–
Enhancement of tumour response	+	–

Key points

1. The processes by which the addition of chemotherapy to radiotherapy may lead to an improvement in therapeutic result may be classified as *interactive* or *non-interactive*.
2. Non-interactive processes include *spatial cooperation* and *independent cell kill*. These can be clearly demonstrated in experimental animals and are probably responsible for the gains that have so far been claimed for clinical combined modality therapy.
3. *Synergism* or *supra-additivity* is an intricate concept in the combined modality field; non-linear dose-response curves may give rise to spurious evidence for synergism.
4. Interactions between cytotoxic drugs and radiation tend often to be time-dependent. This is especially the case in normal tissues, less so in tumours. The evidence from studies on experimental animals is therefore that concurrent treatment is bad, in terms of therapeutic index. Longer time intervals between drugs and radiation (or *vice versa*) are safer, and still allow potential benefit from the non-interactive processes.

Bibliography

Bleyer WA and Poplack DG (1985). Prophylaxis and treatment of leukemia in the central nervous system and other sanctuaries. *Sem Oncol* 12:131-148.

Collis CH (1981). The response of the lung to ionizing radiation and cytotoxic drugs. Thesis, University of London.

Collis CH and Steel GG (1983). Lung damage in mice from cyclophosphamide and thoracic irradiation: the effect of timing. *Int J Radiat Oncol Biol Phys* 9:685-689.

Hedley DW, Millar JL, McElwain TJ and Gordon MY (1978). Acceleration of bone-marrow recovery by pre-treatment with cyclophosphamide in patients receiving high-dose melphalan. *Lancet* 4 November:966-967.

Kelland LR and Steel GG (1988a). Inhibition of recovery from damage induced by ionizing radiation in mammalian cells. *Radiother Oncol* 13:285-299.

Kelland LR and Steel GG (1988b). Modification of radiation dose-rate sparing effects in a human carcinoma of the cervix cell line by inhibitors of DNA repair. *Int J Radiat Biol* 54:229-244.

van der Kogel AJ and Sissingh HA (1985). Effects of intrathecal methotrexate and cytosine arabinoside on the radiation tolerance of the rat spinal cord. *Radiother Oncol* 4:239-251.

von der Maase H (1986). Experimental studies on interactions of radiation and cancer chemotherapeutic drugs in normal tissues and a solid tumour. *Radiother Oncol* 7:47-68.

Mauro F and Madoc-Jones H (1970). Age response of cultured mammalian cells to cytotoxic drugs. *Cancer Res* 30:1397-1408.

Millar JL, Blackett NM and Hudspith BN (1978). Enhanced post-irradiation recovery of the haemopoietic system in animals pretreated with a variety of cytotoxic agents. *Cell Tissue Kinet* 11:543-553.

Millar JL and McElwain TJ (1978). Combinations of cytotoxic agents that have less than expected toxicity on normal tissues in mice. In: *Antibiotics and Chemotherapy*, pp. 271-282. (Ed) Schonfeld H. Karger; Basel.

Pearson AE and Steel GG (1984). Chemotherapy in combination with pelvic irradiation: A time dependence study in mice. *Radiother Oncol* 2:49-55.

Phelps TA and Blackett NM (1979). Protection of intestinal damage by pretreatment with cytarabine (cytosine arabinoside). *Int J Radiat Oncol Biol Phys* 5:1617-1620.

Rosen G, Wollner N, Wu SJ *et al* (1974). Disease-free survival in children with Ewing's sarcoma treated with radiation therapy and adjuvant four-drug sequential chemotherapy. *Cancer* 33:384-393.

Steel GG (1977). *The Growth Kinetics of Tumours*. Oxford University Press; Oxford.

Steel GG (1979). Terminology in the description of drug-radiation interactions. *Int J Radiat*

Oncol Biol Phys 5:1145-1150.

Steel GG, Adams K and Peckham MJ (1979). Lung damage in C57Bl mice following thoracic irradiation: enhancement by chemotherapy. *Br J Radiol* 52:741-747.

Steel GG, Hill RP and Peckham MJ (1978). Combined radiotherapy-chemotherapy of Lewis lung carcinoma. *Int J Radiat Oncol Biol Phys* 4:49-52.

Tubiana M, Frindel E and Vassort F (1975). Critical survey of experimental data on *in vivo* synchronisation by hydroxyurea. In: *Recent Results in Cancer Research* (Eds) Grundman E and Groos R, pp. 187-205. Springer-Verlag; Berlin.

Vietti T, Eggerding F and Valeriote F (1971). Combined effect of x-radiation and 5-fluorouracil on survival of transplanted leukemic cells. *J Nat Cancer Inst* 47:865-870.

Withers HR, Taylor JMG and Maciejewski B (1988). The hazard of accelerated tumor clonogen repopulation during radiotherapy. *Acta Oncol* 27:131-146.

Yarnold JR, Horwich A, Duchesne G *et al* (1983). Chemotherapy and radiotherapy for advanced testicular non-seminoma. *Radiother Oncol* 1:91-99.

Further reading

Phillips T and Fu KK (1976). Quantification of combined radiation therapy and chemotherapy effects on critical normal tissues. *Cancer* 37:1186-1200.

Steel GG (1988). The search for therapeutic gain in the combination of radiotherapy and chemotherapy. *Radiother Oncol* 11:31-53.

Steel GG and Peckham MJ (1979). Exploitable mechanisms in combined radiotherapy-chemotherapy: The concept of additivity. *Int J Radiat Oncol Biol Phys* 5:85-91.

Tannock IF (1989). Combined modality treatment with radiotherapy and chemotherapy. *Radiother Oncol* 16:83-101.

Tubiana M (1989). The combination of radiotherapy and chemotherapy: a review. *Int J Radiat Biol* 55:497-511.

19

Overcoming hypoxic cell radio-resistance

Jens Overgaard and Michael R. Horsman

19.1 Introduction

There are two principal ways to overcome the radiobiological problem of tumour hypoxia: by increasing the delivery of oxygen or oxygen-mimicking agents to the cells, or by exploiting the special environmental conditions of hypoxic cells using agents that exercise their toxicity under those conditions. The first approach has been applied in radiotherapy by use of hyperbaric or normobaric oxygen, by attempts to increase blood flow, or by the application of hypoxic cell radiosensitizers. Past experience has shown that even in tumours that have the same histology and degree of differentiation there may be substantial heterogeneity in hypoxia; thus, the identification of those tumours in which hypoxic radioresistance is a serious problem is currently a major goal of research. The second approach is illustrated by the use of bioreductive drugs or hyperthermia to destroy radioresistant hypoxic cells. This can be intensified by temporarily *increasing* the hypoxic state using agents such as hydralazine that *reduce* blood flow.

19.2 Hyperbaric oxygen

Following the identification of hypoxia as a potential source of tumour radioresistance, intensive efforts were made to overcome this problem especially by the use of hyperbaric oxygen therapy (Churchill-Davidson, 1968). Most trials were small and suffered from the use of unconventional fractionation schemes, but hyperbaric oxygen therapy did appear to be superior to radiotherapy given in air (Table 19.1), especially when

a few large fractions were applied (Overgaard, 1989). Whether this gain also occurs with conventional fractionation has been the subject of considerable debate. However, the largest multicentre clinical trials of hyperbaric oxygen (those by the British Medical Research Council, MRC) showed both in uterine cervix and in advanced head and neck cancer a significant benefit in local tumour control and in subsequent survival. The same was not observed in bladder cancer, nor was this result confirmed by a number of smaller studies (Dische, 1985; Overgaard, 1989). The exploration of hyperbaric oxygen therapy was discontinued partly because of problems with patient compliance and partly due to the introduction of chemical radiosensitizers; in retrospect this may have been somewhat premature.

19.3 Hypoxic cell radiosensitizers

The concept of chemical radiosensitization of hypoxic cells was introduced by Adams (1977) and his coworkers. The largest group of sensitizing agents are the electron-affinic radiosensitizers, so-called because their efficiency of sensitization is directly related to their electron affinity. The rationale for their use is that they diffuse out of the tumour blood supply and are absorbed by, and thus sensitize, distant hypoxic cells. In principle, these drugs mimic the sensitizing effect of oxygen and therefore do not increase the radiation response of well-oxygenated cells, for instance in surrounding normal tissues.

The first electron-affinic compounds to show radiosensitization were the nitro-benzenes. They were followed by the nitro-furans and finally

Table 19.1 Multicentre randomized trials with hyperbaric oxygen (HBO)

Site and reference	No. of patients	Endpoint	HBO		Air
Head and Neck Carcinoma					
MRC (1st trial) (Henk *et al*, 1977)	294	local-regional control (5 yrs)	53%	(p < 0.01)	30%
MRC (2nd trial) (Henk, 1986)	106	local-regional control (5 yrs)	60%	(p < 0.05)	41%
Uterine Cervix Carcinoma					
MRC (Watson *et al*, 1978)	320	local-regional control (5 yrs)	67%	(p < 0.001)	47%
Bronchogenic Carcinoma					
MRC (60 Gy/40 fx) (Cade and McEwen, 1978)	51	survival (2 yrs)	15%	(n.s.)	8%
MRC (36 Gy/6 fx) (Cade and McEwen, 1978)	123	survival (2 yrs)	25%	(p > 0.05)	12%
Carcinoma of the Bladder					
MRC (Cade *et al*, 1978)	241	survival (5 yrs)	28%	(n.s.)	30%

n.s. = not significant.
See Overgaard (1989) for references.

nitro-imidazoles, the most potent of which was found to be the 2-nitro-imidazole, *misonidazole*. Its *in vitro* activity is illustrated in Figure 19.1. Note that in these experiments misonidazole is radiation dose-modifying: the survival curves have the same extrapolation number (i.e. 4). The radiation response of hypoxic cells can thus be enhanced substantially by irradiating the cells in the presence of misonidazole. In fact, at a drug concentration of 10 mM the radiosensitivity of hypoxic cells approaches that of aerated cells. The response of the aerated cells is unaffected.

Radiosensitizers such as misonidazole also enhance radiation damage in experimental tumours *in vivo*, as shown in Figure 19.2. The magnitude of the sensitizing effect is usually expressed by the Sensitizer Enhancement Ratio (SER):

$$\text{Sensitizer Enhancement Ratio} = \frac{\text{Radiation dose } without \text{ sensitizer}}{\text{Radiation dose } with \text{ sensitizer}}$$

for the same biological effect. Large enhancement ratios (> 2.0) have been found in a variety of animal tumours following single-dose irradiation. Since the problem of tumour hypoxia increases with increasing fraction size, the benefits of radiosensitizers are clearest when tested by single-dose treatment. When misonidazole was

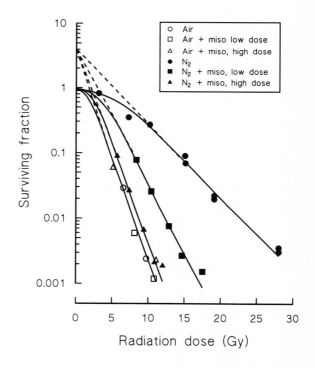

Figure 19.1 Survival curves for aerated and hypoxic Chinese hamster cells irradiated in the presence or absence of misonidazole. Low dose: 1 mM; high dose: 10 mM. From Adams (1977), with permission.

combined with *fractionated* radiation, the SER values were smaller. This probably results from reoxygenation between radiation fractions reducing the therapeutic impact of hypoxia. Also shown in Figure 19.2 is the effect of giving misonidazole *after* irradiation, where a small but significant enhancement is seen. This obviously cannot be due to hypoxic cell radiosensitization; it is probably due to the well-demonstrated observation that mizonidazole is directly toxic to hypoxic cells, the level of cell killing increasing considerably with the *duration* of exposure to the sensitizer.

Following encouraging laboratory studies, misonidazole was introduced into clinical trials. As will be discussed in the next section, the results have been disappointing. This may largely be attributed to the fact that doses were limited to inadequate levels because of neurotoxicity. Figure 19.3 summarizes the evidence in mice for sensitization by misonidazole, in comparison with *in vitro* results. The maximum-tolerated dose of this drug that can be given with standard clinical fractionated radiotherapy is around 0.5 g/m², which results in a tumour concentration of only about 15 µg/g, and it is clear from the laboratory animal data that such a dose could only be expected to yield a small sensitizer enhancement ratio.

The difficulty of achieving sufficiently large

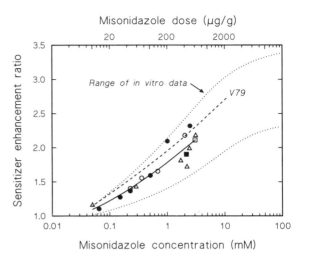

Figure 19.3 Sensitizer enhancement ratios determined *in vivo* using large single radiation doses as a function of misonidazole dose (upper scale). The symbols indicate different tumour types. The solid line shows the best fit to the *in vivo* results. The dotted lines enclose the range of *in vitro* data (lower scale); data on V79 cells indicated by the dashed line. From Brown (1989), with permission.

clinical doses of misonidazole has led to a search for better radiosensitizing drugs (EORTC, 1991). Of the many compounds synthesized and tested, some of the most promising are etanidazole, pimonidazole and RSU-1069 (Figure 19.4). Etanidazole was selected as being superior to misonidazole for two reasons. Firstly, although it has a sensitizing efficiency equivalent to misonidazole, it does have a shorter half-life *in vivo*, which should reduce its toxicity. Secondly, it also has a reduced lipophilicity (a lower octanol/water partition coefficient) and thus is less readily taken up in neural tissue. This tends to reduce neurotoxicity which was dose-limiting for misonidazole. Pimonidazole contains a side-chain with a weakly basic piperidine group. This compound is more electron-affinic than misonidazole and thus is more effective as a radiosensitizer; it is also uncharged at acid pH and this promotes its accumulation in ischaemic regions of tumours.

These new hypoxic cell sensitizers may be more potent than misonidazole but unfortunately they have a variety of side-effects that may hamper their clinical use. Another strategy was to search for a less toxic drug that could be given in high doses. On this basis, nimorazole was evaluated (Figure 19.4; Overgaard *et al*, 1991). Although its

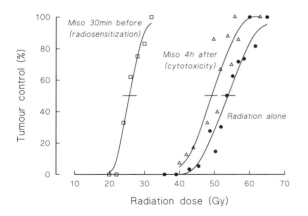

Figure 19.2 Local tumour control in C3H mouse mammary carcinomas measured 120 days after tumour irradiation. Mice were given misonidazole (1 g/kg, ip) either 30 min before or 4 h after irradiation. The TCD_{50} dose was reduced from 54 Gy in control animals to 26 Gy in the misonidazole-pretreated mice, equivalent to an enhancement ratio (SER) of 2.1. Misonidazole given 4 hours *after* irradiation gave a TCD_{50} of 49 Gy, an SER of 1.1.

sensitizing ability is less than theoretically can be achieved by misonidazole, the drug shows a flat dose-response curve so that at clinically relevant doses the SER is approximately 1.3. Furthermore, the drug can be given in association with a conventional radiation therapy schedule and is therefore amenable to clinical use.

RSU-1069 and its pro-drug RB-6145 (Adams *et al*, 1991) are dual-functional radiosensitizers because the presence of the nitro group confers radiosensitization while the aziridine group in the side-chain allows it to act also as cytotoxic alkylating agent. RSU-1069 is a more active radiosensitizer *in vivo* than any other nitroheterocyclic compound so far investigated and it also displays a particularly high cytotoxic activity towards hypoxic cells. Unfortunately RSU-1069 is also rather toxic to patients.

19.4 Hypoxic cell radio-sensitizers: clinical studies

Initial clinical studies using metronidazole in brain tumours generated enthusiasm for chemical radiosensitizers and these were followed by the widespread introduction of misonidazole. The late 1970s then saw a boom in clinical trials exploring the potential of misonidazole (Dische, 1985; Overgaard, 1989). Table 19.2 reviews the results of some of the larger multicentre studies. Overall, there was no clinical benefit and the general conclusion from the misonidazole era must be that this drug was unable to generate significant improvement in the results of radiotherapy. Dose-dependent peripheral neuropathy was a significant limiting factor.

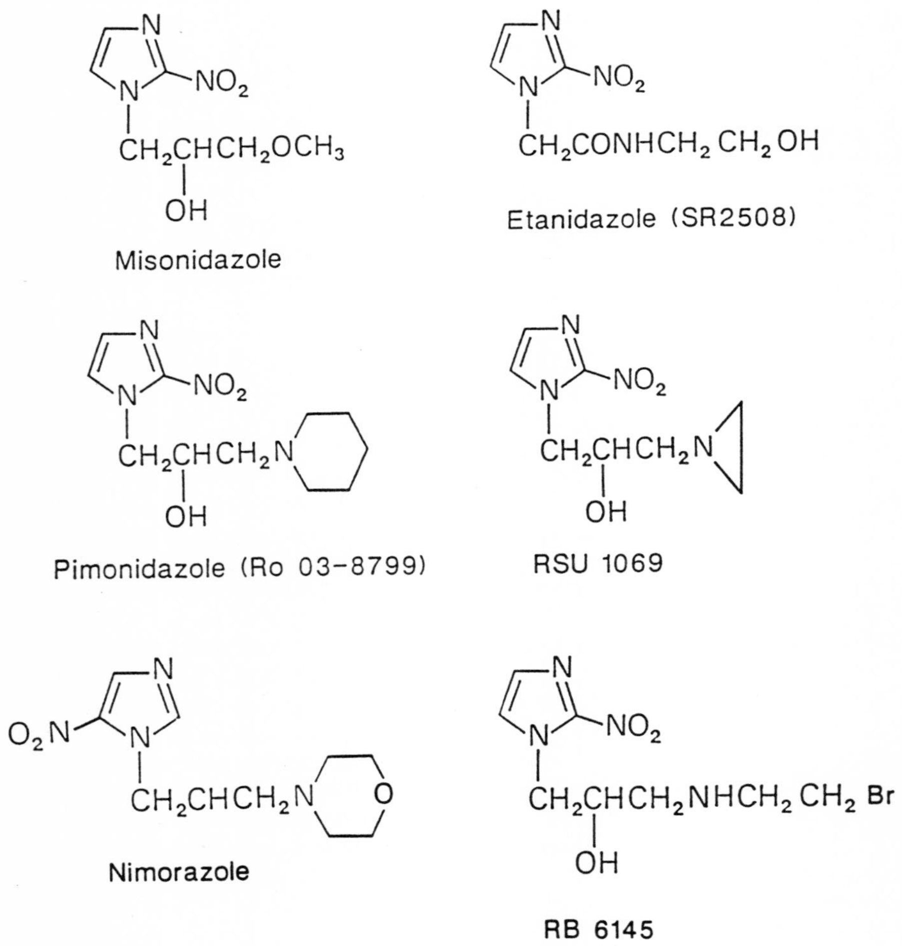

Figure 19.4 Structure of misonidazole and structurally related radiation sensitizers currently undergoing clinical testing. From Adams *et al* (1991), with permission.

Table 19.2 Multicentre randomized trials with misonidazole

Site and reference	No. of patients	Endpoint	RT+ Miso*	RT alone
Head and Neck Carcinoma				
DAHANCA 2 (Overgaard et al, 1989)	626	local-regional control (5 yrs)	41%	34%
MRC (1984)	267	local-regional control (>2 yrs)	40%	36%
EORTC (1986)	163	local-regional control (3 yrs)	52%	44%
RTOG (Fazekas et al, 1987)	306	local-regional control (3 yrs)	19%	24%
RTOG 79-04 (Fazekas et al, 1987)	42	local-regional control (2 yrs)	17%	10%
Uterine Cervix Carcinoma				
Scandinavian study (Overgaard et al, 1989)	331	local-regional control (5 yrs)	50%	54%
MRC (1984)	153	local-regional control (>2 yrs)	59%	58%
RTOG (Leibel et al, 1987)	119	local-regional control (3 yrs)	53%	54%
Glioblastoma				
Scandinavian study (Hatlevoll et al, 1985)	244	median survival (months)	10	10
MRC (1983)	384	median survival (months)	8	9
EORTC (1983)	163	median survival (months)	11	12
RTOG (Nelson et al, 1986)	318	median survival (months)	11	13
Bronchogenic Carcinoma				
RTOG (Simpson et al, 1987)	117	median survival (months)	7	7
RTOG (Simpson et al, 1989)	268	median survival (months)	7	8

* None of the radiation plus misonidazole groups was significantly different from radiation alone.
See Overgaard (1989) for references.

Some trials did show improvement in certain subgroups of treated patients. This was especially prominent in the Danish head and neck cancer trial, DAHANCA 2 (Figure 19.5), which despite an overall insignificant effect of misonidazole showed a highly significant improvement in pharynx tumours. In contrast, the prognostically better glottic carcinomas showed no influence of misonidazole.

The overall impression of the misonidazole era is that problems related to hypoxia have not been overcome. The development of more efficient or less toxic hypoxic sensitizers has therefore continued and currently there are several promising options (Coleman, 1988; EORTC, 1991). Experience from the misonidazole trials has led to the selection of more homogeneous tumour populations in which hypoxia is more likely to be a problem. The pimonidazole trial in uterine cervix has been disappointing, but nimorazole in patients with supraglottic and pharynx carcinomas (DAHANCA 5) has shown a highly significant improvement in loco-regional tumour control and survival (Figure 19.6; Overgaard et al, 1991).

19.5 Meta-analysis of controlled clinical trials of modified tumour hypoxia

The clinical role of hypoxia is one of the most thoroughly addressed issues in radiotherapy and has been under investigation for over two decades. Numerous clinical trials have been conducted, but most have been inconclusive. This may either be because no true difference exists among the treatment groups or because the trials have been too small to detect it. Meta-analysis seeks to distinguish between these alternatives: the results from *all* relevant trials are combined and analyzed together.

A literature survey has identified 9315 patients treated in 72 randomized clinical trials. The median number of patients per trial was 86 (range 14–626). The trials were directed at hyperbaric oxygen (25 trials), hypoxic cell radiosensitizers (43 trials), oxygen- or carbogen-breathing (3 trials), and blood transfusion (1 trial). The tumour sites were bladder (12 trials), uterine cervix (14 trials), CNS (13 trials), head and neck (19 trials), lung (9 trials), and mixed (2 trials). The trials were analyzed with regard to local tumour control (44 trials), survival (59 trials), distant metastases (13 trials) and complications resulting from radiotherapy (21 trials). The overall results are given in Table 19.3. The most relevant endpoint was considered to be local control, in view of the local nature of the radiation treatment, and this showed an improvement by 6.6% (51.5-44.9%; p < 0.001). This improvement persisted when the trials were evaluated separately for radiosensitizer or hyperbaric oxygen treatment. When analyzed according to site, only head and neck cancer showed a significant improvement (8.5%, p < 0.001). No other tumour sites demonstrated significant improvement.

Figure 19.7 shows the distribution of the statistical parameter Z in the 44 trials that gave local control data. Each point represents the results of a particular trial and the clear tendency for these to lie to the left of the zero value indicates the benefit of reducing the problem of tumour hypoxia. The overall survival probability also showed significant reduction (p < 0.05), once again dominated by head and neck tumours. No significant difference was observed in the incidence of distant metastases or radiotherapy complications.

Meta-analysis has thus demonstrated significant improvement from the manipulation of the hypoxic status of tumours of the head and neck. This indicates that the underlying biological rationale is probably sound, at least in the case of squamous cell carcinoma of the head and neck. It would be logical, therefore, to direct future clinical studies of the hypoxic problem at this tumour type and site.

19.6 Improving the oxygen supply to tumours

The relationship between haemoglobin concentration and local tumour control, which appears to be most pronounced in larger tumours, raises the possibility of improving tumour control by manipulation of the haemoglobin concentration or, in a broader sense, the *oxygen unloading capacity* of the blood. Haemoglobin levels have been increased by blood transfusion prior to radiotherapy in a number of studies (Overgaard, 1989) and a small randomized study in the uterine cervix has shown that this led to a significant improvement of local tumour control probability (Bush, 1986). Transfusion is also part of the DAHANCA 5 trial (Overgaard *et al*, 1991). Although local tumour control may be associated with haemoglobin concentration, its association with the transfusion is complex. Nevertheless, the clinical results in patients with low haemoglobin who received both transfusion and hyperbaric oxygen are impressive (Overgaard, 1989).

Other approaches to the improvement of tumour oxygenation by manipulating the oxygen-unloading capacity of the blood are also being made. These include the use of artificial blood substances, such as perfluorocarbons, or manipulation of the oxy-haemoglobin dissociation curve (Coleman, 1988; Hirst, 1986; Horsman, 1993).

Smoking is clearly an important factor influencing tumour oxygenation, especially in patients with head and neck or lung cancer who are known to smoke during their treatment. Smoking may lead to the loss of more than 30% of the oxygen-unloading capacity of the blood and this could lead to a significantly reduced tumour oxygenation (Overgaard *et al*, 1992). Patients should be strongly encouraged to quit smoking, at least during radiotherapy.

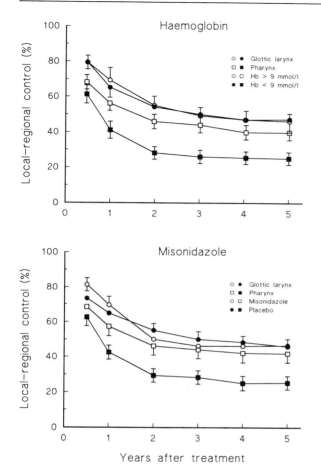

Figure 19.5 Results from the DAHANCA 2 study. Effect of misonidazole and haemoglobin concentration on loco-regional tumour control in males with glottic larynx and pharynx carcinomas. From Overgaard *et al* (1989), with permission.

19.7 Overcoming acute hypoxia in tumours

Although several of the procedures that have been used in patients to combat radiation resistance due to hypoxic cells have met with some success, the results are far from satisfactory. One explanation is that most of the procedures so far used clinically operate against diffusion-limited chronic hypoxia, and they have little or no influence on acute hypoxia (Section 11.2). Several years ago it was demonstrated that nicotinamide, a vitamin B3 analogue, could enhance radiation damage in a

variety of murine tumour models (Horsman *et al*, 1989; Figure 19.8). Nicotinamide seems primarily to prevent the transient fluctuations in tumour blood flow that lead to the development of acute hypoxia (Horsman *et al*, 1990). It can be given in clinically effective doses and clinical studies are now under way.

It could be that the optimal approach to the hypoxic problem in human tumours is to combine treatments which independently attack chronic and acute hypoxia. Nicotinamide has been

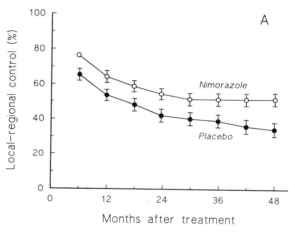

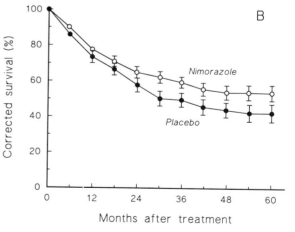

Figure 19.6 Results from the DAHANCA 5 study. Actuarial loco-regional tumour control (A) and corrected survival (B) in patients randomized to receive nimorazole (219 patients) or placebo (195 patients) in conjunction with radiotherapy for carcinoma of the pharynx and supraglottic larynx. From Overgaard *et al* (1991, 1992), with permission.

Table 19.3   Summary of meta-analysis of clinical modification of tumour hypoxia

Endpoint	Treatment	Control	(O - E)	VAR	Z	Odds ratio*
Loco-regional failure	1414/3152 (44.9%)	1638/3178 (51.5%)	−106	395	−5.32	1.31 (1.21–1.41)
Death	2602/4036 (64.5%)	2685/4032 (66.6%)	−43	456	−2.01	1.10 (1.01–1.19)
Distant metastasis	331/1611 (20.5%)	344/1604 (21.4%)	−7	133	−0.63	1.06 (0.89–1.23)
Complications to radiation	237/1548 (15.3%)	203/1424 (14.3%)	8	94	0.81	0.92 (0.72–1.12)

* with 95% confidence interval.

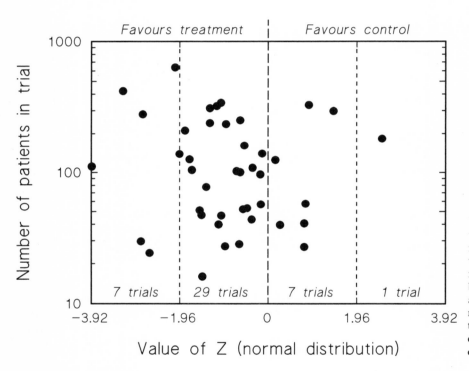

Figure 19.7 Meta-analysis of 44 randomized trials of radiotherapy combined with a treatment to modify tumour hypoxia, using the end-point of loco-regional control. The value of Z represents the observed-minus-expected control rates divided by a measure of the uncertainty of this difference. Negative values denote results that favour the treatment arm, while positive values favour radiation alone. Results falling between 0 to ±1.96 indicate a tendency towards improvement and from ±1.96 to ±3.92 this difference becomes significant. (Overgaard, unpublished observations).

shown in experimental systems to improve tumour radiosensitization induced by hyperthermia, by the use of a perfluorochemical emulsion, and by normobaric carbogen or oxygen breathing (Kjellen *et al*, 1991; Horsman, 1991). Preliminary clinical testing is now being undertaken with nicotinamide in combination with carbogen.

19.8 Exploiting tumour hypoxia

Although hypoxic cells are resistant to radiotherapy, they are *sensitive* to a number of other modalities, especially to bioreductive drugs (Adams *et al*, 1991) and to hyperthermia (Section 20.2). Both of these agents can directly sensitize hypoxic cells to radiation or specifically kill them. In the case of hyperthermia, cytotoxicity is not a consequence of hypoxia *per se*, but rather due to cellular metabolic changes leading to an increase in acidity, which is the result of prolonged oxygen deprivation (EORTC, 1991).

Rather than seeking to reduce hypoxia in tumours, some studies suggest that it might be beneficial to *increase* the level of tumour hypoxia before subsequent exposure to agents

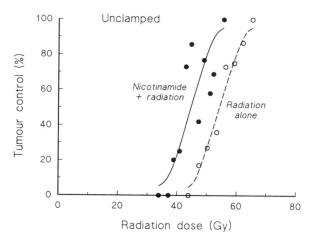 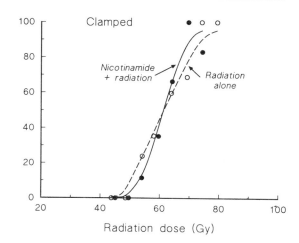

Figure 19.8 Effect of nicotinamide (1 g/kg ip 30 min before radiation) on the radiation response of a mouse mammary carcinoma. The left-hand panel shows that nicotinamide enhanced the radiation response of tumours treated under ambient conditions. When tumours were made fully hypoxic by clamping (right panel) no effect of nicotinamide was seen, indicating that the effect is due to hypoxic modification. Adapted from Horsman *et al* (1990), with permission.

that specifically kill hypoxic cells. There are a number of ways in which tumour hypoxia can be increased experimentally. One is to modify the oxygen-carrying capacity of the blood using either carbon monoxide-breathing or haemoglobin-oxygen affinity-modifying drugs like BW12C. Alternatively, tumour blood flow can be lowered using physiological modifiers like hydralazine or glucose, or by destroying tumour blood vessels by photodynamic therapy or with drugs like flavone acetic acid. These and similar agents have been shown both to improve the radiation response of solid tumours and also to enhance (or act additionally with) the antitumour activity either of bioreductive drugs or hyperthermia (EORTC, 1991; Horsman, 1993).

Key points

1. Hypoxic cell radioresistance is a significant cause of failure in the local control of tumours, in particular carcinomas of the head and neck.
2. Chemical radiosensitizers work well in experimental animal studies but they have been disappointing in clinical trials. The search for improved agents is under way.
3. Pharmacological modification of tumour blood flow shows promise in experimental systems. Examples are nicotinamide, which appears to reduce the problem of acute (i.e. transient) hypoxia in tumours, and hydralazine which *increases* tumour hypoxia and can enhance the activity of some bioreductive drugs that are toxic to hypoxic cells.

Bibliography

Adams GE (1977). Hypoxic cell sensitizers for radiotherapy. In: *Cancer* Vol 6. Ed. FF Becker. Plenum Press, New York.

Adams GE, Bremner J, Stratford IJ *et al* (1991). Nitroheterocyclic compounds as radiosensitizers and bioreductive drugs. *Radiother Oncol* 20 (Suppl 1):85-91.

Bush RS (1986). The significance of anemia in

clinical radiation therapy. *Int J Radiat Oncol Biol Phys* 12:2047-2050.

Churchill-Davidson I (1968). The oxygen effect in radiotherapy–historical review. *Front Radiat Ther Oncol* 1:1-15.

Coleman CN (1988). Hypoxia in tumours: a paradigm for the approach to biochemical and physiological heterogeneity. *J Natl Cancer Inst* 80:310-317.

Hirst DG (1986). Anemia: A problem or an opportunity in radiotherapy? *Int J Radiat Oncol Biol Phys* 12:2009-2017.

Horsman, MR (1991). Nicotinamide and the hypoxia problem. *Radiother Oncol* 22:79-80.

Horsman MR, Hansen PV and Overgaard J (1989). Radiosensitization by nicotinamide in tumors and normal tissues: the importance of tissue oxygenation status. *Int J Radiat Oncol Biol Phys* 16:1273-1276.

Horsman MR, Chaplin DJ and Overgaard J (1990). Combination of nicotinamide and hyperthermia to eliminate radioresistant chronically and acutely hypoxic tumor cells. *Cancer Res* 50:7430-7436.

Kjellen E, Joiner MC, Collier JM *et al* (1991). A therapeutic benefit from combining normobaric carbogen or oxygen with nicotinamide in fractionated x-ray treatments. *Radiother Oncol* 22:81-91.

Overgaard J, Sand Hansen H, Andersen AP *et al* (1989). Misonidazole combined with split-course radiotherapy in the treatment of invasive carcinoma of larynx and pharynx. Final report from the DAHANCA 2 study. *Int J Radiat Oncol Biol Phys* 16:1065-1068.

Overgaard J, Sand Hansen H, Lindeløv B *et al* (1991). Nimorazole as a hypoxic radiosensitizer in the treatment of supraglottic larynx and pharynx carcinoma. First Report from the Danish Head and Neck Cancer Study (DAHANCA) Protocol 5-85. *Radiother Oncol* 20 (Suppl 1):143-150.

Overgaard J, Sand Hansen H, Overgaard M *et al* (1992). The Danish Head and Neck Cancer Study Group (DAHANCA) randomized trials with radiosensitizers in carcinoma of the larynx and pharynx. In: *Radiation Research. A Twentieth-Century Perspective*, Vol II, pp. 573-577. (Eds) Dewey WC *et al*. Academic Press; New York.

Further reading

Brown JM (1989). Hypoxic cell radiosensitizers: where next? *Int J Radiat Oncol Biol Phys* 16:987-993.

Dische S (1985). Chemical sensitizers for hypoxic cells: A decade of experience in clinical radiotherapy. *Radiother Oncol* 3:97-115.

EORTC Cooperative Group for Radiotherapy (1991). Consensus Meeting on Tumour Hypoxia. *Radiother Oncol* 20 (Suppl 1):1-159.

Horsman, MR (1993). Hypoxia in tumours: its relevance, identification and modification. In: *Current Topics in Clinical Radiobiology of Tumours*. (Ed) Beck-Bornholdt HP. Springer Verlag; Berlin. (In press).

Overgaard J (1989). Sensitization of hypoxic tumour cells–clinical experience. *Int J Rad Biol* 56:801-811.

20

Hyperthermia

Jens Overgaard and Michael R. Horsman

20.1 History and background

Knowledge of the effects of heat treatment on tumours is as old as the oldest written text in medicine. The Edwin Smith Surgical papyrus, which was probably the first medical textbook, dating back more than 5,000 years, gives a description of a patient with a tumour in the breast treated with hyperthermia (i.e. cautery). Similar procedures have subsequently been used throughout history. In the last decades of the nineteenth century hyperthermia underwent a renaissance, triggered by the observation that patients with high fever due to erysipelas in some instances demonstrated spontaneous regression of tumours. This led the New York surgeon William B. Coley to develop his 'Mixed Bacterial Toxin' and thereby he became the father both of the modern use of hyperthermia and nonspecific immunotherapy for the treatment of cancer. Concurrent with Coley's interest, a more direct local application of hyperthermia was performed by others who demonstrated that moderately elevated temperatures (up to 45°C) could induce significant regression and even disappearance of tumours.

This treatment principle developed throughout the first part of the present century, not only as a modality by itself, but also in combination with radiotherapy. The combination with radiotherapy was initially triggered by the belief that increased blood flow resulted in a more pronounced radiation response. Since heat was known to enhance blood flow in the skin, it was used to obtain a better penetrating effect of low-voltage external-beam radiation. This principle of 'thermal penetration' of x-rays was indeed shown to be beneficial (Müller, 1912), although the biological mechanism of this combined effect was later found to be other than by a change in blood flow. Hyperthermia has also been applied in combination with chemotherapy, especially in association with whole-body heating or the regional perfusion of limbs. Most recently it has been applied in the treatment of advanced local tumours as a part of a multi-modality strategy, or when other more conventional modalities have been ruled out.

The Achilles heel of hyperthermia treatment of malignant tumours is the problem of achieving adequate heating of deep-seated tumours. Current technology only allows reasonably satisfactory heating of superficial lesions. The technology for superficial heating has become easily available and hyperthermia has increasingly been applied in the treatment of various superficial tumours, either alone or in various combined approaches.

In spite of the lack of large-scale controlled clinical trials, hyperthermia has been considered by some to be an established therapy. This is not the case: there is a need for further clinical studies and until these have been performed hyperthermia must still be considered to be an experimental modality.

The present chapter gives an overview of the biological rationale and clinical experience with local hyperthermia, especially in combination with radiation. Based on present knowledge we will also outline the indications for hyperthermia in current oncological practice.

20.2 Biological effects of hyperthermia

Heat Alone

Moderate heat treatment (temperatures of 41 to 44°C) is able to destroy malignant and normal cells *in vitro*. The mechanisms of destruction by heat are complex and involve damage to cell nuclei, to membranes and to other cytoplasmic components.

Sensitivity to hyperthermia varies greatly among different cell lines but as a whole there is no differentially enhanced sensitivity in malignant cells. Most experimental studies have been performed with rodent cell lines which in general seem to be somewhat more sensitive to hyperthermia than human cells, but they do not seem to differ in a qualitative way.

Thermal damage to cells depends on two main factors: temperature and the heating time. This is illustrated in Figure 20.1 which shows that the growth delay of mouse mammary tumours increased linearly with heating time and that the slope of the relationship was highly dependent upon temperature in the range 41–44.5°C. Data of this type can be summarized in an Arrhenius plot, an example of which is given as an inset to Figure 20.1. This is an iso-effect plot in which the logarithm of the heating time for a given level of effect is plotted against temperature. Arrhenius

plots are often linear up to around 42.5° at which point the slope abruptly changes (in the direction of *longer* heating time at the higher temperature). It is possible to calculate from the slope of such plots the activation energy (μ) associated with the effect (Westra and Dewey, 1971). The change in slope that occurs in Figure 20.1 implies that above 42.5° a different biological process is being inactivated. In this case the activation energies correspond with damage to proteins and membranes rather than to DNA.

The sensitivity of cells to heat-induced cell killing varies through the cell cycle. A number of studies have shown that cells in the S-phase tend to be the most sensitive, in contrast to the situation with radiation cell killing. This has been proposed as one rationale for combining these two treatments (see below).

Thermotolerance

Thermotolerance is the phenomenon by which one heat treatment induces temporary resistance against subsequent heating. If two heat treatments are separated by a short interval, thermotolerance may lead to the second having little effect. In the clinical application of hyperthermia, for instance in combination with radiotherapy, it may be necessary to deliver repeated heat treatments and thus thermotolerance is of considerable practical importance.

The magnitude and kinetics of thermotolerance depend on the intensity of the priming treatment and the effects differ among various tumours and normal tissues. An example is shown in Figure 20.2. Mouse mammary tumours were given a 30 minute preheating at a temperature between 42.5° and 44.5°. They were then reheated after various time intervals and the extent of protection (the *thermotolerance ratio*) was determined. The ratio increased linearly with time interval up to a peak, the height of which was very temperature-dependent and occurred between 12–48 hours after preheating; thereafter the protection declined and became negligible at intervals of 4–6 days.

Thermotolerance is a large effect which is important in determining the response to multiple heat treatments. It has been observed in all tissues where it has been sought and it must therefore be considered a general phenomenon. Its extent and timing vary from one tissue to another which makes it difficult to predict precisely.

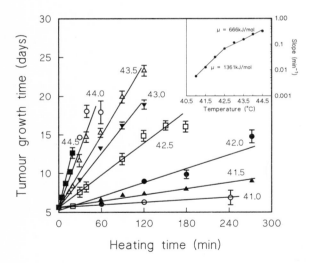

Figure 20.1 Tumour growth time as a function of heating time for a solid mouse mammary carcinoma heated *in vivo* in the range 41.0–44.5°C. Tumour growth time was the time taken for tumours to regrow to five times their treatment volume.

Inset: Time-temperature plot showing the slope of the dose-response curves as a function of heating temperature. Based on the slope values, the activation energy (μ) was calculated by Arrhenius analysis. From Lindegaard and Overgaard (1987), with permission.

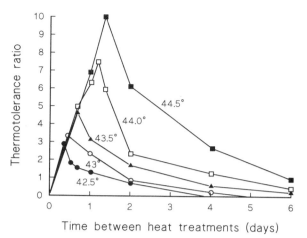

Figure 20.2 Kinetics and magnitude of thermal tolerance in C3H mammary carcinomas. An initial 30 min heating was followed by treatment at the same temperature for various times, but with different time intervals between the two treatments. Thermotolerance ratio is the ratio of heating times for a fixed level of tumour response. From Overgaard *et al* (1987), with permission.

Environmental and Vascular Effects

Heat-induced damage is also strongly influenced by the extracellular environment. Thus an environment characterized by deprived nutritional conditions including chronic hypoxia, increased acidity and starvation, promotes hyperthermic damage. This is not, as with radiation, an oxygen effect. In fact, acute hypoxia or hypoxic conditions that persist for a limited time in an otherwise normal environment do not seem to influence the degree of hyperthermic damage.

The main factor responsible for enhanced cell death within ischaemic tissues is probably the increased acidity (Figure 20.3). Since such a deprived environment usually exists only within solid tumours (and not in normal tissues), this enhancement of sensitivity is a major factor in the rationale for applying hyperthermia in the treatment of cancer. Specific hyperthermic cytotoxicity is seen as direct heat killing of cells in a deprived micro-environment, characterized by insufficient blood supply, which leads to poor nutrition and increased acidity due to anaerobic metabolism and accumulation of lactic acid and other waste products. Cells situated in such an area are highly sensitive to hyperthermia and can be destroyed by a heat treatment that does not cause significant damage to cells in a normal environment.

A further and important effect of the reduced blood flow to ischaemic tissues is that they will experience less cooling and therefore for any given energy input they will rise to a higher temperature. As a result, heat treatment of superficial tumours often results in a higher temperature in the tumour than in the surrounding tissue. In experimental systems this has been shown to lead to a differential response between tumour and normal tissue. Whereas most tumours show a tendency for collapse of the blood vessels at a relatively low temperature, normal tissues sometimes react by *increasing* their blood flow and thus reaching a lower temperature than would otherwise be the

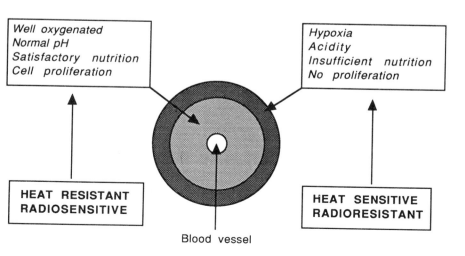

Figure 20.3 The micro-environment in tumours leads to regions that differ in a number of important respects. *See* also Figure 11.5.

case (Figure 20.4). This *physical* effect of blood flow is perhaps the most important factor leading to differential cell killing between tumours and normal tissues.

Direct cell killing by heat occurs rapidly. Heated cells die within hours both *in vitro* and *in vivo*, in contrast to cell killing after irradiation which may take some days to appear (Law *et al*, 1978). Cell kill after irradiation usually occurs in mitosis, but after hyperthermic treatments the cells die within interphase. This rapid necrotic process occurs even faster in tumours with a deprived environment and is probably due to accelerated cytoplasmic and membrane damage. Thermal damage is invariably *acute*: late effects are uncommon and where they have been observed they are thought to be the result of excessive acute tissue damage.

Interaction with Radiation

In addition to direct cell killing, hyperthermia enhances the effect of radiation on cells.

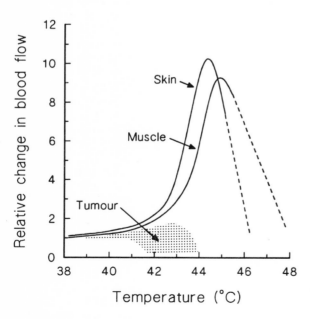

Figure 20.4 Relative changes in blood flow in tumours and normal tissues heated at different temperatures. The stippled area shows the range of values obtained for a variety of animal tumours heated at various temperatures for 30 to 40 minutes. The normal-tissue data are from blood flow measurements in skin and muscle of SD rats heated for the same time periods. Adapted from Song (1984), with permission.

Hyperthermic radiosensitization occurs primarily when the radiation is delivered *during* hyperthermia, i.e. for simultaneous treatment. An interval between the two treatments reduces the effect. The enhancement is expressed as a quantitative increase in the radiation effect but without qualitative changes. The effect is complex, involving both an increased direct radiosensitivity depending on temperature and heating time, and a reduced accumulation of sublethal damage resulting in a smaller shoulder on the survival curve. Variation in radiosensitivity through the cell cycle is less pronounced, since the effect of heating tends to be greatest in cell-cycle phases that are most resistant to radiation. The repair of potentially lethal damage can also be reduced by additional heat treatment. Interestingly, the oxygen effect does not seem to be affected, for the radiation response of oxygenated and acutely hypoxic cells are often equally sensitized by hyperthermia.

The contrast between direct cell killing by heat and hyperthermic radiosensitization is illustrated in Table 20.1.

The extent of hyperthermic radiosensitization is usually expressed as the thermal enhancement ratio:

$$\text{Thermal Enhancement Ratio (TER)} = \frac{\text{Radiation dose without heating}}{\text{Radiation dose with heating}}$$

to produce the same level of effect. The measurement of the TER value for mouse mammary tumours is illustrated in Figure 20.5.

TER values tend to be high for *simultaneous* heat and radiation treatment but of similar magnitude in tumour and normal tissues. Such a treatment will therefore not improve the therapeutic ratio unless the tumour is heated to a higher temperature than the normal tissue. An example of the time-dependence of hyperthermic radiosensitization is shown in Figure 20.6. Mouse mammary tumours were heated to 42.5°C and tumour control was documented as a function of radiation dose. This allowed TER values to be calculated for each selected time interval between the treatments. In parallel experiments skin damage was also measured. It can be seen that effects on both tumour and skin peaked for simultaneous treatment, the TER values reaching 2.5 in each case. For intervals of up to 24 hours between the treatments the tumour data gave a symmetrical curve, falling to a TER of 1.5. In

Table 20.1   Contrast between hyperthermic cytotoxicity and hyperthermic radiosensitization

Hyperthermic cytotoxicity	Hyperthermic radiosensitization
Increased under environmental conditions such as: • Nutritional deprivation • Chronic hypoxia • Acidity (most important)	• Direct radiosensitization • Reduced repair of sublethal damage • Increased sensitivity of cells in radioresistant phases of the cell cycle • Reduced repair of potentially lethal damage • No change in OER • Strongest with truly simultaneous application

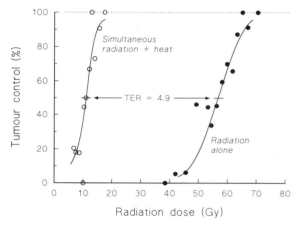

Figure 20.5 Dose-response curves for tumour control in a C3H mammary carcinoma by radiation alone or combined with hyperthermia (43.5°C for 60 min), illustrating the determination of a thermal enhancement ratio. From Overgaard *et al* (1987), with permission.

the skin, there was evidence for sensitization with heat before radiation, but not *vice versa*. In this experimental situation there was therefore a therapeutic advantage in post-radiation heating. This advantage may be expressed as:

Therapeutic Gain Factor (TGF) =

$$\frac{\text{TER for tumour response}}{\text{TER for normal-tissue damage}}$$

In experimental systems it is possible to distinguish the effects of direct hyperthermic cytotoxicity from hyperthermic sensitization. This is illustrated in Figure 20.7. Mouse mammary tumours were either heated simultaneously with radiation treatment or the treatments were given sequentially. Thermal enhancement ratios were

determined for the two situations. Whereas the simultaneous treatment resulted in a linear increase in TER with heat dose, the sequential treatment led to a plateau at a TER of approximately 2.0, with no increase by further heating.

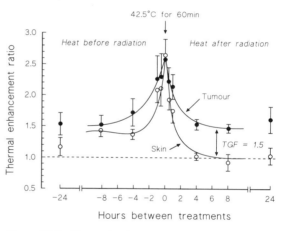

Figure 20.6 Thermal enhancement ratio (TER) as a function of time interval and sequence between hyperthermia and radiation treatment of C3H mammary carcinomas and the surrounding skin. Maximum TER values were observed after simultaneous treatment and any interval reduced the thermal sensitization. From Overgaard *et al* (1987), with permission.

20.3 Clinical hyperthermia

Hyperthermia has been used extensively in the treatment of cancer. The use of heat as an *adjuvant* to radiation in the treatment of local and regional disease is the area where it currently seems to offer the greatest advantages. There is now abundant evidence from clinical Phase I and II studies of combined heat and radiation showing that heat may enhance radiation effects on tumours to a significant degree (Figure 20.8 and Table 20.2).

More recently a number of randomized studies have been completed, and although most have involved a relatively small number of patients they all show the same trend towards a beneficial effect of adjuvant hyperthermia. Table 20.3 shows the results of a meta-analysis of these studies. Overall there is evidence for a highly significant improvement in tumour response.

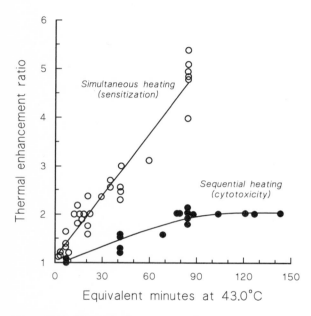

Figure 20.7 Thermal enhancement ratio as a function of heat treatment in a mouse mammary carcinoma exposed either to simultaneous *(radiosensitization)* or sequential *(cytotoxicity)* radiation and hyperthermia (heat 4 hours after radiation). From Overgaard (1989), with permission.

Indications for Hyperthermia in Radiotherapy

The indications for hyperthermia in clinical radiotherapy are two-fold. Firstly, hyperthermia may be included in the primary treatment of locally advanced tumours where improved local control is expected to result in improved cure rate and survival. Secondly, hyperthermia has an evident role in palliation, especially of recurrent tumours in previously irradiated areas. Both in the curative and in the palliative situations clinical experience

is limited by the difficulties of heat delivery; it remains a major technical problem how to deliver homogeneous heating to a defined tumour volume. This is especially the case for other than superficial tumours.

Patients with a relatively long life expectancy are particularly in need of optimal primary treatment. Hyperthermia should here be considered as adjuvant to radiation treatment schedules that are already known to be as effective as possible. It is essential that the adjuvant hyperthermia should not sensitize the normal tissues to radiation treatment, for in this situation the radiation dose will already be at tolerance. The treatment principle should therefore be based on optimal radiotherapy using a standard daily fractionation schedule and adding a heat treatment once or twice a week. The argument for this approach has been discussed in detail, especially with regard to the development of thermal tolerance and the interval between the hyperthermic fractions (Overgaard and Nielsen, 1983).

If normal-tissue heating can be avoided, the heat treatment should be given immediately after radiation, as some degree of radiosensitization may add further to the tumour-destructive effect. Otherwise, an interval of approximately 3 to 4 hours is recommended between radiation and hyperthermia to avoid any sensitization of radiation damage to normal tissues.

Treatment Strategy

The two biological effects of hyperthermia, direct cytotoxicity and radiosensitization, present two alternative strategies for applying hyperthermia as an adjuvant to radiotherapy. The first is primarily as a radiosensitizing agent, enhancing the effect of ionizing radiation in heated tissues. This strategy is only valid if hyperthermia and radiation are applied simultaneously. The second strategy utilizes the specific cytotoxic effect against radioresistant cells and is achieved by sequential treatment. From a practical point of view, truly simultaneous treatment with external heating is difficult to achieve in the clinic and the major effect of the combined treatment will probably be direct hyperthermic cytotoxicity.

The quantitative difference between the simultaneous and sequential treatments appears to be less for clinical studies than expected from animal studies. However, recent studies have indicated

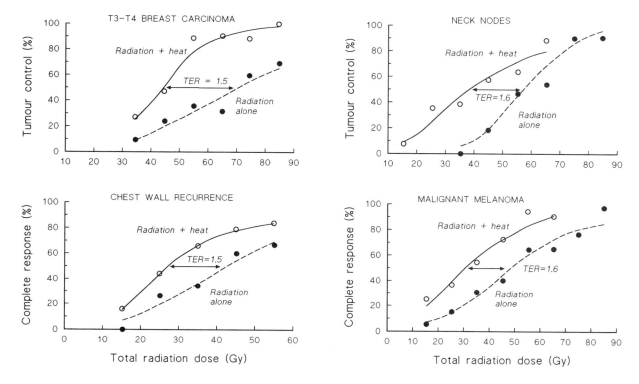

Figure 20.8 Dose-response relationships for advanced breast carcinoma, recurrent breast carcinoma, advanced neck nodes, and malignant melanoma treated with radiation or combined radiation and hyperthermia. The total radiation doses were normalized to daily fractions of 2 Gy using an α/β ratio of 25 Gy for breast and head and neck carcinomas and 2.5 Gy for malignant melanoma. From Overgaard (1989), with permission.

that this is probably again due to the fact that truly simultaneous treatments have not been used in the clinical situation. As shown in Figure 20.9, only a small interval of a few minutes between heat and radiation, or even placing the radiation early or late in the heating session, reduces the amount of hyperthermic radiosensitization. Therefore, if up to half an hour is allowed between radiation and hyperthermia, the major effect of such treatment will be dominated by direct hyperthermic cytotoxicity, although some radiosensitization may persist both in tumour and normal tissues.

20.4 Prognostic parameters and other factors of importance

The effect of heat combined with radiotherapy depends on a number of factors relating to the tumour, the patient, and the choice of treatment:

Volume

Tumour size is probably the most important parameter for the outcome of hyperthermic treatment. It is difficult to heat large tumours. However, provided sufficient hyperthermia can be applied there is a general tendency for combined therapy to show less volume dependence than is the case with radiation alone. This is illustrated in Figure 20.10 for three tumour sites; as tumour volume increases the results are relatively better following combined therapy.

Radiation Dose

It has been reported that the effect of hyperthermia is especially seen when combined with low radiation doses. This is probably an artefact based on studies using iso-dose comparisons, rather than based on iso-effect. Nevertheless, hyperthermia

Table 20.2   Tumour response after treatment with the same radiation dose given either alone or combined with heat

	No. of tumours	Complete response rate§		
		Radiation alone %	Radiation and heat %	Ratio of response rates
Chest Wall Recurrence in Breast Cancer				
Perez *et al* (1986)	35	43	86	2.00
van der Zee *et al* (1985)	40	0	24	>1
Scott *et al* (1984)	34	47	94	2.00
Gonzalez *et al* (1988)	18	33	78	2.36
Lindholm *et al* (1989)	66	35	70	2.00
Li *et al* (1985)	42	36	73	2.03
Dunlop *et al* (1986)	32	67	82	1.22
Overgaard (1988)	14	40	78	1.94
* Perez *et al* (RTOG) (1991)	74	26	33	1.27
* Egawa *et al* (1989)	19	40	67	1.68
Malignant Melanoma				
Overgaard *et al* (1987)	63	57	90	1.58
Gonzales *et al* (1986)	24	17	83	4.88
Kim *et al* (1977-84)	149	43	67	1.56
Arcangeli *et al* (1984)	38	53	76	1.43
Valdagni *et al* (unpublished)	35	20	80	4.00
Emami *et al* (1988)	116	24	59	1.94
Shidnia *et al* (1987)	185	33	64	1.94
Primary Advanced Breast				
Morita *et al* (1988)	22	50	100	2.00
Head and Neck				
Arcangeli *et al* (1985)	81	42	79	1.88
Scott *et al* (1984)	18	22	88	4.00
Marchal *et al* (1986)	54	7	41	5.86
* Valdagni *et al* (1988)	36	37	82	2.22
Emami *et al* (1988)	160	13	38	2.92
Goldobenko *et al* (1987)	65	86	100	1.16
* Datta *et al* (1990)	65	32	55	1.72
* Perez *et al* (RTOG) (1991)	106	33	34	1.03
* Egawa *et al* (1989)	33	44	47	1.07
* Svetitsky (1990)#	54	0	30	>1
* Krishnamurthi *et al* (1990)#	67	61	69	1.13
Uterine Cervix				
Hornback *et al* (1986)	66	35	72	2.06
* Datta *et al* (1987)	53	58	74	1.18
Morita *et al* (1988)	24	71	90	1.26
* Sharma *et al* (1989)	50	50	70	1.40
Gastro-Intestinal				
Muratkhodzhaev *et al* (1987)	313	25	63	2.52
Hiraoka *et al* (1984)	24	10+	43+	4.30
Goldobenko *et al* (1987)	48	0	11	>1
Mentesjasjvili *et al* (1987)	117	33+	69+	2.09
Kai *et al* (1988)	100	3	19	6.33
* Berdov *et al* (1990)	115	2	16	8.00

§   CR if otherwise not indicated
+   PR
*   randomized
#   radiation and chemotherapy

For references see Overgaard and Bach Andersen (1993).

Table 20.3 Meta analysis of radiation + heat *versus* radiation alone

Reference	Site	Total pts.	Rad + Heat		Rad alone		Z	Odds ratio*
			No.	Failures	No.	Failures		
ESHO 3-85	Melanoma	124	61	25	63	42	−2.86	2.9 ± 0.7
Valdagni *et al* (1988)	Head and Neck	40	18	3	22	15	−3.22	10.7 ± 1.5
RTOG 81-04	Mixed	236	119	87	117	95	−1.48	1.6 ± 0.6
Egawa *et al* (1989)	Mixed	24	15	8	18	10	−0.13	1.1 ± 1.4
Datta *et al* (1990)	Head and Neck	65	33	22	32	26	−1.33	2.2 ± 1.2
Datta *et al* (1987)	Cervix	52	27	9	25	14	−1.63	2.6 ± 1.1
Sharma *et al* (1989)	Cervix	42	20	6	22	11	−1.30	2.3 ± 1.3
Berdov *et al* (1990)	Rectal	115	56	47	59	58	−2.72	11.1 ± 2.1
Krishnamurthi *et al* (1990)	Head and Neck	67	36	11	31	12	−0.70	1.4 ± 1.0
Svetitsky (1990)	Head and Neck	54	26	18	28	28	−3.15	> 50
	ALL	828	411	234 (57.4%)	417	311 (74.6%)	−5.61	2.2 ± 0.3

* With 95% confidence interval.
For references see Overgaard and Bach Andersen (1983).

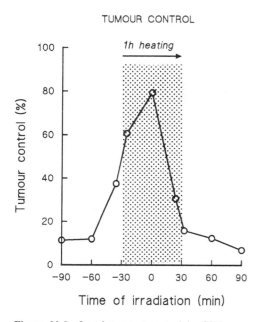
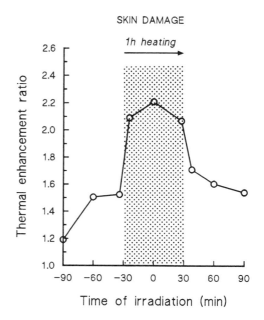

Figure 20.9 Local tumour control in C3H mouse mammary carcinomas and damage to surrounding skin as a function of sequence and interval between hyperthermia and radiation. Tumours were irradiated with 26 Gy at various times before, during or after heating to 42.5°C for 60 min; tumour control was determined 120 days after treatment. From Overgaard *et al* (1987), with permission.

combined with palliative doses of radiotherapy has in some instances resulted in persistent tumour control.

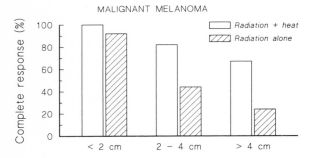

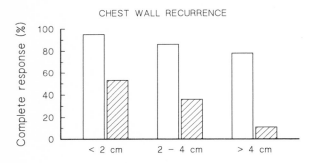

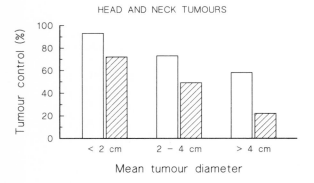

Figure 20.10 Relationship between tumour volume and response to radiotherapy, given alone or combined with hyperthermia, in melanoma, recurrent carcinoma of the breast, and head and neck cancer. Total radiation doses were respectively 18–27 Gy, 40 Gy and 60 Gy. The volume dependence is most pronounced for treatment with radiotherapy alone. Adapted from Overgaard (1990), with permission.

Sequence and Interval

As indicated above, the effect of combined treatment depends on the interval between the two modalities. If hyperthermia is applied simultaneously with every radiation fraction the optimal effect will be obtained provided sufficient spacing is allowed between the fractions. This is a highly complex situation because it may demand a less than optimal radiation schedule. For this reason, most of the current treatment schedules apply hyperthermia once or twice per week. This is less than optimal from a biological point of view, but appears at present to be the most feasible approach.

Number of Heat Treatments

Increasing the number of heat treatments does not result in an improved response. This may be explained either by the heterogeneous distribution of hyperthermia in the tumour, or by thermotolerance. A detailed discussion of thermotolerance in clinical hyperthermia has been given by Overgaard and Nielsen (1983). The conclusion of this analysis was that in clinical treatments where tumours are heated heterogeneously, thermotolerance will also develop in a heterogeneous way, namely to a different extent in different parts of a tumour depending on the degree of heating. The overall outcome of a fractionated treatment in a heterogeneously heated tumour will depend on the heat dose per fraction and on the fractionation interval. Due to dose-dependent variations in the magnitude and time-course of thermotolerance, the parts of the tumour given the highest physical amount of heat may not necessarily be subjected to the greatest biological heat damage and *vice versa*. This will occur if a relatively large heat trauma is applied with the first fraction, which subsequently makes the tissue thermotolerant. Additional physical heat deposition in subsequent fractions given over short intervals thus may not add to the biological damage.

With our current knowledge and technical ability it appears that a single good heat treatment may be biologically satisfactory (Overgaard, 1989). However, several heating attempts may be required in order to secure such a single sufficient treatment. It should be noted that, with few exceptions, there is no apparent correlation between the number of heat treatments and response.

Time-temperature Relationship ('Thermal dose')

Long heating time, high temperature and large heated volume are all parameters of good prognostic value. Thermal dose is a means of expressing a biological heat trauma in equivalent minutes at a given temperature (e.g. 43°C), based on a well-defined Arrhenius relationship for a time-temperature isoeffect (Field and Morris, 1983). Although the concept is theoretically attractive, problems of uniformity of heating and thermotolerance make it difficult to apply in practical clinical therapy. Nevertheless, many attempts have been made to establish a generally acceptable thermal iso-effect dose concept. A variety of correlations have been made, with minimal and maximal temperature, mean temperature, in a single treatment or all treatments, or with the area of the tumour heated above a certain temperature, etc. These attempts have not yet led to a uniform approach.

Several clinical studies have shown a relationship between tumour response and heat dose, but this probably just indicates that good heating (i.e. a relatively large thermal dose) is better than poor heating (a small heat dose), which is in agreement with the idea of needing at least one good heating. It has never been demonstrated that the heat dose concept is more than extremely crude and semi-quantitative. The clinical usefulness of a heat dose concept derived from rodent cells and tissue has been challenged by Hahn *et al* (1989). Certainly more knowledge is required to settle this issue. Since the problem of the physical and biological definition of thermal dose is far from solved, it is important not to convert time-temperature relationships into simple equivalent thermal dose values without keeping the original data on file for later analysis.

Other Prognostic Parameters

Several other factors have been shown to influence the response. These include the site of the tumour (differing in heating feasibility), histopathology, tumour-cell environment and blood flow, primary or recurrent lesion, and other more speculative parameters such as the intrinsic heat sensitivity of the tumour cells.

Key points

1. Tissue damage by hyperthermia depends on two main factors: temperature and heating time. Cell killing rises steeply for temperatures above 41°C and is increased by an acidic environment.
2. One heat treatment reduces the effect of a second, given up to 48 hours later: the phenomenon of *thermotolerance*.
3. In ischaemic tissues the reduced blood flow leads to less cooling and therefore to higher temperatures, for a given energy input. This is an important factor in tumour effects.
4. Hyperthermia enhances the effects of radiotherapy by two mechanisms: direct cell killing, and radiosensitization.
5. The interaction between hyperthermia and radiation is very time-dependent. Maximum cell killing is produced by simultaneous treatment.
6. Significant clinical benefits from combined hyperthermia and radiotherapy have been reported but until large-scale clinical trials have been made, this should be considered to be an experimental therapy.

Bibliography

Field SB and Morris CC (1983). The relationship between heating time and temperature: its relevance to clinical hyperthermia. *Radiother Oncol* 1:179-186.

Hahn GM, Ning SC, Elizaga M *et al* (1989). A comparison of thermal responses of human and rodent cells. *Int J Radiat Biol* 56:817-825.

Law MP, Ahier RG and Field SB (1978). The response of the mouse ear to heat applied alone or combined with x-rays. *Brit J Radiol* 51:132-138.

Lindegaard JC and Overgaard J (1987). Factors of importance for the development of the step-down heating effect in a C3H mammary carcinoma *in vivo*. *Int J Hyperthermia* 3:79-91.

Overgaard J (1985). *Hyperthermic Oncology 1984*. Vol. 1-2. Taylor & Francis; London and Philadelphia.

Müller C (1912). Therapeutische Erfahrungen an 100 mit Kombination von Röntgenstrahlen und Hochfrequentz, resp. Diathermie behandelten bösartigen Neubildungen. *Medizinische Wochenschrift* 59:1546-1549.

Overgaard J (1989). The current and potential role of hyperthermia in radiotherapy. *Int J Radiat Oncol Biol Phys* 16:535-549.

Overgaard J (1990). The rationale for clinical trials in hyperthermia. In: *An Introduction to the Practical Aspects of Clinical hyperthermia.* (Eds) Field SB and Franconi C, NATO ASI Series E: Applied Sciences, No 127, Martinus Nijhoff Publishers, Dordrecht, Boston.

Overgaard J and Bach Andersen J (1993). Hyperthermia. In: *Oxford Textbook of Oncology.* Oxford University Press; Oxford (in press).

Overgaard J and Nielsen O S (1983). The importance of thermotolerance for the clinical treatment with hyperthermia. *Radiother Oncol* 1:167-178.

Overgaard J, Nielsen OS and Lindegaard JC (1987). Biological basis for rational design of clinical treatment with combined hyperthermia and radiation. In: *An Introduction to the Practical Aspects of Clinical hyperthermia.* (Eds) Field SB and Franconi C, NATO ASI Series E: Applied Sciences, No 127, Martinus Nijhoff Publishers, Dordrecht, Boston.

Song CW (1984). Effect of local hyperthermia on blood flow and microenvironment: A review. *Cancer Res* 44:4721s-4730s.

Westra A and Dewey WC (1971). Sensitivity to heat shock of Chinese hamster cells. *Int J Radiat Biol* 19:467-477.

Further reading

Field SB and Hand JW (1990). *Practical Aspects of Clinical Hyperthermia*. Taylor & Francis, London and Philadelphia.

Gerner EW and Cetas TC (1992). *Hyperthermic Oncology 1992*. Vol. 1-2. Taylor & Francis; London and Philadelphia.

Sugahara T and Saito M (1989). *Hyperthermic Oncology 1988*. Vol. 1-2. Taylor & Francis; London, New York, Philadelphia.

Urano M and Douple E (1988). *Hyperthermia and Oncology*. Vol. 1. VSP BV; Utrecht.

Urano M and Douple E (1989). *Hyperthermia and Oncology*. Vol. 2. VSP BV; Utrecht.

Vaupel P and Kallinowski F (1987). Physiological effect of hyperthermia. *Recent Results Cancer Res* 104:71-109.

21

Targeted radiotherapy

Thomas E. Wheldon

21.1 Introduction

Targeted radiotherapy means using biological differences between tumour cells and normal tissues to deliver radionuclide atoms selectively, so that the tumour receives a higher radiation dose than normal tissues. The ultimate goal is to sterilize all the tumour cells by delivering to them a sufficiently high radiation dose, without exceeding the tolerance of any critical tissue. As with other forms of radiotherapy, its effectiveness will be determined both by physical and by radiobiological factors. Targeted radiotherapy has some similarities to low dose-rate brachytherapy. Both modalities achieve preferential cell kill by placing radionuclides close to tumour cells. In brachytherapy this is done by physical implantation, while with targeted radiotherapy it is the biological properties of the tumour that provide the basis for selective irradiation. In principle, targeted radiotherapy has the advantage that it may be capable of sterilizing metastases or micrometastases anywhere within the body, whether the individual tumours can be visualized or not. In practice, targeted radiotherapy is still at an early stage of development and has a long way to go before it achieves its full potential.

21.2 Targeting agents

The most immediate problem is to identify targeting agents or 'vehicles' that can be used to convey radionuclides selectively to tumour cells. Historically, the first clinical example of the targeted radiotherapy principle in oncology was the use of iodine-131 in the treatment of well-differentiated thyroid carcinomas. Unfortunately, no other tumour types exist for which so simple a targeting agent can be used.

In recent years a major impetus for both laboratory and clinical work on targeted radiotherapy has been the development of monoclonal antibody technology (Vaeth and Meyer, 1990). Monoclonal antibodies hold out the possibility of selectively targeting quite small molecular groups (i.e. epitopes) on the surface of cancer cells which, it is hoped, will be sufficiently different from corresponding epitopes on normal cells. Disappointingly, no really dramatic differences between normal and cancer cell surfaces have yet been found. Differences do exist, but these are usually quantitative rather than qualitative, so that monoclonal antibodies directed against the corresponding epitopes often show some degree of cross-reaction with histologically similar normal tissues. It is also recognized that antibodies, which are large molecules, may penetrate rather poorly into some tumours and also that not every cell of a tumour will have equal avidity for the antibody (the tumour heterogeneity problem).

There is considerable current interest in other kinds of molecules as potential targeting agents. One of the most promising of these is the catecholamine precursor analogue meta-iodo-benzylguanidine (mIBG) which is preferentially taken up by the catecholamine-synthesizing cells of certain tumour types such as neuroblastoma and phaeochromocytoma. The hormone somatostatin is also attracting attention as a way of targeting some neuro-endocrine tumours. These are smaller molecules than antibodies and it is likely that problems of tumour penetration will be less. Problems resulting from normal tissue cross-reaction and tumour heterogeneity of uptake are likely to remain. Many other putative targeting agents are now being studied. These include a variety of growth factors that might be used against tumours whose cells have been found to over-express the receptor for the appropriate growth factor (Capala and Carlsson, 1991; Mairs *et al*, 1991). Some actual and potential targeting agents are listed in Table 21.1.

21.3 Radionuclides for targeted therapy

Many radionuclides have been proposed or explored for use in targeted therapy but only a few have reached the point of clinical use. Important considerations in choosing a radionuclide include the nature of the particle emitted, its energy and mean range, its physical half-life and the ease and feasibility of conjugating it to appropriate targeting agents. Table 21.2 summarizes some properties of radionuclides of current interest. Generally, the radionuclides may be divided into long-range β-emitters, short range β-emitters and emitters of α-particles and Auger electrons of still shorter range. Generally, clinical experience to date has been confined to the long-range β-emitters (^{131}I and ^{90}Y). Ultra-short range Auger electrons are capable of direct cell kill only when targeted to DNA itself. Physical half-lives of a few days, comparable with the biological half-lives of most vehicles, are thought to be ideal. Very short half-lives (as with the α-emitters, ^{211}At and ^{212}Bi) may present considerable logistic difficulties. Chemical conjugation to carrier molecules is relatively easy for the halogens and becomes progressively more difficult with radiometals which tend to detach from the biological carrier molecule. Recently a group of 'macrocycle' compounds has been investigated and shown to bind radiometals firmly. It is possible that these compounds will further extend the list of usable radionuclides.

Long-range β-emitters have the property of irradiating untargeted cells by *cross-fire* from adjacent targeted cells. This may be advantageous when tumour heterogeneity leads to non-uniformity of dose delivery (Section 21.4) but it has the disadvantage that adjacent normal tissues may also be irradiated.

21.4 Radiation dosimetry and microdosimetry

In contrast to external beam irradiation, for which dosimetry is a precise science, the dosimetry of radiation delivered by radionuclides involves considerable uncertainties. At present, doses to both tumour and normal tissues can only be estimated approximately. Uncertainties arise from the non-uniformity of radionuclide distribution, its changing pattern with time and its dependence on individual patient pharmacokinetics. The usual approach to dose estimation is to employ the *MIRD Schema*, a set of data published by the US

Table 21.2 Properties of radionuclides of current interest in targeted therapy

Radionuclide	Half-life	Emission	Mean particle range
^{90}Y	2.7 days	β	5 mm
^{131}I	8 days	β	0.8 mm
^{67}Cu	2.5 days	β	0.6 mm
^{199}Au	3.1 days	β	0.3 mm
^{211}At	7 hours	α	0.05 mm
^{212}Bi	1 hour	α	0.05 mm
^{125}I	60 days	Auger	$\approx 1\ \mu$m
^{77}Br	2.4 days	Auger	$\approx 1\ \mu$m

Table 21.1 Targeting agents for radionuclide therapy

Agent	Appropriate tumour type	Clinical use?
Monoclonal antibodies	Wide variety	Yes
Molecular precursors of tumour-associated proteins (miBG, somatostatin)	Neuroblastoma, phaeochromocytoma, neuro-endocrine tumours	Yes
Growth factors (EGF, NGF, TGF α or β)	Tumours over-expressing receptor (e.g. glioma, melanoma, neuroblastoma, squamous-cell carcinomas)	No

Nuclear Medicine Society which provide tables of estimated absorbed dose in various tissues as a function of the radionuclide distribution and its variation with time. Because of the approximate nature of the dose estimates obtained by the MIRD approach, considerable margins of error must be allowed on the tolerances of normal tissues, for which dose-rate effects may also have to be considered (see below).

Despite the imprecision of existing dosimetric methods, sufficient information has been gathered to allow approximate estimates of how effective targeted radiotherapy may be expected to be, in terms of tumour cell kill.

Dosimetry and Radiocurability

Vaughan *et al* (1987) collated published data on the uptake of radiolabelled antibodies into human tumours and on the kinetics of antibody clearance. They observed for systemically injected radioactivity that a tumour uptake of 0.0005% per gram of tumour was typical, and that the concentration of bound antibody usually declined exponentially with a half-life of 2–3 days. These authors then used these parameters in a dosimetric model to calculate the doses that could be delivered to tumours by monoclonal antibody-targeted ^{131}I or ^{90}Y. They concluded that if the total whole-body radiation dose had to be limited to around 2 Gy (in the absence of bone marrow rescue) then it would not be possible to deliver curative doses (say of 60 Gy) to macroscopic solid tumours. To achieve such a dose, better targeting agents would be needed, or targeted therapy would have to be given by

some strategy which was more effective in terms of therapeutic differential than simply injecting radiolabelled antibodies into the bloodstream.

Microdosimetry and Radiocurability

A major difference between external-beam and radionuclide-targeted irradiation relates to microdosimetry, especially the absorption of dose in small tumours where dimensions are less than the mean path length of the particles emitted by the radionuclide (see Table 21.2 for particle path lengths). In the case of ^{131}I, the most commonly used radionuclide in clinical practice, microdosimetric problems arise in tumours whose diameter is less than 1–2 mm. If such microtumours have radionuclide atoms uniformly distributed throughout their volume, the absorption of the emitted energy will be relatively inefficient, with a substantial proportion of nuclear particles escaping into the surrounding tissues (Figure 21.1). Microdosimetric calculations by Humm (1986) have provided estimates of the fraction of emitted energy which would be absorbed by a spherical microtumour as a function of its diameter, for several different radionuclides. However, although the smaller microtumours absorb less dose, they also contain fewer clonogenic cells and therefore less dose is needed to sterilize them. These factors result in a relationship between tumour curability and tumour size which is more complex for targeted radiotherapy than for external-beam irradiation. With conventional radiotherapy, it is well known that the larger a tumour, the lower will be the chance of its being sterilized by any given dose

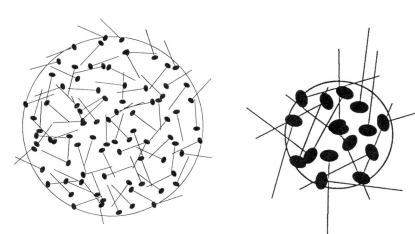

Figure 21.1 The proportion of energy deposited *outside* a radiolabelled metastasis becomes considerable when its diameter is comparable with the mean range of the emitted radiation. Reproduced with permission from Dr. J.A. O'Donoghue.

of radiation (Section 14.4). This is illustrated in Figure 21.2A which shows how at each of several radiation dose levels, tumour cure probability decreases steadily as a function of tumour size. In contrast, Figure 21.2B shows how tumour cure probability changes with tumour size for several activity levels of [131]I. Unlike the external irradiation situation, the family of curves show a rising component (increasing tumour size leading to more efficient absorption of emitted energy), a peak value, and a falling component where the increasing number of cells to be sterilized dominates the response. As a result, for each radionuclide there is an optimal tumour diameter for radiocurability (Table 21.3); both smaller and larger tumours will be less radiocurable than those at the optimal size. The lower radiocurability of very small micrometastases is a unique feature of radionuclide therapy and is one of the reasons why the combination of targeted radiotherapy with external-beam irradiation may be an effective strategy (Wheldon and O'Donoghue, 1990).

21.5 Radiobiological factors in targeted radiotherapy

As with other forms of therapeutic irradiation, the biological effectiveness of targeted radiotherapy will depend on radiobiological factors as well as

on the physics of dose absorption. The *5 Rs* of radiobiology (Section 5.9) will be involved to a greater or lesser extent. *Intrinsic radiosensitivity* is certainly an important factor. Because of the limited uptake and specificity of targeting agents now available, only tumour types with high intrinsic sensitivity (e.g. neuroblastoma, myeloma, seminoma, leukaemia and lymphoma) will have any prospect of being sterilized by targeted radiotherapy alone. *Repair* assumes importance because of the usually low and exponentially-declining dose rate at which most of the treatment will be given. For many tumours, especially those for which the α/β ratio exceeds 10 Gy, the sparing effect of low dose-rate irradiation will probably not be great. Fowler (1990) has calculated that for such a tumour an extra 10–20% dose would have to be given, compared with conventionally fractionated external-beam radiotherapy. However, some tumour types (e.g. glioma, melanoma, osteosarcoma) may have lower α/β ratios and for these considerable sparing could occur. Similarly, for normal tissues, the magnitude of the sparing will be modest for acute-responding tissues (typically with high α/β ratios, Section 8.5) but considerably greater for late-responding tissues (with low α/β ratios). Wheldon and O'Donoghue (1990) have calculated that for biological isoeffect in late-responding tissues, the effectiveness of targeted radiotherapy may be reduced several-fold

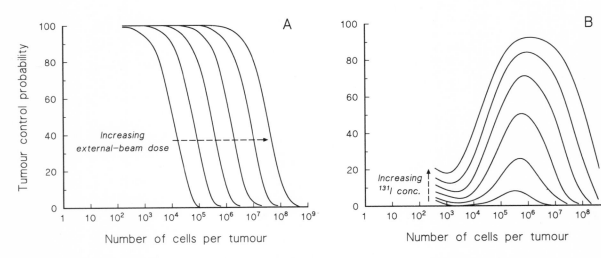

Figure 21.2   Relationship between tumour cure probability and tumour size: for external-beam irradiation at 6 different dose levels (left panel) and for spherical tumours labelled uniformly with various ^{131}I concentrations (right panel). The tumour size for maximum cure rate is a property of the isotope (Table 21.3) but independent of dose.

relative to single-dose irradiation at high dose rate.

Other radiobiological factors are probably of lesser importance. *Redistribution* could be of some significance, because of a possible inverse dose-rate effect. Theoretically, this could result from a gradual recruitment of radiation-inhibited cells into more sensitive phases of the cell cycle, as the dose rate falls. This mechanism would be expected to apply to rapidly proliferating

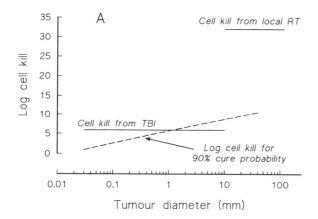

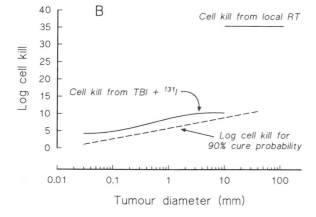

Figure 21.3 Calculated log cell kill for neuroblastoma. **A:** micrometastases (diameter < 10 mm) given 7 × 2 Gy TBI and detectable tumours (diameter > 10 mm) given 30 × 2 Gy local radiotherapy. The 90% isocure line gives the log cell kill that would be necessary for 90% cure at each tumour size and shows that micrometastases in the size range 1–10 mm are most likely to escape sterilization. **B:** log cell kill when one TBI fraction is replaced by targeted ^{131}I therapy sufficient to give 2 Gy whole-body dose (assuming 0.01%/g tumour uptake).

tumour cells and would probably not occur in late-responding tissues, most of whose cells are out of cycle. *Reoxygenation* could be an important cause of resistance, since most of the radiation dose delivered by targeted radiotherapy is usually given within a week, as a result of the biological clearance of the agent and radioactive decay. A week may not be sufficient for complete reoxygenation. However, the clinical efficacy of some forms of brachytherapy (for which the time-scale is similar) and the reduced OER for low dose-rate irradiation argue against this being a serious problem. Nevertheless, hypoxic cell radiosensitizers or bioreductive drugs should be explored in conjunction with targeted radiotherapy in laboratory systems.

Finally, it is unlikely that *repopulation* will be a major factor for a treatment scheme that delivers most of the radiation dose over a few days. It is worth noting, however, that tumour cell proliferation will counteract the modest cell kill achieved by radiation at low dose rates. As a result, when the dose rate falls below 2–3 cGy/hr the treatment is likely to be ineffective (Fowler, 1990).

21.6 Strategies for improved clinical results

It is generally agreed that the specificity of existing targeting agents is insufficient to enable sterilization of macroscopic solid tumours. The number of possible targeting agents is growing, however, and protein engineering techniques are continually being used to shape antibody molecules to give them superior properties.

Several strategies have been developed to improve the therapeutic efficacy of targeted radiotherapy. One approach, pioneered by Epenetos and colleagues, is the use of regionally targeted therapy; radiolabelled antibodies or other agents are injected into a body region or compartment instead of into the general circulation. Obviously, this will not work for widespread cancer but it might be effective in controlling more localized spread. Regional targeting is now being explored clinically for the treatment of carcinoma of the ovary (Stewart *et al*, 1989), also of tumour cells within the cerebro-spinal fluid (Lashford *et al*, 1988), and it may be used in other tumour sites.

Fractionation is also being explored. There is no strong radiobiological case for this, since sparing would not be expected in the fractionation of low dose-rate irradiation. However, there are some non-radiobiological arguments in favour of this, such as the possibility of improving tumour uptake of the agent if all cellular targets had been saturated during the first treatment. Fractionated treatment using antibodies sometimes leads to the development of an immunological response to the antibodies, which are usually of murine origin. Attempts are being made to modify mouse antibodies to make them less antigenic in humans, or to replace portions of the antibody molecule with a human equivalent (*humanization* of antibodies) to overcome the problem of human anti-mouse antibody generation by the host immune system.

There are also theoretical arguments in favour of two-step targeting strategies, to improve the kinetics of the targeting reaction. For example, unlabelled antibodies conjugated to avidin might be injected and allowed to concentrate in the tumour (perhaps over 12–48 hours) before injecting a radiolabelled small molecule (such as biotin) which rapidly targets the avidin component of the conjugate. Two-step targeting strategies could be especially useful with radionuclides with short half-lives, for instance α-emitters such as ^{211}At.

Another strategy is to seek to reduce normal-tissue reactions to the targeted therapy, thus to allow higher doses to be given. At present, myelosuppression due to irradiation of bone marrow is the most important side-effect of targeted radiotherapy. This could be reduced, in selected patients, by the use of bone marrow rescue or, perhaps more widely, by administration of haemopoietic growth factors. Bone marrow rescue is an important component of the strategy of combined modality therapy described below.

21.7 Microdosimetric rationales for combined modality treatment

The future of targeted radiotherapy may be in combination with some other treatment modality. Since targeted radiotherapy is ineffective in treating bulky disease, there is a clear case for combining it with local radiotherapy to sites of known disease, the approach described as *spatial cooperation* (Section 18.2). Combination with chemotherapy might also exploit non-overlapping toxicities. It was suggested some years ago on the basis of macroscopic dosimetry that the combina-

tion of targeted radiotherapy with external-beam irradiation may be therapeutically advantageous (Wessels and Rogus, 1984). Combination treatments are already being employed clinically, mostly on an *ad hoc* basis (Order, 1990). However, the development of microdosimetric modelling has provided new rationales for combination therapy, which now make it seem almost obligatory if cure of disseminated malignant disease is to be achieved.

There are two distinct microdosimetric rationales, one based on the inefficient dose absorption by uniformly targeted microtumours of dimension less than the emitted particle mean range, the other derived from considerations of tumour heterogeneity and consequent non-uniformity of dose distribution within the tumour. Fortunately these rationales lead to the same conclusion.

As indicated in Table 21.3, the most efficient absorption of radiation from ^{131}I occurs in tumours whose diameter is ≈2 mm, which are therefore the most radiocurable by this isotope. Wheldon *et al* (1992) have used these microdosimetric findings in exploring theoretically the clinical implications for treatment of radiosensitive tumours like neuroblastoma or lymphoma. Firstly, note that for local external-beam irradiation it is necessary that a tumour be large enough to be imaged and localized. Generally, this means that the tumour must be at least a few millimetres in diameter. Total-body irradiation (TBI) in conjunction with bone-marrow rescue can be given in 2 Gy fractionated treatments up to a total dose of 14 Gy. This is sufficient to sterilize single cells and small micrometastases of radiosensitive tumours but is insufficient to treat micrometastases approaching millimetre dimensions. Figure 21.3A illustrates this. The dashed line shows the log cell kill necessary to control tumours ranging in size from 0.03 mm diameter (≈10 cells) to 30 mm diameter (≈10^{10} cells). We assume here that 14 Gy (i.e. 7 × 2 Gy) of TBI

Table 21.3 Tumour size for optimal radiocurability by uniformly targeted radionuclides

Radionuclide	Tumour diameter	Cell number
^{90}Y	≈2 cm	≈10^{10}
^{131}I	≈2 mm	≈10^6
^{211}At	≈60 μm	≈10^1
^{125}I (Auger Component)	≈1 μm	≈1

may give 6 logs of cell kill in tumours up to 1 cm diameter and that external-beam radiotherapy confined to larger tumours may give a 32-log cell kill. The diagram shows that this combined treatment would be expected to fail for tumours that are 1–10 mm in diameter. Fortunately, these larger micrometastases are in exactly the right size-class for sterilization by targeted ^{131}I. Figure 21.3B shows the effect of replacing *one* of the TBI fractions with targeted ^{131}I, choosing a dose that might give an equivalent whole-body radiation dose. The result in the intermediate size range is improved. These considerations thus predict benefit from combining external-beam TBI and targeted ^{131}I in treating disseminated malignant disease. Larger tumours should be treated using *localized* high-dose irradiation.

The second microdosimetric rationale derives from the likelihood that dose to cellular targets will be non-uniform, as a result of limited diffusion of targeting agent or intra-tumour gradients due to local absorption of the targeting molecule if not present in excess. In all these circumstances, dose non-uniformity is highly likely, and has been observed in practice (Yorke *et al*, 1987; Griffith *et al*, 1988; Moyes *et al*, 1989). O'Donoghue (1991) has explored theoretically the implications of heterogeneity in targeted radiotherapy. He assumed that a small proportion of cells receive no dose from targeted radiotherapy, a reasonable assumption for targeting by short-range emitters but an approximation for long-range β-emitters where untargeted cells receive some dose from adjacent targeted cells. This led to an important general principle. If a small proportion of cells (say 1 in 10^4) receive no dose from targeting, then it is not useful to apply targeted therapy at treatment intensities that give more than 4 logs of tumour cell kill (i.e. a survival of below 10^{-4}). Otherwise, *overkill* of targeted cells will result, with no advantage in the killing of untargeted cells, yet with an increase in normal-tissue toxicity. This optimal level of targeted treatment would be better combined with sufficiently high levels of some other treatment modality (such as external-beam irradiation or chemotherapy) to sterilize the cells that have escaped the targeting treatment. In a series of model calculations on targeted ^{131}I, TBI and bone marrow rescue, O'Donoghue (1991) showed that the TBI component is obligatory for cure and often forms a high proportion of the total dose given to normal tissues.

These microdosimetric rationales, together with

earlier arguments by Wessels and Rogus (1984), make a strong case for the incorporation of targeted radiotherapy as a component of combined modality treatment. Clinical studies are now under way to determine whether these theoretical predictions are borne out in practice.

21.8 Boron neutron capture therapy (BNCT)

This is a specialized approach to targeted therapy that has been under discussion for many years; it is nevertheless one that holds considerable promise (Barth *et al* 1990). Its title is somewhat misleading in that this is not a form of neutron therapy but a way of generating alpha-particles within the tumour site; it is this secondary radiation that is responsible for any tomouricidal effect. The approach relies on the physical properties of the non-radioactive boron isotope ^{10}B. When exposed to 'slow' neutrons (i.e. with thermal or epithermal energies) this isotope has a large cross-section for neutron capture. A fission reaction ensues in which the boron nucleus splits into ^{7}Li plus ^{4}He, also emitting a pulse of γ-rays. The ^{4}He nucleus is an alpha-particle which produces a densely ionizing track over a range of a few cell diameters. In the absence of boron, fission neutrons at the intensities required for this process produce little biological damage.

BNCT is a two-step strategy: targeting of ^{10}B to tumour cells, followed by fission of the isotope by neutron irradiation (Figure 21.4). The use of an external neutron beam and the fact that ^{10}B itself is a 'cold' isotope gives the therapist more control over the process than is usual in targeted therapy. Boron may accumulate in organ sites (e.g. liver) other than in the tumour, but if these sites are known it may be possible to avoid irradiating them with neutrons. The effectiveness of this treatment requires sufficient difference in uptake between the tumour and *local* normal tissues. Alpha-particle radiation is very damaging to targeted cells and even the most resistant cell types will be efficiently sterilized. Research effort is being given to the production of filtered beams of epithermal neutrons which have superior penetration properties compared with thermal neutrons. In Europe, this effort is concentrated at the Nuclear Reactor Facility at Petten in the Netherlands with the initial objective of treating intracranial disease.

Thermal or Epithermal
Neutrons

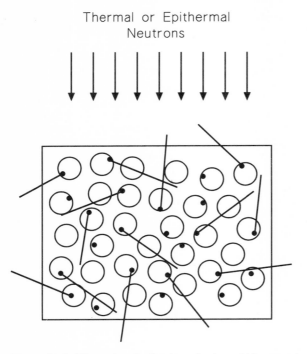

Figure 21.4 Illustrating the local production within a smal volume of tissue of isotropic alpha-particle radiation by neutron-induced fission of boron atoms. (○ cells; ● ^{10}B atoms; —— α-tracks).

As with any form of targeted therapy, success depends critically on the availability of a suitable targeting agent, in this case one that will carry boron into tumour cells to a higher concentration than in local normal tissues. The search for such compounds is under way (Barth *et al* 1990; Nguyen *et al* 1993). Monoclonal antibodies are an obvious candidate, but whether these are capable of carrying sufficient boron is yet to be ascertained. The use of boron-conjugated EGF to target tumours that over-express the EGF receptor is also being considered (Andersson *et al* 1992). Oligonucleotides conjugated to boron are further potential candidates for exploiting specific abnormal DNA sequences in malignamt tumours and these may have the advantage of requiring less boron incorporation for cell killing by BNCT.

Although unique in some respects, BNCT may well be limited by factors that are common to all radioactive targeting methods. Its therapeutic effectiveness will depend on the selectivity of uptake of boron into the tumour. The alpha-particles generated by BNCT have a short range and the level of cell killing will depend on the homogeneity of boron uptake among tumour cells. For this reason, the combination of BNCT and external-beam treatment, as described in the previous section, may be necessary.

Key points

1. Targeted radiotherapy is the irradiation of tumours by means of radionuclides that are selectively delivered by tumour-seeking molecules (*targeting agents*).
2. Targeting agents may be monoclonal antibodies, molecular precursors of tumour-associated proteins, hormones or growth factors. Many radionuclides are under consideration for targeting but only the β-emitters ^{131}I and ^{90}Y have been used clinically to any extent.
3. The most important radiobiological factors governing the success of targeted radiotherapy will be intrinsic radiosensitivity of the tumour cells and the repair capacity of cells in tumours and in critical normal tissues.
4. The major problems of targeted radiotherapy are insufficient selectivity of tumour uptake, limited penetration of the targeting agent into solid tumours, and heterogeneous expression of cellular targets leading to non-uniformity of absorbed dose. When long-range β-emitting radionuclides are used, microtumours whose dimensions are less than the β-particle mean range will be spared due to low absorption of the radiation energy. Some killing of untargeted cells will however result from *cross-fire* from adjacent targeted cells.
5. Clinical strategies to overcome these problems include the use of targeting agents of low molecular weight, regional targeting, two-stage targeting procedures and the combination of targeted radiotherapy with other treatments.
6. Radiobiological modelling studies suggest that the combination of targeted radiotherapy with external-beam irradiation (local and systemic) may be the optimal strategy for those targeting agents which are presently available.

Bibliography

Andersson A, Andersson J, Burgman JO *et al* (1992). Program for BNCT with accelerator keV neutrons and related chemical and biological studies. In: *Progress in Neutron Capture Therapy for Cancer.* (Eds) Allen BJ, Moore DE and Harrington BV; Plenum press, New York, pp41-52.

Capala J and Carlsson J (1991). Influence of chloroquine and lidocaine on retention and cytotoxic effects of ^{131}I-EGF: studies on cultured glioma cells. *Int J Radiat Biol* 60:497-510.

Griffith MH, Yorke ED and Wessels BW (1988). Direct dose confirmation of quantitative autoradiography with micro-TLD measurements for radioimmunotherapy. *J Nuc Med* 29:1795-1809.

Lashford LS, Davies AG, Richardson RB *et al* (1988). A pilot study of ^{131}I monoclonal antibodies in the therapy of lepto meningeal tumours. *Cancer* 61:857-868.

Mairs RJ, Angerson W, Gaze MN *et al* (1991). The distribution of alternative agents for targeted radiotherapy within human neuroblastoma spheroids. *Br J Cancer* 63:404-409.

Moyes JSE, Babich JW, Carter R *et al* (1989). A quantitative study of meta-iodobenzyl-guanidine (mIBG) in children with neuroblastoma: correlation with tumour histopathology. *J Nuc Med* 30:474-480.

Nguyen T, Brownwell GL, Holden SA *et al* (1993). Subcellular distribution of various boron compounds and implications for their efficacy in boron neutron capture therapy by Monte Carlo simulations. *Radiat Res* 133:33-40.

O'Donoghue JA (1991). Optimal scheduling of biologically targeted radiotherapy and total body irradiation for the treatment of systemic malignant disease. *Int J Radiat Oncol Biol Phys* 21:1587-1594.

Stewart JSW, Hird V, Snook D *et al* (1989). Intraperitoneal radioimmunotherapy for ovarian cancer: pharmacokinetics, toxicity and efficacy of ^{131}I labelled monoclonal antibodies. *Int J Radiat Oncol Biol Phys* 16:405-413.

Wessels BW and Rogus KD (1984). Radionuclide selection and model absorbed dose calculations for radiolabelled tumour associated antibodies. *Med Phys* 11:638-644.

Wheldon TE and O'Donoghue JA (1990). The radiobiology of targeted radiotherapy. *Int J Radiat Biol* 58:1-21.

Yorke ED, Griffith ML and Wessels BW (1987). Quantitative autoradiography and micro-TLD measurements in radioimmunotherapy. *J Nuc Med* 28:617.

Further reading

Barth RF, Soloway AH and Fairchild RG (1990). Boron neutron therapy of cancer. *Cancer Res* 50:1061-1070.

Fowler JF (1990). Radiobiological aspects of low dose rates in radioimmunotherapy. *Int J Radiat Oncol Biol Phys* 18:1261-1269.

Humm JL (1986). Dosimetric aspects of radiolabelled antibodies for tumour therapy. *J Nuc Med* 27:1490-1497.

Order SE (1990). Perspectives in radio-immunoglobulin therapy. In: *The Present and Future Role of Monoclonal Antibodies in the Management of Cancer* (Eds) Vaeth JM and Meyers JL. *Frontiers of Radiation Therapy and Oncology, Vol 24.* Karger; Basel.

Vaeth JM and Meyer JL (Eds) (1990). *The Present and Future Role of Monoclonal Antibodies in the Management of Cancer. Frontiers of Radiation Therapy Vol 24.* Karger; Basel.

Vaughan ATM, Anderson P, Dykes P and Bradwell AR (1987). Limitations to killing of tumours using radiolabelled antibodies. *Br J Radiol* 60:567-578.

Wheldon TE, Amin AE, O'Donoghue JA and Barrett A (1992). Radiocurability of disseminated malignant disease by external beam irradiation and targeted radionuclide therapy. In: *Advances in the Applications of Monoclonal Antibodies in Clinical Oncology*, 8th International Hammersmith Meeting. (Ed) Epenetos AE. John Wiley; London.

22

Photodyamic therapy

Fiona A. Stewart and Nico van Zandwijk

22.1 Mechanisms of photodynamic therapy

Photodynamic therapy (PDT) is a relatively new cancer treatment modality which aims to selectively destroy cancerous tissue by an interaction between absorbed light and a photosensitizing agent. The basic principle of PDT consists of systemic administration of the photosensitizer, followed by local illumination of the tumour with light of a suitable wavelength to activate the sensitizer.

Photochemical and Sub-cellular Effects

The majority of PDT studies have used the photosensitizer haematoporphyrin ether (Photofrin II). This compound is a mixture of monomeric, dimeric and oligomeric species with 5 major absorption peaks at 400 nm (strongest absorption) to 630 nm (weakest absorption). The haematoporphyrins are not toxic in the absence of light but can be excited by light of a wavelength corresponding to one of the absorption peaks. The excited sensitizer molecule can then undergo two types of reaction with surrounding molecules (Figure 22.1). An electron-transfer process may occur, in which the sensitizer interacts with biomolecular substrates generating free radicals which in turn react with molecular oxygen to form oxidized products (*type I reaction*). Alternatively, the excited sensitizer may transfer its energy directly to molecular oxygen, yielding singlet oxygen (*type II reaction*). PDT-induced cytotoxicity is thought to be due mainly to singlet oxygen production. The competition between these two types of reaction is influenced by the relative amounts of oxygen, photo-oxidizable target, and pH. Electron donors (e.g. cysteine and glutathione) can compete with molecular oxygen as quenchers for the excited triplet-state sensitizer, so that at low oxygen tensions the formation of free radicals may be an important mechanism of PDT damage. Low pH has also been shown to favour a type I mechanism. For both type I and type II reactions there is a requirement for the presence of oxygen.

The radicals produced by the photochemical reaction are highly reactive, and therefore most of the resultant damage occurs near the site of production. Damage to a wide range of subcellular organelles and biomolecules has been observed, including the plasma membrane, mitochondrial and nuclear membranes, lysosomes and microsomes. DNA damage can also occur (single-strand breaks and alkaline labile lesions) but nuclear damage is not generally considered to be a major consequence of PDT.

Cellular Effects

In vitro cell survival studies have demonstrated that cell killing by PDT depends on the concentra-

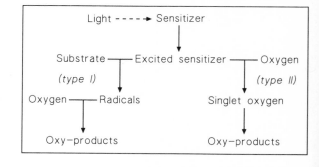

Figure 22.1 Two types of photo-oxidation reaction involving the excitation of a sensitizer molecule by light.

tion of sensitizer and the light dose (joules/cm²), but not strongly on dose rate (watts/cm²), providing that thermal effects are avoided. At non-thermal power settings, light alone does not cause cell killing. The shape of the *in vitro* light-dose survival curves is generally a shouldered exponential, with a threshold at low light doses followed by exponential killing at higher doses (Figure 22.2). Repair of sublethal PDT damage has been demonstrated from split-dose experiments in which the surviving fraction increased as the time between treatments was increased from 0 to 9 hours. Repair of potentially lethal damage has also been demonstrated by repair inhibition experiments involving holding cells at 4°C or treating with caffeine immediately after exposure to light.

Cell killing by PDT can only occur in the presence of oxygen, which interacts directly with the excited triplet-state sensitizer yielding singlet oxygen, or with free radicals formed as an intermediate step by interaction between the excited sensitizer and biomolecular substrate. *In vitro* studies have demonstrated that cell inactivation by PDT does not occur in the absence of oxygen (Figure 22.3) and that reduction of oxygen tension to 1% decreases photoactivation by 50%.

In Vivo Effects

The absolute requirement for the presence of oxygen for direct cell killing by PDT might suggest that the usefulness of PDT would be severely limited when treating solid tumours that contain areas of hypoxia or low oxygen tension. However, it is now clear that PDT damage *in vivo* occurs largely *via the vasculature*, with direct damage to the endothelial cells leading to secondary tumour cell death as the result of vascular constriction and occlusion. Obstruction of tumour blood flow occurs within minutes of PDT, followed by vascular stasis, haemorrhage and extravasation of red blood cells. Damage to endothelial cells in tumours has been observed after PDT, also very high concentrations of porphyrin sensitizers have been measured in endothelial cells. However, it is not certain whether the observed effects represent direct endothelial-cell toxicity or an indirect effect via damage to mast cells or platelets.

Whatever the initial mechanism, much of the PDT-induced damage seen *in vivo* is mediated through damage to the vasculature. Henderson *et al* (1985) showed that when EMT6 or RIF1

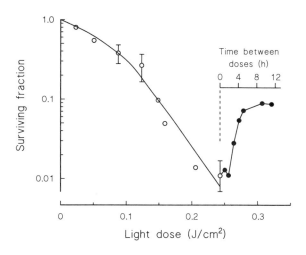

Figure 22.2 Surviving fraction of EJ cells (a subline of the T-24 bladder carcinoma) treated with a haematoporphyrin-derivative sensitizer before graded single doses of red light (○) or 2 equal doses of red light (0.12 J/cm²) separated by 0 to 12 h in the dark (●). Survival increased with increasing interval between light doses, with maximal recovery by 4 to 9 hours. From Bellnier and Lin (1985), with permission.

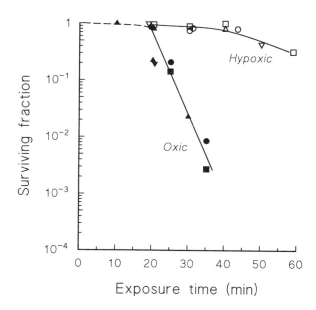

Figure 22.3 Survival of Chinese hamster cells treated with haematoporphyrin derivative and exposed to red light under aerated (closed symbols) or hypoxic conditions (open symbols). From Mitchell *et al* (1985), with permission.

tumour cells were treated *in vivo* and subsequently plated *in vitro* there was little cell killing if the cells were excised and plated immediately. Much more cell killing was observed when the cells were left *in situ* for 24 hours after treatment (Figure 22.4). These results are consistent with an extensive amount of indirect tumour cell kill due to vascular damage.

Measurements of oxygen levels in animal tumours before and after PDT have demonstrated a significant decrease in pO_2 occurring within minutes of treatment and persisting for at least 24 hours (Figure 22.5). Experimental studies have therefore demonstrated a marked influence of PDT on tumour vasculature and oxygenation and have led to the general conclusion that tumour cell death *in vivo* occurs largely as a secondary phenomenon due to vascular collapse. It is likely that PDT will only lead to tumour cure if the vasculature of the tumour and surrounding normal tissue is destroyed.

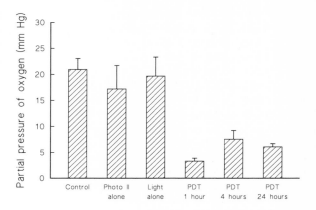

Figure 22.5   The mean pO_2 levels in a rat chondrosarcoma decreased from 1 to 24 hours after PDT (Photofrin II before 120 J/cm² light). Sensitizer or light alone had no effect on pO_2. From Reed *et al* (1989), with permission.

Drug Uptake

The mechanisms by which photosensitizers accumulate in tumours are not clear but may be related to the micro-environment of tumours. High vascular permeability and low lymphatic drainage cause trapping of protein-bound drugs in the interstitial spaces in tumours. Many photosensitizers, such as Photofrin II, do not show preferential uptake in tumours but there are differences in metabolism between cancerous and normal cells which can lead to less rapid clearing of the drugs from tumours, allowing selective therapy if illumination is delayed for several hours or days after drug administration.

Tumour Illumination in PDT

Illumination of the tumour area is nearly always carried out with powerful laser light (for instance produced by argon-pumped dye lasers) and delivered to the tumour by fibre optics. Superficial illumination can be performed with special lens tips to spread the light over the tumour area, or interstitial tumour illumination may be performed using fibres with cylindrical diffusing tips.

One major limitation of PDT with haematoporphyrin sensitizers is that the longest wavelength of light suitable for excitation of the sensitizer is 630 nm. Light of this wavelength penetrates poorly into solid tissues, in fact to a maximum

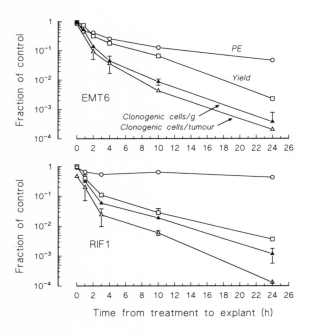

Figure 22.4   Cell survival after *in vivo* PDT of EMT6 or RIF1 tumours (Photofrin II, 24 h prior to illumination with 200 J/cm²) decreased with increasing time between illumination and plating. Plating efficiency (○ and yield of viable cells per gram ● are shown, as well as the resultant clonogenic cells/g (▲) and clonogenic cells per tumour (△). From Henderson *et al* (1985), with permission.

depth of 8 to 10 mm. Light of lower wavelengths, corresponding to the strongest absorption peaks of these sensitizers, is completely unsuitable for PDT of solid tumours due to its even more limited light penetration. At 630 nm, tumours larger than 8–10 mm cannot be effectively treated with a single fibre, either by interstitial or superficial illumination. For small tumours, a significant delay in tumour growth, also cure, can be achieved using interstitial light doses in the range of 200 to 500 J/cm fibre length (Figure 22.6). New second-generation photosensitizers (e.g. phthalocyanines) are currently being developed for PDT. These compounds have strong absorption peaks above 650 nm, which will give better light penetration and distribution with the tumour.

Power settings used for *in vivo* PDT are generally in the range 100 to 400 mW. Remembering that 1 joule = 1 watt second, a power of 200 mW dissipated over an area of 1 cm^2 requires an exposure time of 1000 seconds to deliver a light dose of 200 J/cm^2. At intensities exceeding 200 mW/cm^2 hyperthermia is induced which may contribute to the total cell killing effect.

22.2 Clinical application of photodynamic therapy

During the last 15 years photodynamic therapy has attracted increasing interest as an alternative

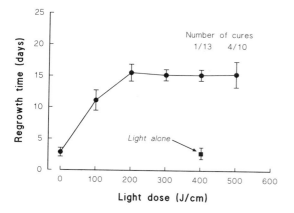

Figure 22.6 Tumour growth delay after *in vivo* PDT of 5 mm RIF1 tumours (● Photofrin II given 24 h before interstitial illumination). Growth delay increased with increasing light dose between 100 and 200 J/cm. At higher light doses some tumours did not regrow. From P. Baas, unpublished, with permission.

treatment modality for small superficial tumours in sites where adequate local surgery is difficult, e.g. carcinoma of bronchus, oesophagus, bladder, head and neck, cervix and the eye. In many cases, particularly in tumours of the bronchus and cervix, a general anaesthetic is not required and treatments can be completed within 30 minutes with minimal patient discomfort. Typical treatment protocols currently involve intravenous administration of 2 mg/kg Photofrin II at 24 to 48 h before illumination of the tumour with laser light at 630 nm. For illumination of individual tumours (e.g. non-small-cell tumours of the bronchus) light doses of 150 to 400 J/cm^2 are typically applied, depending on tumour size. For illumination of the whole bladder, in treating multiple small and occult lesions, lower doses of 15 to 30 J/cm^2 (non-scattered light) are used.

Patients treated to date with PDT have mainly been advanced cases with recurrent tumours or tumours that failed to respond to conventional treatment regimes. Consequently, there is a lack of long-term follow-up information to fully evaluate the efficacy of clinical PDT but experience so far indicates local responses in as many as 60–80% of patients in this heterogeneous and poor-prognosis group. Randomized trials have now been initiated for both obstructive bronchial cancer and carcinoma *in situ* of the bladder. Promising results are being achieved for early-stage lung cancer, with complete responses of 80% and follow-up of over 5 years in some trials (Table 22.1).

22.3 Skin photosensitivity

The only significant toxicity that has been documented for the porphyrin sensitizers is a generalized and long-lasting skin photosensitivity. This reaction can be severe and patients are therefore advised to avoid direct sunlight for up to 8 weeks after treatment. Haematoporphyrin derivatives can be activated by light of different wavelengths throughout most of the visible spectrum (400 to 630 nm) and skin protection by commercially available sunscreens is ineffective, since they only block the UV spectrum.

The development of new photosensitizers, such as the phthalocyanines which have shorter half-lives than Photofrin II or show less retention in the skin, should eventually eliminate the problem

Table 22.1   Results of some clinical studies of photodynamic therapy in early (stage 1) non-small-cell lung cancer

Investigator	N	CR*	Recurrences (unrelated deaths)	Follow-up
Kato *et al*, 1989 (Tokyo Medical College Hospital)	26	100%	1 (9)	mean 39.5 months
Edell and Cortese, 1989 (Mayo Clinic)	13	93%	3	2 yr
Sutedja *et al*, 1992 (The Netherlands Cancer Institute)	11	90%	1 (2)	median 1 year

*Complete remissions

of skin photosensitivity. An alternative approach until these new sensitizers are approved for general clinical use is to combine PDT with singlet-oxygen quenchers or radical scavengers.

The radioprotector WR-2721 has been shown to give effective protection against PDT-induced skin damage in mouse skin. The mechanism of protection probably involves radical scavenging as well as a photobleaching effect (i.e. inactivation of the porphyrins). N-acetylcysteine (NAC) is another radical scavenger which has been in clinical use for many years as a mucolytic agent. NAC also appears to have a protective effect against PDT-induced skin damage in mice, with a protection factor of about 1.5 (Figure 22.7). Note that the reaction due to 150 J/cm^2 with NAC is roughly the same as following 100 J/cm^2 alone. NAC may be a suitable drug to prescribe routinely after clinical PDT, since it has very low toxicity and can be taken orally for protracted periods.

22.4 Methods for improving the efficacy of PDT

Adequate light delivery to tumours above 1 cm^3 in volume is a problem when using haematoporphyrin sensitizers which are activated at relatively short (630 nm) wavelengths. Light distribution could be improved by the use of multiple fibres or a combination of interstitial and superficial light. The development of new photosensitizers which have absorption peaks at longer wavelengths will also help overcome this problem.

Light dosimetry for clinical PDT is complex

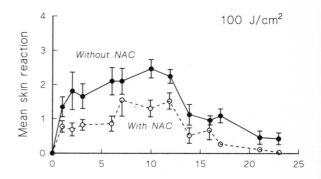

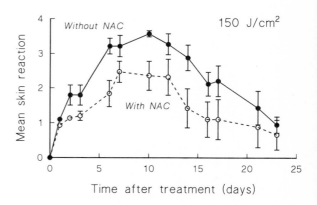

Figure 22.7   Mouse skin reactions after PDT (Photofrin II plus light doses of 100 J/cm^2 (upper panel) or 150 J/cm^2 (lower panel)) increased to a maximum on day 8 to 12, with subsequent healing. Skin reactions were significantly reduced when N-acetylcysteine (2 g/kg) was administered before illumination. Compare with time-course of skin reactions after ionising radiation (Figure 4.4A). From P. Baas, unpublished.

and has so far received insufficient attention. At present, most clinical protocols prescribe the light dose in terms of energy delivered to the tissue. This does not take account of scattered light dose and therefore gives little information on the total fluence of light in the tissue. The contribution of scattered light dose can only be determined if the optical properties of the tissue are known. Accurate dosimetry using phantoms in tissue-equivalent material is required to determine true fluence rate in tissue. Star *et al* (1987) have made such measurements in bladder phantoms and demonstrated that, for the human bladder, the total fluence for whole bladder illumination is about 5 times the incident primary light dose.

One limitation of PDT is that direct cell killing does not occur under hypoxic conditions. However, as indicated above, tumour cells can die as a secondary consequence of PDT-induced vascular damage, leading to a good therapeutic outcome. It may even be possible to exploit PDT-induced hypoxia by combining PDT with bioreductive agents which require metabolic reduction to become toxic. A few experimental studies have demonstrated an improvement in tumour response when PDT was combined with bioreductive drugs (an example is shown in Figure 22.8). This seems a promising approach which needs further investigation to evaluate the potential clinical benefits of photodynamic therapy combined with drug treatment.

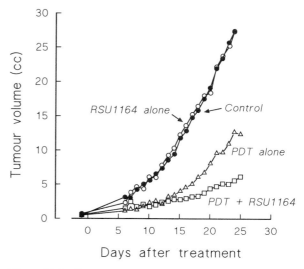

Figure 22.8 Growth of Dunning AT-2 prostate tumours in rats after treatment with PDT alone ($\triangle$: haematoporphyrin derivative before 720 J/cm^2 light) or PDT in combination with the bioreductive agent RSU 1164 ($\square$) Growth curves for untreated tumours ($\bullet$) or tumours treated with RSU 1164 alone ($\circ$) were identical. Tumours treated with combined PDT and RSU-1164 regrew more slowly than those treated with PDT alone. From Henry and Isaacs (1989), with permission.

Key points

1. PDT involves the interaction of a photosensitizer and light of a suitable wavelength. This initiates a photochemical reaction which results in production of free radicals and singlet oxygen, leading to cellular damage.
2. Tumour effects *in vivo* occur mainly by destruction of the vasculature, with secondary tumour cell death as the result of ischaemia. Extensive reduction in tumour blood flow and pO$_2$ are seen within minutes of PDT.
3. Photodynamic therapy is mainly limited by difficulties in adequate light delivery (poor penetration at wavelengths used to excite currently available sensitizers) and light dosimetry.

Bibliography

Bellnier DA and Lin CN (1985). Photosensitization and split dose recovery in cultured human urinary bladder carcinoma cells containing nonexchangeable hematoporphyrin derivative. *Cancer Res* 45:2507-2511.

Edell ES and Cortese DA (1989). Bronchoscopic localization and treatment of occult lung cancer. *Chest* 96:919-924.

Henderson BW, Waldow SM, Mang TS *et al* (1985). Tumor destruction and kinetics of tumor cell death in two experimental mouse tumors following photodynamic therapy. *Cancer Res* 45:572-576.

Henry JM and Isaacs JT (1989). Synergistic enhancement of the efficacy of the bioreductively activated alkylating agent RSU-1164 in the treatment of prostatic cancer by photodynamic therapy. *J Urol* 142:165-170.

Kato H, Kawate N, Kiroshita K *et al* (1989). Photodynamic therapy of early stage lung cancer. In: *Ciba Foundation Symposium 146*, pp. 183-194. (Eds) Bock G and Harnett S. John Wiley & Sons Ltd.; Chichester.

Mitchell JB, McPherson S, De Graff W *et al* (1985). Oxygen dependence of hematoporphyrin derivative-induced photoinactivation of Chinese hamster cells. *Cancer Res* 45:2008-2010.

Reed MWR, Mullins AP, Anderson GL *et al* (1989). The effect of photodynamic therapy on tumor oxygenation. *Surgery* 106:94-99.

Star WM, Marijnissen HPA, Jansen H *et al* (1987). Light dosimetry for photodynamic therapy by whole bladder wall irradiation. *Photochem Photobiol* 46:619-624.

Sutedja T, Baas P, Stewart F *et al* (1992). Photodynamic therapy in patients with inoperable non-small cell lung cancer. A pilot study. *Eur J Cancer* 28A:1370-1373.

Further reading

Gomer CJ, Rucker N, Ferrario A and Wong S (1989). Properties and applications of photodynamic therapy. *Radiat Res* 120:1-18.

Henderson BW and Dougherty TJ (1992). How does photodynamic therapy work? *Photochem Photobiol* 55:145-157.

Kessel D (1986). Photosensitization with derivatives of haematoporphyrin. *Int J Radiat Biol* 49:901-907.

23

Prediction of tumour response

Adrian C. Begg

23.1 Introduction

The most important goal of a predictive assay is to obtain information that can be used to choose a treatment protocol, so that each individual patient will receive optimal treatment. At the present time, the treatment plan is usually based on parameters such as tumour site, histological type, tumour stage and performance status. Within these broad categories, some tumours will show a greater response to radiotherapy than others. If these could be identified before treatment, alternative therapies might be selected which may give a better chance of cure than the standard conventional therapy. The choices may include chemotherapy or surgery in preference to radiotherapy, or non-standard radiotherapy schedules. Predictive assays should be simple, quick and reliable tests for parameters that will predict response to a particular treatment. The assays currently being most intensively investigated for radiotherapy are those for *intrinsic radiosensitivity* and *repopulation rate*. This chapter will therefore mainly concentrate on these.

23.2 Assay types

A wide variety of assays are currently being explored for predicting either the natural history of individual tumours or their response to therapy. Some of these are listed in Table 23.1. Cytogenetic changes and oncogene expression allow subgroups of patients to be identified who potentially may have a different prognosis. These aspects may also provide an indication of treatment response; *ras* oncogene expression, for example, has been associated with both cisplatin and radiation resistance in some cell lines. Other assays are purely designed to indicate treatment response;

for instance, measurement of the number of DNA-drug adducts in tumour cells after chemotherapy can be an indicator of the likelihood of response to treatment (more adducts = greater response). Some assays are direct measures of cell killing (e.g. colony assays) and are applicable to most forms of treatment, while others give an indirect measure of sensitivity (e.g. pO_2 and thiol content for radiation response, DNA adducts and *p*-glycoprotein for drug response). Direct methods are preferable to indirect ones, and measurements directly on biopsy material are preferable to those

Table 23.1 Potential predictors of natural history and treatment response

Parameter	Predictor of	
	Natural history	Treatment response
Proliferation cell kinetics	+	+
Ploidy/cytogenetics	+	?
Surface receptors/antigens	+	?
Proto-oncogene expression	+	?
NK cell activity	+	−
Intrinsic cell sensitivity	−	+
pO_2/pH	−	+
O_2 and heat regulated proteins	−	+
Endogenous thiols	−	+
p-glycoprotein	−	+
DNA-drug adducts	−	+
DNA repair enzymes	−	+
Tumour regression/necrosis	?	+
Host cell infiltrates	?	+
Magnetic resonance imaging or spectroscopy:		
^{32}P	?	+
^{1}H	?	?
Positron-emission tomography	?	?

in which the tumour cells must be treated *in vitro* with radiation or drug, since the response may be different from that *in vivo*. This is not always possible, and *in vitro* treatments can give useful predictive information, as will be illustrated below.

The ideal predictive assay should have the following characteristics:

- Harmless
- Accurate and reliable
- Quick and cheap
- Few false positives or negatives
- Independent predictive power

Within this range of predictive tests that may be of value to clinical radiotherapy there are two that stand out at the present time: the prediction of intrinsic radiosensitivity and of repopulation rate during radiotherapy.

23.3   Intrinsic sensitivity to drug or radiation treatment

Radiosensitivity

Intrinsic radiosensitivity of tumour cells can be measured by colony formation after irradiation *in vitro* (Section 5.4). For these studies, a cell suspension from the biopsy must first be made and the cells grown in dishes or culture tubes. One widely used measure of radiosensitivity is the surviving fraction after 2 Gy (SF_2, Section 14.5). This dose is low enough to indicate the *initial slope* of the survival curve although especially in radioresistant cell lines it is not identical with it. It is also a commonly used dose per fraction in clinical radiotherapy. Although there are many reasons why *in vivo* and *in vitro* responses may differ (e.g. the presence or absence of hypoxic cells, or cell-contact effects), some studies have shown a correlation between *in vitro* radiosensitivity of human tumour cell lines and clinical response (Figure 14.9).

Assays for cell survival can take up to 4 weeks to complete and it is normally inappropriate to delay the start of radiotherapy for this length of time. There is therefore a need for more rapid assays of cellular sensitivity. One approach is to measure growth inhibition of tumour cells plated out *in vitro*: the so-called *growth assays* (Section 5.4). In this type of assay, the change in total cell number in dishes given different treatment doses is measured; the higher the dose the fewer cells are present after a given growth period. This is similar to a growth-delay experiment for tumours *in vivo*. A variety of methods have been used to rapidly determine the number of cells in the cultures at the end of the growth period, including cell counting with the aid of a vital stain for viable cells (the *dye-exclusion method*) and automated colourimetric assays using the *tetrazolium (MTT) method* (Carmichael *et al*, 1987; Mitchell, 1988).

An alternative approach is to measure some parameter of radiation-induced DNA damage as an indicator of radiosensitivity. This is an area of active laboratory research at the present time and it is not yet clear whether a clinically useful assay can be found. The methods described in Section 24.3 are being employed, especially *pulsed-field gel electrophoresis (PFGE)*. These can be used to measure either the initial level of induced DNA damage or the speed and extent of strand-break rejoining. The level of initial damage shows a tendency to be higher in the more radiosensitive cell lines that have been studied, but there are significant exceptions to this. Some investigators have reported that radioresistant cells show faster rejoining of double-strand DNA breaks (Schwartz *et al*, 1988) but this also does not yet provide a practicable assay for routine use.

The measurement of chromosomal damage is another possible approach. Conventional techniques of counting radiation-induced chromosome aberrations in metaphase, the scoring of micronuclei, and newer techniques including *in situ* hybridization and premature chromosome condensation, are being tested. There are encouraging reports of correlations with radiosensitivity but these methods have yet to be applied and validated in the clinic.

Chemosensitivity

Similar techniques can in principle be used to measure cell killing by drugs. Figure 23.1 shows results of a cell population growth assay to assess sensitivity of two human tumours to four different drugs. The tumour cells were primary explants, i.e. grown direct from biopsy material and tested immediately after removal from the patient. Data on two patients are compared and their responses to each of these drugs differed considerably. This illustrates the fact that differences among tumour cell lines to a given cytotoxic drug are probably larger than is the case with radiation. For a given cell line there are also wide differences in the effectiveness of various chemotherapeutic agents (Steel, Courtenay and Peckham, 1983). Perhaps as a result of their more specific biochemical modes of action, drugs are more selective in their cell killing effects. For this reason, prediction of tumour response should be easier to achieve than is the case with radiation. A number of assays have been developed for this purpose but none has yet come into general use. In the late 1970s, S.E. Salmon and his coworkers described the 'human tumor stem-cell assay' (Salmon *et al*, 1978). A suspension of tumour cells was exposed to a range of drug concentrations, after which the cells were

grown in tissue culture medium thickened with agar (to keep the colonies compact and to inhibit growth of fibroblasts). After an appropriate culture period, colonies of more than 40 cells were counted. Although widely used at the time, this assay has not persisted, probably because clumps of cells in the original tumour cell suspensions were sometimes as frequent as the colonies that grew in this system (Selby, Buick and Tannock, 1983).

A general feature of chemosensitivity assays so far described has been that whilst they are variably successful in predicting *sensitivity* they have a high success rate in predicting drug *resistance* (KSST, 1981). In principle, this should be a significant benefit to cancer chemotherapy since

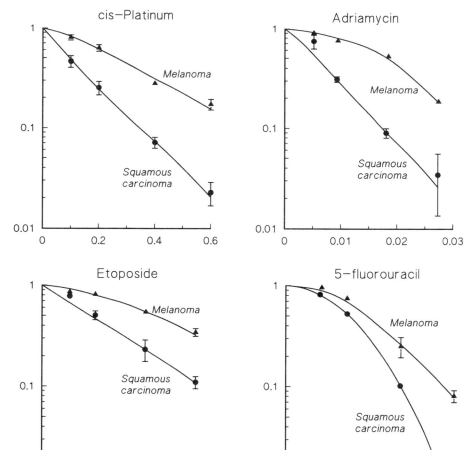

Figure 23.1 Survival curves for a melanoma (▲) and a squamous carcinoma of the lung (●) exposed continuously for 5 days to each of four chemotherapeutic agents and assayed in primary culture using the adhesive tumour cell culture system. The abscissa is drug concentration in μg/ml. From Baker *et al* (1986), with permission.

it will allow patients with resistant disease to be spared the toxicity of ineffective treatment; this potential advance has not, however, been taken up presumably because it is the view of medical oncologists that, even if the likelihood of response is low, the patient should be given the chance of benefiting from chemotherapy.

Cell survival or cell growth assays can also be used to examine the individuality of response to other treatments such as hyperthermia or high-LET radiotherapy. Their main disadvantage remains that the treatment takes place in a culture dish and not in the patient.

Correlation with Outcome

Intrinsic radiosensitivity data for human tumours using a cell-population growth assay are shown in Figure 23.2 (Brock *et al*, 1987). The cumulative plots of the surviving fraction at 2 Gy were obtained from complete *in vitro* survival curves. The slope of each line indicates the extent of inter-tumour variation (flatter = more variable) and the lateral position represents the overall radiosensitivity (left = more radiosensitive). Significant differences between tumour types can be seen in panel **A**. For head and neck tumours treated with surgery followed by radiotherapy, patients with subsequently recurring tumours tended to have more radioresistant tumours (panel **B**), but this difference was not statistically significant.

A similar type of study is shown in Figure 23.3. The *in vitro* radiosensitivity of cervix tumours was measured with a colony assay and compared with the clinical response to radical radiotherapy (West *et al*, 1991). Patients with local recurrence were found to have more radioresistant tumours (panel **A**), a significant difference. The survival of patients with low SF_2 values was significantly better than those with high values (panel **B**). This illustrates the predictive potential of *in vitro* radiosensitivity measurements. An advantage of this study compared with the Houston study (Figure 23.2) was that no surgery was involved, and the radiotherapy was given over a short time (3 weeks), thus minimizing problems of proliferation rate differences between tumours (see below).

23.4 Tumour-cell repopulation

Evidence for Tumour-cell Repopulation

As described in Section 9.3, tumour-cell repopulation during fractionated radiotherapy can reduce the probability of local control. Evidence for the importance of repopulation has come from two main sources: the analysis of clinical data and measurements of the kinetics of cell proliferation in human tumour biopsies.

The clinical evidence has come from the analysis of data on the correlation between local control and overall treatment time. The review by Withers *et al* (1988) gave the first clear indication that

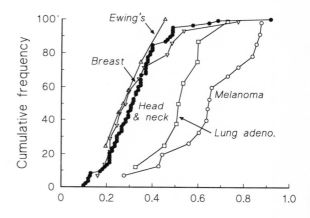

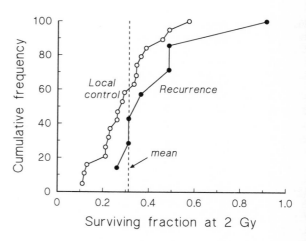

Figure 23.2 Cumulative frequency curves for SF_2 values. **A:** in 5 tumour types. **B:** in relation to the local tumour control of head and neck tumours. From Brock *et al* (1987), with permission.

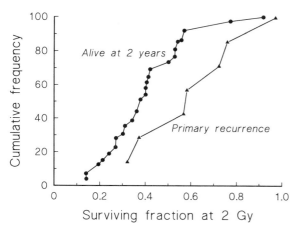

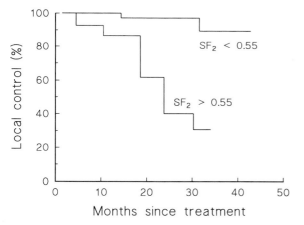

Figure 23.3 SF_2 values as a predictor of outcome in the radiotherapy in cervix carcinoma. **A:** recurrence in relation to SF_2. **B:** recurrence in patients with SF_2 values above or below 0.55; the difference between these groups is significant (p < 0.001; N = 51). From West *et al* (1991), with permission.

clinical data can yield estimates of the doubling time for tumour-cell repopulation. They summarized published estimates of the tumour control dose (TCD_{50}) for head and neck tumours and plotted these against the duration of radiotherapy treatment. Extrapolation of the data was sometimes necessary. Figure 23.4 shows the result of this study. There was a systematic tendency for longer treatments to require a larger total dose for tumour control, although it appeared that there was a lag period of perhaps 25 days before the curve began to rise. The solid lines through the data have a slope of 0.61 Gy/day. Based

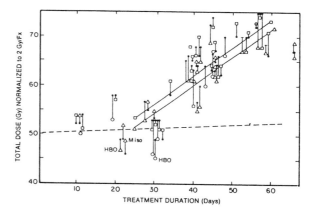

Figure 23.4 TCD_{50} values in relation to overall treatment time, calculated from published data on the local control of head and neck tumours. Total doses were normalised to a 2 Gy per fraction schedule using $\alpha/\beta = 25$ Gy. The dashed line shows the rate of increase in TCD_{50} calculated from a 2-month clonogen doubling time. From Withers *et al* (1988), with permission.

Table 23.2 Effective proliferation rates calculated from clinical radiotherapy results

Tumour	Source	Change in overall time (days)	Result	Effective doubling time (days)
Hodgkin's disease	Friedman	20	TCD increased by 6 Gy	3
Burkitt lymphoma	Norin	7	CR increased by 63%	3
Head and Neck, T2/3	Parsons	21	TCD increased by 16%	6
Larynx	Niederer	15	TCD increased by > 5 Gy	6
Larynx, T3/4	Maciejewski	16	TCD increased by 8 Gy	4
Skin carcinoma	Hliniak	8	TCD increased by 51%	8

TCD: local tumour control dose; CR: complete response.
From Fowler (1986).

on assumptions about the radiosensitivity of the cells, Withers *et al* deduced a clonogen doubling time for head and neck cancers of about 4 days. A subsequent analysis of these data by Bentzen and Thames is shown in Figure 9.4; this confirmed the progressive increase of TCD_{50} with overall treatment time but the existence of a lag period was less clear.

Similar analyses have been made for other tumour types and some of these are listed in Table 23.2. If assumptions are made about tumour cell radiosensitivity, it is possible to calculate effective doubling times during radiotherapy; these values are remarkably short (3–8 days) compared with pretreatment volume doubling times of perhaps 3–15 weeks (Section 2.4).

Proliferation Measurements in Human Tumours

Three of the principal kinetic parameters in tumours are cell cycle time, potential doubling time and volume doubling time (Section 3.3). Of these, only the potential doubling time (T_{pot}) can be measured in a patient from a single biopsy . In the *relative movement method*, a non-toxic dose of IUdR or BrUdR is given intravenously and a tumour biopsy is taken several hours later for flow-cytometric analysis. The DNA histogram (Figure 23.5, bottom panel) shows the presence of both normal and malignant cells in the biopsy. Only the aneuploid tumour cells are analyzed. Cells labelled with the anti-IUdR antibody can be seen clearly distinguished from the unlabelled cells (top panel), from which T_{pot} can be calculated using Equation 3.1. A wide range of T_{pot} values have been found by this method in clinical head and neck tumours. Figure 23.6 shows some of these results in head and neck tumours; the values range from 1.5 to over 11 days. It is remarkable that the average value of 4.5 days from this study is similar to that calculated from the clinical tumour control data shown in Figure 23.4. This provides encouraging support for the view that pretreatment T_{pot} values may predict for clonogen repopulation during radiotherapy.

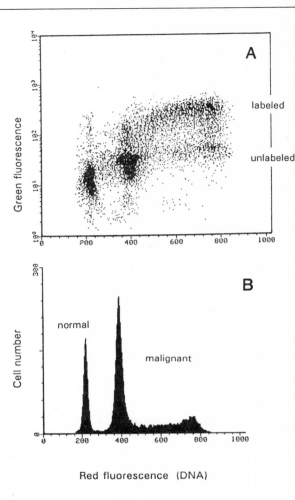

Figure 23.5 Flow cytometry analysis of a human tumour. **A:** a scatter diagram of IUdR content (vertical scale) and DNA content (horizontal scale). **B:** The distribution of DNA content. From Begg, Hofland and Horiot, unpublished.

Correlation of T_{pot} with Treatment Outcome

Pretreatment T_{pot} values have been measured by *in vivo* IUdR labelling within an EORTC randomized phase III trial of conventional versus accelerated fractionation for advanced head and neck tumours. Patients were split into two groups: those with fast- and those with slow-growing tumours, defined by T_{pot} values smaller or larger than 4.5 days (which was the median T_{pot} for this series). Patients whose tumours gave short T_{pot} values had a significantly worse overall survival

(Figure 23.7A). Within this trial, patients with both fast- and slow-growing tumours were randomized to receive either a conventional course of radiotherapy (C) or accelerated treatment (A). The difference in overall treatment time between the two arms was 2 – 2½ weeks. In terms of local tumour control (Figure 23.7B), patients who did the worst had fast-growing tumours and were given the conventional treatment schedule. Those with fast-growing tumours who were given accelerated radiotherapy had a higher level of tumour control. These data provide further valuable support for the hypothesis that pretreatment T_{pot} measurements can predict repopulation rates during fractionated radiotherapy.

A study from the Egyptian National Cancer Institute of postoperative radiotherapy for head and neck cancer has led to similar findings (Awwad, 1992). Tumour biopsy material was labelled *in vitro* with ³H-thymidine and T_{pot} values were calculated from the labelling indices (Equation 3.1), assuming an average value for T_s. The proportion of tumours locally controlled by conventional fractionation was lower when the potential doubling time was short (Table 23.3). No difference was found for patients given accelerated radiotherapy, as might be expected since repopulation is unlikely to be a problem with as short a treatment time as 11 days.

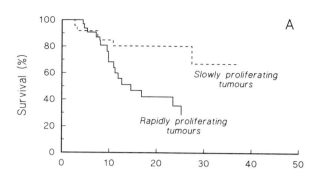

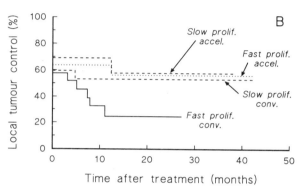

Time after treatment (months)

Figure 23.7 Results of the EORTC 22851 cooperative trial of accelerated radiotherapy in advanced head and neck cancer, analyzed at 36 months. **A:** Survival in relation to T_{pot} value ('rapid proliferation' < 4.5d; 'slow proliferation' > 4.5d). **B:** local tumour control in the accelerated and conventional arms, in relation to proliferation rate. *Conventional*: 72 Gy, 2 Gy per fraction, 1 fraction per day, no split, 7 – 7½ weeks overall time. *Accelerated*: 72 Gy, 1.6 Gy per fraction, 3 fractions per day, 1 week radiotherapy – 2 weeks gap – 2 weeks radiotherapy, 5 weeks overall time. From Begg *et al* (1992), with permission.

Table 23.3 Conventional *versus* accelerated post-operative radiotherapy in head and neck cancer

	Potential doubling time§	Local tumour control
Accelerated*	>4.5d	9/16 (56%)
	<4.5d	4/8 (50%)
Conventional*	>4.5d	11/19 (58%)
	<4.5d	0/9 (0%)

§ By *in vitro* thymidine labelling
* Accelerated: 30 × 1.4 Gy; overall time 11 days
Conventional: 25 × 2.0 Gy; overall time 32 days

From Awwad (1992).

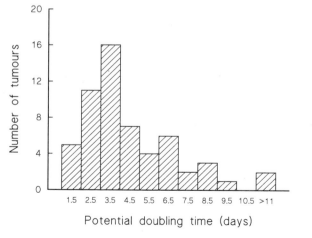

Potential doubling time (days)

Figure 23.6 Distribution of T_{pot} values for head and neck tumours, derived from flow cytometry analysis. The mean potential doubling time is 4.47 days. From Begg, Hofland and Horiot, unpublished.

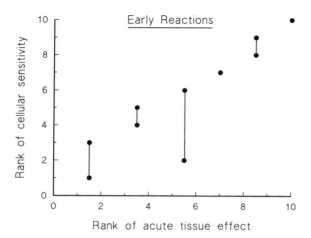

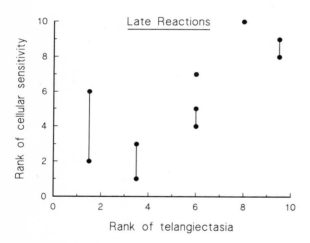

Figure 23.8 Correlation between early or late skin reactions to radiotherapy and the *in vitro* radiosensitivity of skin fibroblasts. The six patients have been ranked in relation to each parameter. Some patients gave two skin biopsies from which two independent sensitivity measurements were made (connected points). Burnet *et al* (1992), with permission.

23.5 Hypoxia

There is strong evidence that tumour hypoxia can reduce radiotherapy cure rates in some sites (*see* Chapters 11, 19). This may not be a problem in all tumours, however, and hypoxic cell sensitizers, hypoxic cytotoxins, high LET radiation, etc., should ideally only be given to patients where hypoxic tumour cells can be demonstrated to present a therapeutic problem.

Methods to detect tumour hypoxia include the use of fine oxygen electrodes, the binding of radiolabelled misonidazole which is selective for hypoxic cells, or the detection of fluorine-labelled misonidazole or its derivatives using positron-emission tomography (PET). Recent studies have shown that nitroimidazole derivatives can also be detected immunologically in hypoxic cells, opening up the possibility of detection by both immunocytochemistry and flow cytometry. These studies require administration of potentially toxic drugs to the patient. They are beginning to be tested in the clinical setting but no large-scale studies have yet been done.

23.6 Prediction of normal-tissue tolerance

Although this chapter is directed at the prediction of tumour response, the complementary approach of seeking to predict for radiation-induced damage to normal tissues must also be mentioned. It is well recognized by radiotherapists that among a group of patients who are given the same radiation treatment some will show more severe reactions than others. The underlying causes of these differences include:

(a) differences in the actual radiation dose delivered to the target cells of the normal tissue in question.

(b) inter-patient differences in the volume of normal tissue irradiated (Section 13.4).

(c) statistics of the survival of clonogenic cells. When irradiation has reduced the number of 'tissue-rescuing units' to critically low levels the failure or continued integrity of the tissue depends upon the survival of one or more of these entities (Section 10.3). The probability of failure is then determined by a Poisson distribution, which in part fixes the maximum slope of the dose-response curve. Dose-response curves for normal-tissue damage in inbred strains of laboratory animals (Figures 13.7, 13.10, 13.13) have a slope that may largely be determined by this factor. Which animals or patients will show damage due to this cause could never be predicted.

(d) inter-patient differences in tissue physiology or tissue biology: for instance in blood flow to the tissue, proliferation rate, etc. Some of these could have a genetic basis, others may depend on the age or environment of the patient. They may also be tissue-dependent, in the sense that not all tissues in an individual may have a higher or lower sensitivity than average.

(e) genetic differences in radiation sensitivity. Predisposition to enhanced radiation sensitivity is known to be associated with a number of rare syndromes (Section 24.5). In addition, there are in the population individuals who are heterozygotes for the genes that give rise to these forms of enhanced sensitivity; they also, but perhaps to a lesser extent, may be more sensitive to radiation treatment than individuals who do not carry those genes. Other predisposing genes may be as yet unrecognized.

All of these sources of variation will contribute to the observed differences in normal-tissue damage observed in radiotherapy patients. If methods of predicting their susceptibility to radiation damage can be developed, then either or both of two courses of action are open: to *reduce* radiation dose for the susceptible patients, thus sparing them the risk of severe tissue damage, or to increase radiation dose for the non-susceptible patients, with the likelihood of improved tumour response. It is causes (d) and (e) above that are likely to be predictable by this approach.

Evidence for the feasibility of predicting normal-tissue damage has come from the work of Burnet *et al* (1992). They obtained skin biopsies from breast carcinoma patients who had been treated with a highly standardized radiotherapy protocol by Dr. I. Turesson and her colleagues at Sahlgren's Hospital, Gothenburg, Sweden. Fibroblasts were grown out of the biopsies and their radiosensitivity determined at high and low dose rate. The results showed a significant correlation with the severity of early and late radiation skin damage (Figure 23.8).

The measurement of fibroblast cell survival is too slow to be used as a predictive assay and efforts are being made to identify rapid and reliable alternatives. Blood lymphocytes are more readily available than skin biopsies and their damage can be assessed soon after a test dose of radiation. The micronucleus test (Streffer, van Beuningen and Molls, 1982) is a rapid method for detecting radiation cell killing and in normal tissues it has potential as a predictive assay. Efforts are also being made to develop tests based on radiation DNA damage. These include the use of single-cell electrophoresis, the so-called 'comet' assay (Olive, Banath and Durand, 1990).

Key points

1. The two most widely investigated predictive assays for tumour response to radiotherapy are those for intrinsic radiosensitivity and clonogen repopulation.
2. Intrinsic radiosensitivity can be measured by cell growth or colony assays after irradiation *in vitro* and there are encouraging signs of a correlation between SF_2 and outcome. A disadvantage of the colony assay is its approximately 4 week duration.
3. Analysis of clinical data indicates that repopulation during radiotherapy limits cure in several tumour types. Tumour potential doubling times measured before treatment using *in vivo* labelling with thymidine analogues are similar to values for repopulation rate calculated from clinical radiotherapy response data. Current clinical trials support the predictive value of pretreatment T_{pot} measurements and favour accelerated radiotherapy for the more rapidly proliferating tumours.
4. Prediction of normal-tissue sensitivity to radiotherapy is also a potentially feasible option which has yet to be fully evaluated.

Bibliography

Awwad HK (1992). Unconventional fractionation studies and T_{pot} correlation. *Semin Oncol* 2:62-66.

Baker F, Spitzer G, Ajani J *et al* (1986). Drug and radiation sensitivity measurements of successful primary monolayer culturing of human tumor cells using cell-adhesive matrix and supplemented medium. *Cancer Res* 46:1263-1274.

Begg AC, Hofland I, van Glabekke M *et al* (1992). Predictive value of potential doubling time for radiotherapy of head and neck tumor patients: results from the EORTC cooperative trial 22851. *Semin Radiat Oncol* 2:22-25.

Brock WA, Bhadkamkar VA, Williams M and Spitzer G (1987). Radiosensitivity testing of primary cultures derived from human tumors. In: *Progress in Radio-Oncology, Vol.III*, pp. 300-306. (Eds) Karcher KH, Kogelnik HD and Szepesi T. Int. Club for Radio-Oncology; Vienna.

Burnet NG, Nyman J, Turesson I *et al* (1992). Potential for improving radiotherapy cure rates by predicting normal tissue tolerance from *in vitro* cellular radiation sensitivity. *Lancet* 339:1570-1571.

Carmichael J, DeGraff WG, Gazdar AF *et al* (1987). Evaluation of a tetrazolium-based semiautomated colorimetric assay: assessment of radiosensitivity. *Cancer Res* 47:943-946.

Fowler JF (1986). Potential for increasing the differential response between tumors and normal tissues: can proliferation rate be used? *Int J Radiat Oncol Biol Phys* 12:641-645.

KSST: Group for Sensitivity Testing of Human Tumors (1981). *In vitro* short-term test to determine the resistance of human tumors to chemotherapy. Cancer 48:2127-2135.

Mitchell JB (1988). Potential applicability of nonclonogenic measurements to clinical oncology. *Radiat Res* 114:401-414.

Olive PL, Banath JP and Durand RE (1990). Heterogeneity in radiation-induced DNA damage and repair in tumour and normal cells measured using the 'comet' assay. *Radiat Res* 122:86-94.

Salmon SE, Hamburger AW, Soehnlen B *et al* (1978). Quantitation of differential sensitivity of human-tumor stem cells to anticancer drugs. *New England J Med* 298:1321 1327.

Schwartz JL, Rotmensch J, Giovanazzi S *et al* (1988). Faster repair of DNA double-strand breaks in radioresistant human tumor cells. *Int J Radiat Oncol Biol Phys* 15:907-912.

Selby P, Buick RN and Tannock I (1983). A critical appraisal of the 'human tumour stem-cell asssay'. *New England J Med* 308:129-134.

Steel GG, Courtenay VD and Peckham MJ (1983). The response to chemotherapy of a variety of human tumour xenografts. *Brit J Cancer* 47:1-13.

Streffer C, van Beuningen D and Molls M (1982). Possibilities of the micronucleus test as an assay in radiotherapy. *Progress in Radiooncology II* Eds. KH Karcher, HD Kogelink and G Reinartz. Raven Press, New York.

West CML, Davidson SE and Hendry JH and Hunter RD (1991). Prediction of cervical carcinoma response to radiotherapy. *Lancet* 338:818.

Withers HR, Taylor JMG and Maciejewski B (1988). The hazard of tumour clonogen repopulation during radiotherapy. *Acta Oncol* 27:131-146.

Further reading

Chapman JD, Peters LJ and Withers HR (Eds) (1989). *Prediction of Tumor Treatment Response*. Pergamon Press; Oxford.

Paliwal BR, Fowler JF, Herbert DE *et al* (1989). *Prediction of Response in Radiation Therapy: Part I, the Physical and Biological Basis*. American Institute of Physics Inc; New York.

Peters LJ, Brock WA, Johnson T *et al* (1986). Potential methods for predicting tumor radiocurability. *Int J Radiat Oncol Biol Phys* 12:459-467.

Trott KR and Kummermehr J (1985). What is known about tumour proliferation rates to choose between accelerated fractionation or hyperfractionation? *Radiother Oncol* 3:1-9.

Tucker SL and Chan KS (1990). The selection of patients for radiotherapy on the basis of tumor growth kinetics and intrinsic radiosensitivity. *Radiother Oncol* 18:197-282.

24

Molecular aspects of radiation biology

Trevor J. McMillan and G. Gordon Steel

This chapter deals with a large and rapidly expanding area of radiobiology that has many points of contact with other aspects of molecular biology. Within the scope of this book it is only possible to indicate some of the more important areas that a radiotherapist should be aware of. A list of further reading is given below.

24.1 Initial processes of radiation damage

Irradiation of a biological system initiates a series of processes that can be classified in terms of the time-scale over which they act (Figure 1.2). The physical, chemical, and biological phases of this process have been described in Section 1.3.

An electron with an energy of 1 MeV has a range in soft tissue of a few millimetres. In the early part of its track the particle moves very quickly and its rate of energy deposition is low; the result is a relatively straight track in which the ionizations may be separated by distances of around 0.1 μm on average. We describe this as radiation with a low Linear Energy Transfer (*low LET*, Section 16.2). As the electron slows down it interacts more strongly with the orbital electrons in the medium. Its rate of energy loss increases, the track becomes more tortuous due to stronger collisions, and the ionization density increases. Figure 24.1A shows a computer simulation of the tracks of 1 keV electrons, representing a very small terminal part of the tracks of 1 MeV electrons. The important feature is the tendency towards *clustering* of the ionization events, each cluster having the size of a few nanometres.

Within each electron track there is opportunity for interactions between the products of separate ionization events and it is thought that, particularly at low dose rate or following acute radiation doses up to a few gray, the main biological effects of radiation (cell killing and cell mutation) are predominantly due to damage that is produced by these 'hot spots'.

Within perhaps 10^{-10} seconds of exposure to either photon or particle beams the irradiated volume will contain atoms that have been ionized and a corresponding number of free electrons, all produced by the cascade of atomic reactions just described and with a rather non-uniform spatial distribution. The numbers of ionizations produced at therapeutic dose levels is very large: approximately 10^5 ionizations per cell per gray. One gray gives roughly 1 *lethal* lesion per cell and the ineffectiveness of most of the ionizations is due to 3 main factors: free-radical scavenging processes, the small number of ionizations that are close enough to DNA to damage it, and cellular repair processes.

Free-Radical Processes

Since biological systems consist largely of water, the bulk of the ionizations produced by irradiation occur in water molecules. Negatively charged free electrons (e^-) that are produced by ionization will rapidly become associated with polar water molecules, greatly reducing their mobility. The configuration of an electron surrounded by water molecules (a 'hydrated electron') has a degree of stability and a lifetime under physiological conditions of a few microseconds. The water molecule that has lost an electron is a highly reactive positively charged ion. It quickly breaks down to produce a hydrogen ion (H⁺) and an (uncharged) OH radical. OH is a molecule that normally does not exist in water. Oxygen has valency 2, hydrogen 1, and the stable configuration is H_2O. The uncharged OH radical has an unpaired electron ('unattached valency') that makes it highly reactive. We designate it as a free radical thus: OH•. Free radicals are simply fragments of broken molecules. OH• is different from OH⁺ which is a positively charged *ion*: the OH radical has equal numbers of protons and orbital electrons but because of the unpaired electron it is chemically reactive (note that some ions may also be radicals, for example a water molecule that has lost an electron is actually H_2O^{+}•, a radical cation). Similarly, H⁺ is a bare proton, positively charged, whilst H• is a proton plus an electron (neutral charge) but again highly reactive because the stable form of hydrogen is H_2.

Around 10^{-10} seconds after irradiation there will be 3 principal radiolysis products:

$$e^{-}_{aq} \quad H• \quad OH•$$

These highly reactive species will go on to take part in further reactions. An important one is

$$OH• + OH• \rightarrow H_2O_2$$

– the production of hydrogen peroxide. Oxygen, if present, plays an important part in the free radical reactions that follow irradiation. Molecular oxygen has a high affinity for free radicals (R•):

$$R• + O_2 \rightarrow RO_2•$$

giving rise to further reactive products and acting to *fix* the free-radical damage. The oxygen effect in radiation cell killing has often been explained in terms of this type of process.

In biological systems the free radicals produced in water may react with essential macromolecules. A vast range of reactions take place, most of which are unimportant for the survival and functioning of the cell. The important reactions are those with DNA, because of the uniqueness of the function of many parts of this molecule. Damage to DNA from free radicals produced in water is called the *indirect* effect of radiation; ionization of atoms that are part of the DNA molecule is the *direct* effect.

Compounds containing sulphydryl (-SH) groups have a particular affinity for free radicals. Their

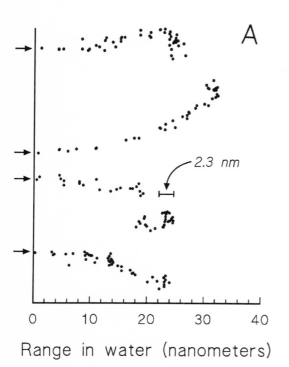

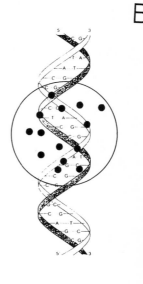

Figure 24.1 **A**: Computer-simulated tracks of 1 keV electrons. Note the scale in relation to the 2.3 nm diameter of the DNA double helix (adapted from Chapman and Gillespie, 1981). **B**: Illustrating the concept of a Local Multiply-Damaged Site produced by a cluster of ionizations impinging on DNA.

Range in water (nanometers)

presence within the cell may therefore act to 'mop up' a proportion of radicals, thus decreasing radiation effects. The principal non-protein thiols in mammalian cells are:

Cysteine   – a natural amino acid
Cysteamine – decarboxylated cysteine
Glutathione – the commonest non-protein thiol

Administration of these compounds to animals or to cells in tissue culture immediately before irradiation reduces the extent of damage. The radiation dose required to produce a given level of damage can go up by as much as a factor of 2.0.

During the first millisecond after radiation exposure a competition takes place between damage-fixing and scavenging reactions for radicals in key target molecules. There is considerable interest in the possibility of manipulating the levels of cellular thiols either to protect normal tissues or, by depressing thiol levels, to increase the radiosensitivity of tumour cells. Thiol depression can be achieved experimentally by blocking the synthesis of glutathione using such agents as diamide or buthionine sulphoximine (BSO).

The development and radiobiological properties of hypoxic-cell radiosensitizers are dealt with in Section 19.3. The most important class of sensitizers are the electron-affinic compounds, principally the nitroimidazoles, which act like oxygen in promoting the fixation of free radical damage. Since they are less rapidly metabolized than oxygen, they can diffuse further in tumour tissue and thus reach hypoxic cells.

24.2 Radiation damage to DNA

The Structure of DNA

Deoxyribonucleic acid (DNA) is a large molecule that has a characteristic double-helix structure consisting of two strands, each made up of a sequence of nucleotides (Figure 24.2). A nucleotide is a subunit in which a 'base' is linked through a sugar group to a phosphate group. The sugar is deoxyribose which has a 5-atom ring: 4 carbons and one oxygen. The 'backbone' of the molecule

consists of alternating sugar-phosphate groups. Note that by the conventional numbering system the connection points of the phosphates to the sugar ring are labelled 3' and 5': this leads to the ends of a sequence of nucleotides also being labelled in this way and it defines the direction in which the sequence is read during transcription. There are 4 different bases. Two are single-ring groups (pyrimidines): thymine and cytosine. Two are double-ring groups (purines): adenine and guanine. It is the order of these bases along the molecule that specifies the genetic code.

The two strands of the double helix are held together by hydrogen bonding between the bases. These bonds are formed between thymine and adenine, and between cytosine and guanine. The bases are paired in this way along the length of the DNA molecule. During the S-phase of the cell cycle DNA synthesis takes place – the process of *replication* – in which every base is accurately duplicated.

The first stage in the manufacture of proteins is the construction by the process of *transcription* of a messenger RNA (labelled *mRNA*) that has a similar structure to DNA except that the sugar

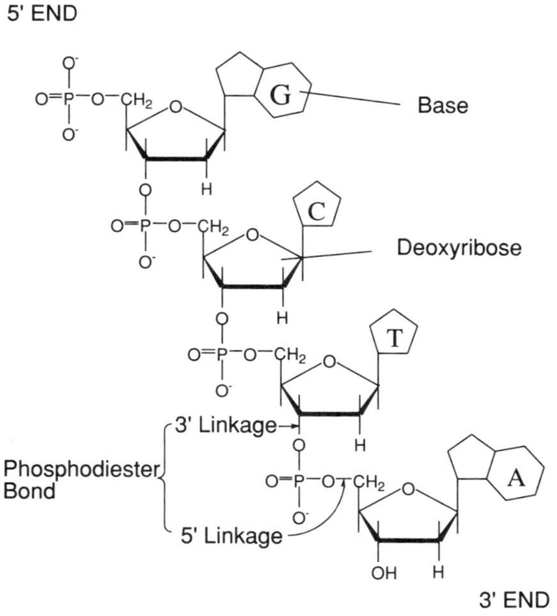

Figure 24.2 The structure of DNA, in which the 4 bases (G, C, T, A) are linked by sugar groups to the phosphate backbone.

groups are ribose in place of deoxyribose, and thymine is replaced by uracil. The decoding is based on the pairing of bases: A→U, C→G, G→C, T→A. Transcription is performed by RNA polymerases which bind to DNA and generate the corresponding RNA. The control of transcription is not yet well understood but specific DNA sequences at the beginning and ends of genes seem to be involved. Within the *coding region* of the gene there may be several stretches of DNA that are not required for mRNA. These are called *introns* (the required regions are *exons*) and they need to be removed at some point prior to the translation of the mRNA into protein. Protein production occurs at ribosomes where transfer RNA (*tRNA*) with an amino acid attached recognizes groups of three bases in the mRNA (*codons*) and in this way the amino acids are lined up in the correct sequence for the protein.

The very long DNA double-helix molecule, together with nuclear proteins, is organized within the cell through a number of levels of supercoiling. The DNA double helix (about 2.3 nm in diameter) is first coiled around protein cores to form a bead-like string of nucleosomes, then coiled into a 25 nm fibre, which is further spiralized and becomes visible in the condensed form of a chromosome at mitosis. During interphase and in chromatin that has been gently extracted from cell nuclei, DNA shows a series of loops or *domains* that are attached to the nuclear matrix. A human chromosome may have around 2600 looped domains, each formed from about 0.4 μm of the 25 nm DNA fibre and containing 20,000 to 80,000 base pairs.

Radiation Damage to DNA

Early experiments showed that irradiation leads to a loss of viscosity in DNA solutions. Subsequently this has been shown to result from DNA strand breaks. There are two categories of DNA strand breaks; single-strand (SSB) and double-strand breaks (DSB). The detection of these depends on a study of the size distribution of fragments of DNA after extraction from irradiated cells (Section 24.3). There are a variety of other types of DNA lesion, some of which are important in the cytotoxic action of chemotherapeutic agents (Figure 24.3).

Why do we believe that DNA damage is the critical event in radiation cell killing and mutation?

There are many sources of evidence, including the following:

(i)   microirradiation studies show that to kill cells by irradiation only of the cytoplasm requires far higher radiation doses than irradiation of the nucleus;

(ii) isotopes with short-range emission (such as ^{3}H, ^{125}I) when incorporated into cellular DNA efficiently produce radiation cell killing and DNA damage (Table 24.1);

(iii) the incidence of chromosomal aberrations following irradiation is closely linked to cell killing;

(iv) thymidine analogues such as IUdR or BrUdR when specifically incorporated into chromatin modify radiosensitivity.

The number of lesions induced by radiation in DNA is far greater than those that eventually lead to cell killing. A dose of radiation that induces on average one lethal event per cell will kill 63% and leave 37% still viable (this results from Poisson

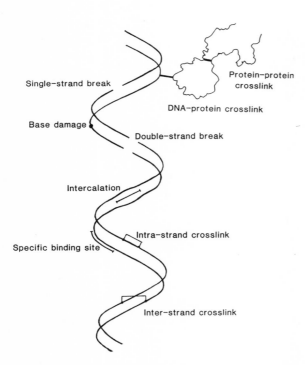

Figure 24.3   Types of damage to DNA produced by radiation and chemical agents.

Table 24.1 Toxicity of radioisotopes depends upon their subcellular distribution

	Subcellular dose* (Gy)		
	to nucleus	to cytoplasm	to membranes
X-ray	3.3	3.3	3.3
^{3}H-thymidine	3.8	0.27	0.01
^{125}I-conconavalin	4.1	24.7	516.7

* For each of these three treatments a dose has been chosen that gives 50% cell killing in CHO cells. The absorbed radiation doses to the nucleus, cytoplasm or membranes have then been calculated. ^{3}H-thymidine is bound to DNA, ^{125}I-conconavalin to cell membranes. It is the *nuclear* dose that is constant and thus correlates with cell killing, not the cytoplasmic or membrane doses.
From Warters *et al* (1977).

statistics) and we call this the D_o dose (Section 6.3). D_o values for oxic mammalian cells are usually in the region of 1–2 Gy. The numbers of DNA lesions that are detected immediately after such a dose have been estimated to be approximately:

	Events per D_o
Base damage	> 1000
Single-strand breaks	≈ 1000
Double-strand breaks	≈ 40

together with cross-links between DNA strands and with nuclear proteins. Irradiation at clinically used doses thus induces a vast amount of DNA damage, most of which is successfully repaired by the cell. In a variety of experimental situations it has been found that the incidence of cell killing fails to correlate with the number of SSB induced, but relates better to the incidence of DSB (Table 24.2). Furthermore, a dose of hydrogen peroxide that induces many SSB produces little cell killing and few DSB. On this basis it is generally believed that DSB are the critical lesions for radiation cell killing, although as the next paragraph indicates it may be only *some* DSB that are important.

The realization that low-LET radiation produces 'hot-spots' in which clusters of ionizations may occur within a diameter of a few nanometres (Section 24.1) has led to the notion that such an event may produce a particularly severe lesion if it impinges on the DNA molecule. This lesion might consist of one or more DSB together with a number of SSB, and also DNA base damage, etc. Ward (1986) has termed this a

Local Multiply-Damaged Site (Figure 24.1B). The importance of these hypothetical lesions derives from the fact mentioned above that the great majority of DNA lesions are repaired. Any difference in repair among DSB will lead to lethality being associated with the rare lesion that fails to repair, which may *inherently* be difficult to repair. An LMDS, which will be recognized by a strand-break assay as merely one DSB, may have a low repair probability and high probability of leading to cell death.

The importance of the initial slope of cell survival curves for clinical radiotherapy has been described in Sections 14.5 and 15.2; the concept of a linear component of cell killing is also essential to the linear-quadratic and LPL models of cell killing (Sections 6.5 and 6.6). LMDS are a type of radiation-induced lesion that could cause single-hit cell killing and therefore conceivably could give rise to the linear component.

Even strand-breaks induced by single events may be heterogeneous. Over 20 products of thymine have been detected using gas chromatography/mass spectrometry. It is therefore highly likely that the chemical residues on the edges of a strand-break vary markedly. The biological consequences of this are not yet known.

Radiation-induced Mutations

Some damage induced by radiation may be insufficient to stop cell division but enough to lead to mutation. Mutations arise by a non-lethal alteration in the base sequence in DNA. They may be qualitative where bases are inserted, altered or deleted or they may be quantitative where genes are increased in number. Mutations result in the expression of an altered protein or in the increase or decrease in the level of a normal protein.

The frequency of radiation-induced mutations usually increases in a dose-dependent manner in the range of doses per fraction commonly used in fractionated radiotherapy. At higher radiation doses lethal events may predominate and the frequency of mutations will fall. The biological consequences of mutations depend on where they occur. Cellular resistance to cytotoxic agents can arise by mutation of the enzyme to which the drug is targeted. Cellular transformation can occur if a mutated gene leads to a decrease in the normal control mechanisms of cell proliferation. Each of these examples has obvious implications for the

Table 24.2 Double-strand DNA breaks correlate best with cell killing

Modifier	Cell kill	DSB	SSB	Base damage	DNA-protein cross-links
High-LET radiation	↑	↑	↓	↓	–
Hypoxia	↓	↓	↓	0	
Thiols	↓	↓	↓	0	↓
Hyperthermia	↑	↑	0	0	0
Hydrogen peroxide	0	0	↑	↑	–

↑ increased; ↓ decreased; 0 little or no effect; – not known.
See Frankenburg-Schwager (1989) for further information on these relationships.

use of radiation in therapy and for the effects of environmental exposure to radiation.

The molecular analysis of non-lethal mutations has allowed a detailed examination of the results of radiation-induced DNA damage. A wide spectrum of types of damage has been detected and an interesting observation is that ionizing radiation tends to produce a higher proportion of large deletions relative to simple base changes when compared with mutations that have arisen spontaneously (Yandell *et al*, 1990).

24.3 Methods for detecting DNA damage

Since it is widely believed that strand-breaks are the critical lesion produced by ionizing radiation a large amount of effort has gone into producing methods by which they can be measured. These include:

Sucrose Gradient Sedimentation.

Sucrose solutions are prepared within plastic centrifuge tubes with a sucrose concentration that varies continuously from around 30% at the bottom to 5% at the top. Cells are exposed to ^{14}C-thymidine for a sufficient period to label most of the DNA. They are then mixed with a solution that induces cell *lysis* and releases the DNA. Some solutions (such as 0.2M NaOH) release DNA in a single-stranded form; at lower (i.e. less strongly alkaline) pH the double-stranded structure is retained. The mixture is floated on the top of the gradient. When the tubes are spun in a high-speed centrifuge at around 30,000 rpm the large DNA fragments travel further and the profile down the

gradient reflects the amount of DNA damage. This is detected by piercing the bottom of the centrifuge tube, collecting fractions of the fluid, and assaying for ^{14}C. The strand-break frequency is then deduced from the distribution of fragment sizes.

Neutral Filter Elution.

Cells whose DNA has been made radioactive are lysed on the top of a filter whose pore size is about 2 μm (remember that the DNA fibre has a diameter of $\approx$25 nm, 100 times smaller). A flow of elution buffer washes DNA fragments through the membrane and the rate of elution of DNA is related to the size of the DNA molecules on the membrane. To measure DSB the elution buffer is at pH 7.4 or 9.6. The use of pH 9.6 increases the sensitivity of the technique but also allows the detection of *alkali-labile sites* that are not actual DSB at physiological pH. Comparison of the two buffers has rarely led to different answers to biological questions. Increasing pH even further to 12.3 leads to denaturation of the two strands of the DNA and allows the measurement of SSB.

Nucleoid Sedimentation Technique.

The lysis of cells at neutral pH in the presence of high salt concentration and a non-ionic detergent allows the interphase nucleus to open up and reveal the tangled mass of chromatin. The resulting structures, often called *nucleoids*, consist of supercoiled DNA still retaining attachment to residual protein structures. The sedimentation of these structures in a sucrose gradient is influenced by the induction of SSB which allow the domains to relax and therefore enlarge. Two adaptations of this technique are in use, each of which allows radiation effects in single cells to be documented. The *halo* method assesses the expansion of nucleoids by incorporating a fluorescent dye (usually ethidium bromide) into the DNA and measuring the size of halos by microscopy. The concentration of the intercalating dye greatly influences the degree of unwinding of the domains, and the relationship between halo size and dye concentration gives information about the chromatin structure in the nucleoid. The *comet* assay measures radiation-induced relaxation of chromatin domains by exposing the nucleoids to an electric field which stretches the DNA into a tail. The length of the tail is related to the number of strand breaks. An adaptation of the comet assay involves a more rigorous lysis of the nucleus of single cells embedded in agar so that naked DNA, rather than nucleoid structures, are left. When exposed to an electric field the migration of the DNA is proportional to the number of strand breaks. Unlike the basic comet method, this assay is dominated by DSB at neutral pH; it can also be used to measure SSB by increasing the pH.

Pulsed Field Gel Electrophoresis.

Fragments of DNA carry a net negative charge and when incorporated into an agarose gel they generally migrate under an electric field at a speed that is inversely related to their size. In order to detect the movement of the DNA, this is either made radioactive (in the live cells prior to lysis) or is stained with a DNA-specific fluorescent dye after electrophoresis. The separation of fragments is improved by pulsing the electric field and alternating it, for instance between directions at 30° to the axis of migration. This technique overcomes problems of anomalous movement of large DNA molecules in an electric field so that their separation can be translated into a measure of strand breakage produced by small radiation doses. DNA of known molecular weight (for instance intact yeast chromosomes) is used to calibrate the movement of irradiated DNA in the gels.

24.4 Chromosome aberrations

One of the most obvious cytological effects of irradiation is the production of damage to chromosomes. Irradiation induces a dose-dependent delay in the entry of cells into mitosis and when cells that were irradiated while in interphase begin to divide, some of them reveal chromosome aberrations. Whilst the most serious of these will lead to early cell death, some aberrations can be carried through many divisions. Some of the main types of aberration are illustrated in Figure 24.4. They consist of a variety of exchanges and deletions: fragments may be exchanged between chromosomes, between the arms of a single chromosome, or even within a single arm. This can lead to chromosomes in which arm-lengths are abnormal, also to chromosomes sticking together and forming X or O structures, or to dicentric chromosomes containing two centromeres plus a chromosome fragment.

Aberrations may also be classified as chroma*tid* or chromo*some* aberrations. The irradiation of cells in the G_2 phase leads mainly to chroma*tid* damage; radiation damage in G_1, if unrepaired, will lead to defects involving both chromatids and thus to chromo*some* aberrations. Irradiation of cells in the S-phase can lead to either type, depending on whether the affected chromosome sites themselves had undergone replication.

What is the relationship between chromosome aberrations and cell viability? Cells do seem to be able to tolerate a variety of structural chromosomal changes and in irradiated individuals some changes persist throughout life. Tumours are characterized by chromosomal instability (both in terms of chromosome structure and number of chromosomes) and irradiation increases the extent of this. But some chromosome changes tend to be lethal. In general terms, the lethal events are those that eventually lead to the loss of a substantial part of the genome. Any rearrangement that leads to a portion of a chromosome lacking a centromere (an *acentric fragment*) will usually lead to its eventual loss from the cell. This may be seen in a subsequent interphase as a *micronucleus*. In diploid cells the formation of a micronucleus signals cell death. This has been exploited in the *micronucleus assay* for cell survival (Section 5.4).

The Technique of Premature Chromosome Condensation.

The morphological signs of chromosome damage are only visible when cells undergo mitosis. Cells irradiated early in the cell cycle take some hours

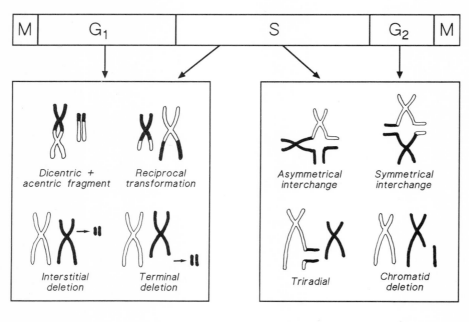

Figure 24.4 Significant types of radiation-induced chromosome aberration. From Bedford (1991), with permission.

to enter mitosis and therefore the chromosome breaks that are observed are those that have failed to rejoin during this period. However, if an interphase cell is fused with a mitotic cell it is found that the interphase cell undergoes a process of *premature chromosome condensation (PCC)* in which the chromosomes become visible. The mitotic cell can be of a different cell type and its chromatin can be labelled with BrUdR so that within the binucleate fusion it is possible to identify the chromosomes of the target cell. This technique enables breaks in chromatin to be scored within 10–15 minutes of irradiation; the speed of their rejoining can also be determined.

The analysis of both chromosome aberrations and PCC has been greatly facilitated by the development of chromosome-specific lengths of DNA (i.e. probes) that can be used in *fluorescence in situ hybridization (FISH)*. In this technique the chromosomes are spread and fixed on microscope slides, then heated so that much of their DNA becomes single-stranded. The specimens are incubated with labelled probe DNA and the probe binds to those regions of the chromsomal DNA with which it is homologous. The bound probe is detected with a fluorescent ligand that binds to the probe and may be seen under fluorescence

microscopy. This technique has made the identification of individual chromosomes and translocations between chromosomes much easier.

24.5 Mechanisms by which DNA damage is 'processed'

The use of the word 'processed' reflects the current view that damage induced in DNA is modified by a series of enzymic processes that may lead either to successful repair or to fixation of damage (i.e. *misrepair*). The outcome depends not only on the speed and efficiency of repair but also on the competition between these two processes.

The nature of repair processes depends to a large degree on the type of lesion that is being repaired. Where damage involves simply a change in one of the DNA bases, it can be removed by a simple *excision-repair* process. This involves the nicking of the DNA on either side of the lesion, the removal of a few bases around the point of damage, synthesis of new DNA within the damaged region, and finally ligation of the newly synthesized DNA to the original DNA strand (Figure 24.5). This process has been well characterized in the repair of damage induced by

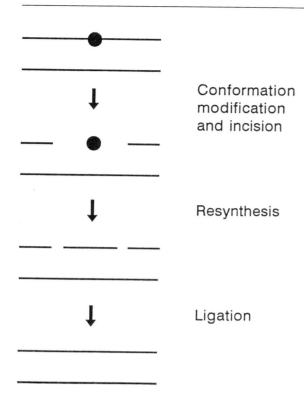

Conformation
modification
and incision

Resynthesis

Ligation

Figure 24.5 Excision-repair of damage in a single strand of DNA. The damage is recognized, the DNA unwound and the DNA strand nicked around the damage site. Following removal of the damaged bases, DNA is resynthesized using the opposite strand as a template and finally the new piece is ligated back into the DNA molecule.

ultra-violet light and some of the genes that are involved have been identified.

Repair of other types of lesion is based essentially on this simple scenario but with some variations. Cytotoxic drugs often produce specific lesions (Figure 24.3) and unique enzymes may be required to recognize and remove their particular adducts. Where both strands of the DNA are involved there may be a loss of information either directly as a result of the damage or during the excision stage. In this situation a strand of DNA with a homologous sequence can be used as a template in what is known as *recombination repair*. After these processes are over there may still be some loss of sequence information and this may be one way in which misrepair occurs. The extent of damage may not be sufficient to compromise the

viability of the cell but the genetic code has been disrupted and the resulting message translated into RNA and protein may be erroneous (i.e. a mutation has occurred).

Radiosensitive Human Syndromes

Abnormally severe normal-tissue reactions to radiotherapy are not only a practical problem to the radiotherapist but are also of great interest from the point of view of the molecular nature of the underlying genetic abnormality. In some cases patients who show such a response have been identified as exhibiting the traits of specific inherited syndromes (Table 24.3). It should be stressed, however, that it is only in the case of *ataxia-telangiectasia (A-T)* that cells taken from the patient have frequently been found to be more radiosensitive than normal, and even in this case there are examples of clinically diagnosed A-T patients who do not exhibit the laboratory radiosensitivity test of increased chromosomal damage following treatment with ionizing radiation. A-T is an autosomal recessive syndrome which presents clinically as oculo-cutaneous telangiectasia and progressive cerebellar ataxia. Immunodeficiency and a high frequency of neoplasia are also associated with this disease. An excessive degree of normal-tissue reaction following radiotherapy was the first indication that these patients may have an increased sensitivity to ionizing radiation. This has been confirmed subsequently in the laboratory through experiments on lymphocytes and fibroblasts from A-T patients (Figure 24.6). The cellular defect in A-T cells has yet to be identified conclusively. There is one report of a decrease in DSB rejoining; another study has indicated that the cells may have a reduced fidelity of repair, leading to an increased incidence of misrepair of double-strand breaks. A-T cells have been found

Table 24.3 Some human syndromes in which there have been reports of increased sensitivity to ionizing radiation

Ataxia-telangiectasia
Basal Cell Nevoid Syndrome
Cockayne's Syndrome
Gardner's Syndrome
Fanconi's Anaemia
Down's Syndrome
Nijmegen Breakage Syndrome
Usher's Syndrome

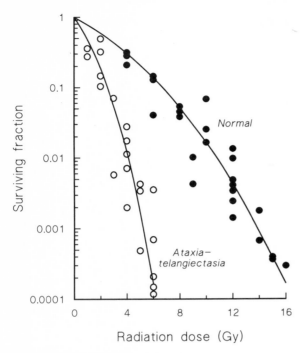

Figure 24.6 Examples of clonogenic survival curves for transformed fibroblasts taken from a normal individual and a patient with *ataxia-telangiectasia (A-T)*.

to lack a radiation-induced arrest at the G_1–S boundary, which may allow replication of damaged DNA, damage that normally would have had time to repair during the period of arrest. Interest in A-T extends beyond the response of these individuals to radiation, as it has been reported that those who are heterozygous at the A-T locus may have an increased susceptibility to cancer. It has been estimated that as many as 15% of breast cancer patients may be A-T heterozygotes.

Radiosensitive Mutants of Established Cell Lines

Radiosensitive mutants isolated from cell lines maintained in the laboratory are playing an important role in the investigation of mechanisms of cellular radiosensitivity. A large number of such mutants are now available, especially in rodent cell systems. By investigating the nature of the underlying DNA lesion it is possible to identify critical stages in the pathway that leads to radiation cell killing (*see* next section).

24.6 The sequence of events that lead to cell death

The complex sequence of processes that follow the initial induction of free-radical damage to DNA and may eventually lead to cell death or mutation are illustrated in Figure 24.7. This sequence may be divided into three main sections: *induction*, *processing* and *manifestation*, each of which has been described in the foregoing sections of this chapter.

At what points in this sequence is radiosensitivity determined? There is no single answer to this question. Mammalian cells that are more than usually sensitive to ionizing radiation fall into a number of different categories, including:

(i)   Stem-cells of certain radiosensitive normal tissues (e.g. lymphocytes, spermatocytes);

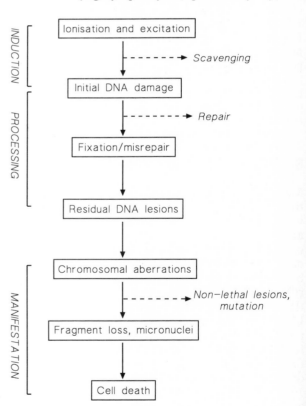

Figure 24.7 The sequence of processes that take place in cells following exposure to ionising radiation, which may lead eventually to cell death. They can be divided into three main phases, as described in the text.

(ii) Cells from patients with inherited hypersensitive syndromes (e.g. A-T);
(iii) Radiosensitive tumour types (e.g. lymphomas, neuroblastomas);
(iv) Radiosensitive mutants of established cell lines (e.g. xrs, L5178Y-S).

Current evidence suggests that the mechanisms of sensitivity differ among these categories, although the picture is in many respects not yet clear.

Initial DNA damage

There is evidence that the radiosensitivity of mammalian cells may to a considerable extent be determined during the *induction* phase (Figure 24.7). Radford (1985, 1986) measured initial DNA damage in V79 and other cell lines irradiated under a variety of conditions; the cells were irradiated at 4°C and assayed immediately for DSB, thus preventing enzymatic processing. He found a good correlation between initial damage and cellular radiosensitivity. McMillan *et al* (1990) performed a similar study on a range of human tumour cell lines (category iii above); the correlation was not as good as that found by Radford, although initial damage was clearly an important factor.

Rate, Extent, and Fidelity of Repair

Many studies have detected a correlation between the rejoining of DNA strand breaks and cell survival. In some cases it is the *speed* of rejoining that appears to be important (Schwartz *et al*, 1988), in others it is the *residual level* of unrepaired DNA damage. These two parameters may of course be linked. It has also been appreciated that the rejoining of a DSB does not necessarily mean that the function of damaged genes has been restored. Using endonuclease-induced strand breaks in plasmid DNA, it has been possible to probe for the ability of mammalian cells to restore gene function and thus to gain a measure of the *fidelity* of repair of these lesions (Powell and McMillan, 1991). There was evidence that fidelity of repair was lower in more radiosensitive human tumour cell lines.

In addition to the processes directly involved in the induction and repair of damage following irradiation, the following factors can indirectly alter these processes:

Chromatin Structure:

DNA in the cell is associated with a variety of proteins, together making up the chromatin. The nature of DNA-protein interactions may influence both the enzymatic repair of the DNA lesions as well as the chemical modification of the radiation-induced free radicals which do the damage. This has been well characterized following UV-irradiation where it has been shown that transcribing regions of DNA are repaired more readily than non-transcribing regions. Indeed, it has also been shown that the *transcribing strand* may be more repairable than its opposite DNA strand.

Membrane Structure:

It was suggested some years ago by Alper that not all of the effects of radiation can be explained by a simple direct action on DNA itself. She and others have postulated that damage to cell membranes, perhaps at the point of attachment between DNA and the nuclear membrane, may also be important in some situations.

Precursor Pools:

The levels of deoxyribonucleotide triphosphates in *E. coli* and other eukaryotes have been shown to affect DNA repair and other closely related processes. In mammalian cell mutants with an altered pool balance the accuracy with which DNA polymerases incorporate nucleosides during replication is reduced and this can lead to an increased rate of mutation. These imbalances have been shown to alter the response to ethylmethane sulphonate (EMS) and there have been claims that radiation sensitivity may be linked to differences in the level of deoxynucleotide triphosphates and enzymes associated with their production.

24.7 Genetic control of radiosensivity

Complementation Analysis

In view of the many factors involved in the determination of radiosensitivity it is likely that many genes are involved. A first estimate of this number can be obtained by complementation analysis in which two sensitive cells are fused together. If the resulting hybrid is also sensitive, then this suggests that the two cell lines are deficient in the same gene. On the other hand, if the hybrid is resistant, then this implies that the two cell lines have different defective genes and therefore that at least two genes are involved in radiation sensitivity. Among rodent cell lines that are sensitive to ionizing radiation, at least 8 or 9 complementation groups have been identified; three of these groups have been characterized as having a reduced ability to rejoin DNA double-strand breaks. Multiple complementation groups have also been identified in cells from patients with radiosensitive syndromes. The UV-sensitive cells from *xeroderma pigmentosum* fall into 7 complementation groups and *ataxia-telangiectasia* cells are known at the present time to have at least 4 complementation groups.

Isolation of "Radiosensitivity" Genes

A large number of genes have been isolated from prokaryotes and lower eukaryotes, such as yeast, which influence sensitivity either to UV or ionizing radiation. The cloning of radiosensitivity genes from humans has largely come about through complementation by human DNA of defects in radiosensitive rodent cell mutants. A number of genes have been isolated that are involved in the repair of UV-induced damage in mammalian cells, including at least 3 that are involved in *xeroderma pigmentosum*. To date only one mammalian gene involved in the repair of ionizing radiation-induced damage has been isolated: the *XRCC1* gene which was obtained by complementation of a single-strand break repair defect in a rodent cell mutant (Thompson *et al*, 1990). The location of other radiosensitivity genes within the genome has been identified but as yet these have not been cloned.

Oncogenic Transformation and Radiosensitivity

Recent data from several laboratories have linked oncogenes with the development of radioresistance. For example, transformation of primary rat embryo cells with a combination of *c-ras* and *v-myc* has been found to lead to radiation resistance (McKenna *et al*, 1992). Radioresistance in human tumour cells has in one instance been associated with the *raf* oncogene. The mechanisms underlying the effects of these oncogenes are not clear but there is some doubt whether they are associated with alterations in the induction or repair of DNA double-strand breaks. Some investigators believe that the oncogenes may exert their effects via cell-cycle control following irradiation. Radiation is known to induce cell-cycle progression delay at a number of points in the cell cycle (especially in G_2 or at the G_1–S boundary) and in *ataxia-telangiectasia* cells this is usually modified in parallel with radiosensitivity. The known effects of oncogenes on cell-cycle control pathways therefore make this a potentially important factor in the determination of radiosensitivity.

Epigenetic Modulation of Radiation Sensitivity

Epigenetic processes are those that alter gene expression without modifying the sequence of bases in DNA. Differentiation, for example, is largely an epigenetic process because it involves the switching on and off of specific genes at given times during cellular development. Within an individual not all cells have the same sensitivity. Bone marrow stem cells, for example, are more radiosensitive than fibroblasts or the stem cells of some epithelia. Little is known of what determines these differences but epigenetic processes no doubt play an important role. Some of the determinants of radiosensitivity in normal cells probably carry over into the neoplastic cells that derive from them, as evidenced by the radiosensitivity of leukaemias and some lymphomas.

One example in the laboratory where switching off a critical gene leads to an increase in radiosensitivity is in *xrs* mutants of Chinese hamster ovary cells. Treatment of these radiosensitive mutants with 5-azacytidine tends to abolish their increased radiosensitivity (Jeggo and Holliday, 1986). This drug is known to increase gene expression by reducing the methylation status of DNA, and the observed increase in resistance is believed to be due to the switching back on of a gene involved in DNA double-strand break rejoining.

Inducible Responses to Irradiation

Bacteria sometimes respond to DNA-damaging agents by increasing the expression of proteins that subsequently promote DNA repair. In mammalian cells there is also a limited amount of evidence for this process of *inducible repair*. For example, if a mammalian cell is irradiated and then exposed to irradiated virus, the virus may be repaired to a greater degree than if the mammalian cell had not been pre-irradiated (Jeeves and Rainbow, 1979). Pre-irradiation appears to have induced the repair of the viral DNA damage. The significance of these observations for radiation therapy is still a matter of debate. There is,

however, increasing evidence for gene activation by exposure to low doses of ionizing radiation. The genes that are switched on are diverse and include growth factors such as the fibroblast growth factor *(FGF)*, nuclear signal transducers and natural cytotoxins like tumour necrosis factor *(TNF–α)*. These genes are potentially involved in many biological responses to radiation, including repopulation, fibrosis, repair, and indeed cell killing.

Key points

1. A therapeutic dose of low-LET radiation produces in every cell a large number of ionizations. Some of these give rise to direct damage to DNA; others to free radicals that react with DNA. Most of this damage is repaired by rapid chemical reactions. The remaining lesions in DNA are very effectively repaired by enzymatic reactions. Some of them fail to repair and become fixed, and it is these that lead to cell lethality.
2. The death of most cells is associated with certain types of chromosomal aberrations, in particular those aberrations that lead to the loss of a substantial chromosome fragment in the form of a micronucleus.
3. Techniques of molecular genetics are beginning to throw light on the processes of cell killing and mutation. These involve both genetic and epigenetic mechanisms.

Bibliography

Bedford JS (1991). Sublethal damage, potentially lethal damage, and chromosomal aberrations in mammalian cells exposed to ionising radiations. *Int. J. Radiat. Oncol. Biol. Phys.* 21:1457-1469.

Chapman JD and Gillespie CJ (1981). Radiation-induced events and their time-scale in mammalian cells. *Adv. Radiat. Biol.* 9:143-198.

Friedberg EC (1985). *DNA Repair.* WH Freeman & Co.; New York.

Jeeves WP and Rainbow AJ (1979). Gamma-ray enhanced reactivation of gamma-irradiated adenovirus in human cells. *Biochem Biophys Res Commun* 90:567-574.

Jeggo PA and Holliday R (1986). Azacytidine-induced reactivation of a DNA repair gene in Chinese hamster ovary cells. *Mol Cell Biol* 6:2944-2949.

McKenna WG, Iliakis G and Muschel RJ (1992). Mechanism of radioresistance in oncogene transfected cell lines. In *Radiation Research: A Twentieth Century Perspective*, pp. 392-397.

(Eds) Dewey WC *et al.* Academic Press Inc; San Diego.

McMillan TJ, Cassoni AM, Edwards S *et al* (1990). The relationship of DNA double-strand break induction to radiosensitivity in human tumour cell lines. *Int J Radiat Biol* 58:427-438.

Powell S and McMillan TJ (1991). Clonal variation of DNA repair in a human glioma cell line. *Radiother Oncol* 21:225-232.

Radford IR (1985). The level of induced DNA double-strand breakage correlates with cell kiling after X-irradiation. *Int J Radiat Biol* 48:45-54.

Radford IR (1986). Evidence for a general relationship between the induced level of DNA double-strand breakage and cell killing after X-irradiation of mammalian cells. *Int J Radiat Biol* 49:611-620.

Schwartz JL, Rotmensch J, Giovanazzi S *et al* (1988). Faster repair of DNA double-strand breaks in radioresistant human tumor cells. *Int J Rad Oncol Biol Phys* 15:907-912.

Thompson LH, Brookman KW, Jones NJ *et al*

(1990). Molecular cloning of the human *XRCC1* gene, which corrects defective DNA strand break repair and sister chromatid exchange. *Mol Cell Biol* 10:6160-6171.

Warters RL, Hofer KG, Harris CR and Smith JM (1977). Radionuclide toxicity in cultured mammalian cells: elucidation of the primary site of radiation damage. *Curr Top Radiat Res Q* 12:389-407.

Yandell DW, Dryja TP and Little JB (1990). Molecular genetic analysis of recessive mutations at a heterozygous autosomal locus in human cells. *Mutation Research* 229:89-102.

Further reading

Frankenburg-Schwager M (1989). Review of repair kinetics for DNA damage induced in eukaryotic cells in vitro by ionising radiation. *Radiother Oncol* 14:307-320.

Lehmann AR, Hoeijmakers JHJ, van Zeeland AA *et al* (1992). Workshop on DNA repair. *Mutat Res* 273:1-28.

Powell SN and McMillan TJ (1990). DNA damage and repair following treatment with ionizing radiation. *Radiother Oncol* 19:95-108.

Von Sonntag C (1987). *The Chemical Basis of Radiation Biology*. Taylor & Francis; London.

Ward JF (1986). Mechanisms of DNA repair and their potential modification for radiotherapy. *Int J Radiat Oncol Biol Phys* 12:1027-1032.

Whitaker SJ, Powell SN and McMillan TJ (1991). Molecular assays of radiation-induced DNA damage. *Eur J Cancer* 27:922-928.

Yarnold JR, Stratton M and McMillan TJ (1993). *Molecular Biology for Oncologists*. Elsevier Science Publishers; Amsterdam.

Glossary of terms in radiation biology

α/β ratio: The ratio of the parameters α and β in the linear-quadratic model.

Accelerated fractionation: Reduction in overall treatment time without a significant change in dose per fraction or total dose.

Additive: A situation in which the effect of a combination is the sum of the effects of the separate treatments (= 'independent cell kill').

Apoptosis: A mode of cell death principally seen in embryonic cells, lymphocytes and lymphoid tumour cells. It has distinctive morphological features and DNA is degraded into inter-nucleosomal fragments.

Autoradiography: Use of a photographic emulsion to detect radioactivity in a tissue specimen.

Brachytherapy: Radiotherapy using radioactive sources inserted into a body cavity or through needles into tissues.

Biologically-effective dose (BED): In fractionated radiotherapy, the total dose that would be required in very small dose fractions or at infinitely low dose rate, as indicated by the linear-quadratic equation. Otherwise known as Extrapolated Total Dose (ETD). BED values calculated for different α/β ratios are not strictly comparable.

Cell-cycle time: The time between one mitosis and the next.

Cell loss factor (φ): The rate of cell loss from a tumour, as a proportion of the rate which cells are being added to the tumour by mitosis. Usually calculated by the relation: $\phi = 1 - T_{pot}/T_d$, where T_{pot} is potential doubling time and T_d is the cell population doubling time.

Chronic hypoxia: Persistent low oxygen concentrations such as exist in viable tumour cells close to necrosis.

Clonogenic cells: Cells that have the capacity to produce an expanding family of descendants (usually at least 50). Also called 'colony-forming cells' or 'clonogens'.

Colony: Aggregate or small family of cells derived from a single cell.

Compton effect: Scattering of photons by free electrons in matter. Contrast with the photoelectric effect in which the scattering is from bound electrons.

D_o: A parameter of radiosensitivity in the multitarget equation: the radiation dose which reduces survival to e^{-1} (i.e. 0.37) of its previous value on the exponential portion of the survival curve.

Direct action: Ionization or excitation of atoms within DNA, as distinct from the reaction with DNA of free radicals formed in nearby water molecules.

Dose-modifying factor (DMF): When a chemical or other agent acts as if to change the dose of radiation, DMF indicates the ratio: (dose without/dose with) the agent for the same level of effect. Similarly:
Dose-reduction factor (DRF): or **Sensitizer enhancement ratio (SER).**

Dose-rate effect: Change of radiation response with decreasing radiation dose rate.

Doubling time: Time for a cell population or tumour volume to double its size.

'Early' responses: Radiation-induced normal-tissue damage that is expressed within weeks to a few months after exposure. Generally due to damage to parenchymal cells. α/β ratio tends to be large.

Elkind repair: Recovery of the shoulder on a survival curve when irradiation follows several hours after a priming dose.

Equivalent photon dose: Dose × RBE, for high – LET radiations.

Exponential growth: Growth according to an exponential equation: $V = V_0 \exp(kt)$. The volume doubling time is constant ($= \ln2/k$).

Extrapolated total dose (ETD): Calculated isoeffect dose when the dose rate is very low, or when fraction size is very small. (*see* Biologically Effective Dose).

Extrapolation number: A parameter in the multitarget equation: the point on the survival scale to which the straight part of the curve back-extrapolates.

Field-size effect: The dependence of normal-tissue damage on the size of the irradiated area; also known as the 'volume effect'.

'Flexible' tissues: Non-hierarchical cell populations in which function and proliferation take place in the same cells.

Flow cytometry: Analysis of cell suspensions in which a dilute stream of cells is passed through a laser beam. DNA content and other properties are measured by light scattering and fluorescence following staining with dyes or labelled antibodies.

Free radical: A broken molecule: fragments that contain an unpaired electron and are therefore very reactive.

gray (Gy): Unit of absorbed dose. 1 gray = 1 joule per kg (= 100 rad).

Growth delay: Extra time required for a treated tumour to reach a given size, compared with an untreated control.

Growth fraction: The proportion of cells in cycle in a population.

'Hierarchical' tissues: Cell populations comprising a lineage of stem cells, proliferating cells, and mature cells. The mature cells do not divide.

Hyperbaric oxygen (HBO): The use of high oxygen pressures (2–3 atmospheres) to enhance oxygen availability in radiotherapy.

Hyperfractionation: Increase in number of fractions and reduction in dose per fraction, within a similar overall time.

Hyperthermia: The use of heat treatments in excess of 42°C to treat cancer.

Hypofractionation: A reduction in the number of fractions, increase in fraction size, within a similar overall time.

Hypoxia: Low oxygen tension; usually the very low levels that are required to make cells maximally radioresistant. Sometimes used to mean **Anoxia** (= literally, the complete absence of oxygen).

Incomplete repair model: A model that deals with the increased effectiveness of radiotherapy when fractions are too close together to allow complete recovery.

Indirect action: Damage to DNA by free radicals formed through the ionisation of nearby water molecules.

Initial slope: The steepness of the initial part of the cell survival curve, sometimes indicated by the surviving fraction at 2 Gy.

Interphase death: The death of irradiated cells before they reach mitosis.

Isoeffect plot: A graph of the total dose for a given effect (e.g. ED_{50}) plotted, for instance, against number of fractions, dose per fraction or dose rate.

$LD_{50/30}$: Dose to produce lethality in 50% of subjects by 30 days; similarly $LD_{50/7}$ *etc*.

Labelling index: Proportion or percentage of cells within the S-phase, and therefore labelled by ^{3}H-thymidine or bromo-deoxyuridine.

'Late' responses: Radiation-induced normal-tissue damage that is expressed months to years after exposure. Generally due to damage to connective-tissue cells. α/β ratio tends to be small.

Latent period or Latency interval: Time between irradiation and expression of injury.

Linear energy transfer (LET): The rate of energy loss along the track of an ionizing particle. Usually expressed in keV/μm.

Linear-quadratic model (LQ model): Model in which the effect (E) is a linear-quadratic function of dose (d): $E = \alpha d + \beta d^2$. For cell survival: $S = \exp(-\alpha d - \beta d^2)$.

Log-phase culture: A cell culture growing exponentially.

Mitotic death: Cell death during mitosis.

Mitotic delay: Delay of entry into mitosis, or accumulation in G_2, as a result of treatment.

Mitotic index: Proportion or percentage of cells in mitosis at any given time.

Multitarget equation: Model that assumes the presence of a number of critical targets in a cell, all of which require inactivation to kill the cell. Survival is given by:
$S = 1 - [1 - \exp(D/D_o)]^n$.

Non-stochastic effect: An effect where severity increases with increasing dose after a threshold region (*see* Stochastic effect).

NSD: Nominal standard dose in the Ellis formula.

Oxygen enhancement ratio (OER): The ratio of radiation dose given under anoxic conditions to the dose resulting in the same effect when given under oxic conditions.

Photodynamic therapy: Cancer treatment using light to activate a photosensitizing agent.

Plateau-phase cultures: Cell cultures grown to confluence so that proliferation is markedly reduced (= 'stationary phase').

Plating efficiency: The proportion or percentage of plated cells that form colonies.

Potential doubling time (T_{pot}): The predicted cell population doubling time in the assumed absence of cell loss.

Potentially-lethal damage (PLD): Cellular damage that is recovered during the interval between treatment and assay.

Prodromal phase: Signs and symptoms during the first 48 hours following irradiation.

Quasi-threshold dose (D_q): Point of extrapolation of the exponential portion of a multi-target

survival curve to the level of zero survival: $D_q = D_o \ln(n)$.

Radio-responsiveness: A general term, indicating the overall level of clinical response to radiotherapy.

Radiosensitizer: In general, any agent that increases the sensitivity of cells to radiation. Usually applied to electron-affinic chemicals that mimic oxygen in fixing free-radical damage.

Radiosensitivity: The sensitivity of cells to ionising radiation. Usually indicated by the surviving fraction at 2 Gy (i.e. SF_2) or by the parameters of the linear-quadratic or multitarget equations.

Reassortment or Redistribution: Return towards a more even cell-cycle distribution, following the selective killing of cells in certain phases of the cell cycle.

Recovery: An increase in cell survival or decrease in tissue injury as a function of time during or after irradiation (*see* Repair).

Regression rate: The rate at which a tumour shrinks during or after treatment.

Relative biological effectiveness (RBE): Ratio of dose of a reference radiation quality (usually 250 kV x-rays) and dose of a test radiation that produce equal effect.

Reoxygenation: The process by which surviving clonogenic cells that are hypoxic become better oxygenated.

Repair: Restoration of the integrity of damaged macromolecules (*see* Recovery).

Repair-saturation: Explanation of the shoulder on cell survival curves on the basis of the reduced effectiveness of repair after high radiation doses.

Reproductive integrity: Ability of cells to divide many times.

Sievert (Sv): Dose-equivalent in radiation protection. Dose in grays is multiplied by a quality factor.

Slow repair: Long-term repair which takes place on a time-scale of weeks to months.

Spatial cooperation: The use of radiotherapy and chemotherapy to hit disease in different anatomical sites.

Spheroid: Clump of cells grown together in suspension culture. Not usually a colony.

Split-dose recovery (SLD recovery): Decrease in radiation effect when a single radiation dose is split into two fractions separated by times up to a few hours (= Elkind recovery, or recovery from sublethal damage).

Stathmokinetic method: Study of cell proliferation using agents that block cells in mitosis.

Stem cells: Cells capable of both self-renewal and supply of daughter cells that differentiate to produce all the various types of cells in a lineage.

Stochastic effect: An effect where the incidence, but not the severity, increases with increasing dose.

Sublethal damage: Non-lethal cellular injury that can be repaired, or accumulated with further dose to become lethal.

Supra-additivity or Synergism: A biological effect due to a combination that is greater than would be expected from the addition of the effects of the component agents.

Target cell: A cell whose death contributes to a reduction in tissue growth or function.

Targeted radiotherapy: Treatment of disseminated cancer by means of drugs that localise into tumours and carry therapeutic amounts of radioactivity.

Target theory: The idea that the shoulder on cell survival curves is due to the number of unrepaired lesions per cell.

Therapeutic Index: Tumour response for a fixed level of normal-tissue damage.

Thermal dose: A function of temperature and heating time that is thought to relate to biological effect.

Thermotolerance: The observation that an initial heat treatment reduces the effect of a second heat treatment given shortly afterwards.

Time-dose fractionation relationships: The dependence of isoeffective radiation dose on the duration (and number of fractions) in radiotherapy.

Tissue-rescuing unit (TRU): Hypothetical element of a tissue that is the minimum that is capable of rescuing the tissue from failure.

Tolerance: The maximum level of normal-tissue damage produced by radiotherapy that the therapist judges to be acceptable. Usually indicated in dose units, although the actual values will depend on fractionation, field size, and concomitant treatments.

Transient hypoxia: Low oxygen concentrations associated with the transient closing and opening of blood vessels. Sometimes called *acute* or *cyclical* hypoxia.

Tumour bed effect (TBE): Slower rate of tumour growth after irradiation due to stromal injury in the irradiated 'vascular bed'.

Tumour cord: Sleeve of viable tumour growing around a blood capillary.

Volume doubling time: Time for a tumour to double in size.

Volume effect: Dependence of radiation damage to normal tissues on the volume of tissue irradiated.

Xenografts: Transplants between species; usually applied to the transplantation of human tumours into immune-deficient mice.

Index

[Page numbers in **bold** refer to the Glossary]